PROBLEMS IN
MOVEMENT CONTROL

ADVANCES IN PSYCHOLOGY

74

Editors:

G. E. STELMACH

P. A. VROON

NORTH-HOLLAND
AMSTERDAM • NEW YORK • OXFORD • TOKYO

PROBLEMS IN MOVEMENT CONTROL

Edited by

Greg REID

Department of Physical Education
McGill University
Montreal, Quebec, Canada

1990

NORTH-HOLLAND
AMSTERDAM • NEW YORK • OXFORD • TOKYO

NORTH-HOLLAND
ELSEVIER SCIENCE PUBLISHERS B.V.
Sara Burgerhartstraat 25
P.O. Box 211, 1000 AE Amsterdam, The Netherlands

Distributors for the United States and Canada:
ELSEVIER SCIENCE PUBLISHING COMPANY, INC.
655 Avenue of the Americas
New York, N.Y. 10010, U.S.A.

Library of Congress Cataloging-in-Publication Data

Problems in movement control / edited by Greg Reid.
p. cm. -- (Advances in psychology ; 74)
Includes bibliographical references and indexes.
ISBN 0-444-88093-3
1. Movement disorders. 2. Psychomotor disorders.
3. Developmentally disabled. I. Reid, Greg, 1948- . II. Series:
Advances in psychology (Amsterdam, Netherlands) ; 74.
[DNLM: 1. Movement Disorders--physiopathology. 2. Movement
Disorders--psychology. 3. Movement Disorders--rehabilitation. W1
AD798L v. 74 / WL 390 P962]
RC376.5.P76 1990
616.8'3--dc20
DNLM/DLC
for Library of Congress 90-14091
CIP

ISBN 13: 978-0-444-88093-2

Transferred to Digital Printing 2007

PREFACE

It is generally acknowledged that 10-20% of people in Western countries have some degree of physical, cognitive, emotional or sensory deficit. These conditions may interfere with optimal social, educational, vocational and leisure growth. Despite the large number of persons who are disabled or handicapped in some way, psychological, educational and health professionals have generally been silent in research efforts designed to understand their plight. As Asch (1984, p. 533) argued "We need to know whether existing psychological theories and research methods can account for the experience of disabled people."

Problems in motor behaviour are associated with a variety of disabilities. In fact, difficulty in movement control is the essence of cerebral palsy and other physical disabilities. In areas such as mental retardation, motor and cognitive impairments are linked in ways that have fascinated scholars for a number of years (cf. Wade, 1986). Early research efforts focused on descriptions of specific groups of people who shared some disability (e.g. motor performance of children who are mentally handicapped) or on evaluating the impact of intervention programs. While some of this research must continue, a number of investigators have begun to explore questions from a variety of theoretical positions in an attempt to build a more fundamental understanding of persons with a disability. In addition, some have posited that expanding our motor behaviour knowledge base of disabled persons may advance the understanding of the intact motor system (e.g. Kelso & Tuller, 1981; Reid, 1989). The aim of the present volume is (1) to describe a number of research fronts which have dealt with disabled persons but have not yet been presented in the form of a comprehensive review and (2) to provide an overview of theories and research design issues which presently, or which have the potential to, advance our understanding of special populations.

More specifically, authors have been challenged to critically review their area from a theoretical and applied perspective with emphasis on the former. Furthermore, they have been asked to point to future needs and directions in an attempt to spawn additional research.

Roy and Wall both contribute chapters in the present volume to the first major section, *Research Issues and Views*. Roy examines the issues and limitations inherent in understanding the extent to which knowledge of pathological and nonpathological states advances our view of each regarding the mechanisms involved in the control of movement. Wall explores a number of troublesome research design issues which confront investigators and proposes a more holistic knowledge-based viewpoint to overcome them.

The second major section of the book, *Perspectives*, is an eclectic collection of papers representing several exciting research fronts. Beuter follows a neurophysiological approach in her work on oscillatory processes in tremor and its implications to modelling of neuromotor control. Burton and Wade adopt the action theory perspective (Kugler, Kelso & Turvey, 1982) as they outline the notion of physical constraints as a factor in the movement of disabled performers. A problem solving viewpoint is sketched by Bouffard and Wall as they explain the less efficient movement performance of handicapped persons. Tomporowski and Hayden focus on motor performance in the match between the individual and the demands of work in promoting employment of individuals with developmental disabilities. Finally, Vallerand and Reid follow a cognitive intrinsic motivation approach as they explore the basic tenets of theory and put forth a number of practical suggestions to promote intrinsic motivation toward physical activity by persons with a disability.

Special Populations, the third major section of the book includes four chapters which highlight a specific disability. Elliot chronicles the neuropsychological research of his laboratory which has investigated the cerebral organization of person with Down's Syndrome and the implications of that work to difference and developmental models of mental retardation. Hoover and Horgan critically review the short term memory literature dealing with mental retardation and highlight the remedial studies. Lazarus has a broader focus than Elliot or Hoover and Horgan as she tackles the complete learning disability field from a movement perspective. Finally Wall, Reid and Paton provide an overview of the syndrome of physical awkwardness and describe major research thrusts with this group.

Athletes with Disabilities, the final section, presents two major reviews. DePauw points out that sport for persons with a disability is a relatively new phenomenon with exciting research potential but must be understood in a cultural and historical context. The final chapter is a critical review of the sport psychology literature with disabled athletes; Sherrill arguing that such research is descriptive at present but must expand into sound theory.

This book should be of interest to those currently involved in motor behaviour research with disabled persons such as clinical, developmental and experimental psychologists, physical educators, recreation therapists, physical and occupational therapists and nurses. For the scholar who wishes to begin investigating questions with disabled persons, the reviews will be useful as an introduction, coupled with the opening chapters which deal with broad theoretical and research design questions.

• • • • • • • • • • • • • • • • • • • •

The authors who contributed to this volume did so enthusiastically. This was much appreciated. In addition, sincere thanks is extended to those editorial assistants, typists and word processing specialists who did so much to make this volume a reality: Leslie Levinson, Erin O'Brien and Stanley Rog.

Greg Reid
Montreal
March 1990

References

Asch, A. (1984). The experience of disability: A challenge for psychology. *American Psychologist, 39*, 529-536.

Kelso, J.A.S. & Tuller, B. (1981). Toward a theory of apratic syndromes. *Brain and Language, 12*, 224-245.

Kugler, P., Kelso, J.A.S. & Turvey, M.T. (1982). On the control and co-ordination of naturally developing systems. In J.A.S. Kelso & J.E. Clark (Eds.), *The development of movement control and co-ordination* (pp. 5-78). New York: John Wiley & Sons.

Reid, G. (1989). Ideas about motor behaviour research with special populations. *Adapted Physical Activity Quarterly, 6*, 1-10.

Wade, M.G. (Ed.) (1986). *Motor skill acquisition of the mentally handicapped.* Amsterdam: North Holland.

LIST OF CONTRIBUTORS

Anne **Beuter**	Département de Kinanthropologie Université du Québec à Montréal Centre for Nonlinear Dynamics in Physiology and Medicine McGill University Montreal, Quebec, Canada
Allen W. **Burton**	School of Physical Education and Recreation University of Minnesota Minneapolis, Minnesota, USA
Marcel **Bouffard**	Department of Physical Education and Sport Studies University of Alberta Edmonton, Alberta, Canada
Karen P. **DePauw**	Department of Physical Education, Sport and Leisure Studies Washington State University Pullman, Washington, USA
Digby **Elliott**	School of Physical Education and Athletics McMaster University Hamilton, Ontario, Canada
Alys M. **Hayden**	Department of Psychology University of Alabama Tuscaloosa, Alabama, USA
John H. **Hoover**	School of Education University of South Dakota Vermillion, South Dakota, USA
James S. **Horgan**	College of Health, Physical Education and Recreation University of Illinois - Chicago Chicago, Illinois, USA
Jo-Anne C. **Lazarus**	Department of Physical Education and Dance University of Wisconsin - Madison Madison, Wisconsin, USA

James **Paton** — Department of Physical Education and Sport Studies
University of Alberta
Edmonton, Alberta, Canada

Greg **Reid** — Department of Physical Education
McGill University
Montreal, Quebec, Canada

Eric A. **Roy** — Department of Kinesiology
University of Waterloo
Department of Psychology and Rehabilitation Medicine
University of Toronto
Toronto, Ontario, Canada

Claudine **Sherrill** — Department of Kinesiology
Texas Women's University
Denton, Texas, USA

Phillip **Tomporowski** — Department of Psychology
University of Alabama
Tuscaloosa, Alabama, USA

Robert J. **Vallerand** — Laboratoire de Psychologie Sociale
Université du Québec à Montreal
Montreal, Quebec, Canada

Michael G. **Wade** — School of Physical Education and Recreation
University of Minnesota
Minneapolis, Minnesota, USA

A.E. (Ted) **Wall** — Department of Physical Education
McGill University
Montreal, Quebec, Canada

CONTENTS

SECTION I:

RESEARCH ISSUES AND VIEWS

Problems In Movement Control
G. Reid (editor)

THE INTERFACE BETWEEN NORMALITY AND PATHOLOGY IN UNDERSTANDING MOTOR FUNCTION

Eric A. Roy
Department of Kinesiology
University of Waterloo

and

Departments of Psychology and Rehabilitation Medicine
University of Toronto

The focus of this chapter is on considering how an examination of motor function under both normal and pathological states may yield particularly fruitful insights into the nature of the control processes in movement. In the context of this discussion, pathology refers to various types of damage to the brain which are associated with disruptions to motor control. This question of the relationship between pathology and normality may be viewed as part of the larger question of the relationship between the brain and behaviour. The concept and form of the relationship between brain structure/function and behaviour has changed with advances in knowledge about the two components, brain and behaviour. Marshall (1982, p. 4) argues that "our preferred forms of interpretation constantly change in psychological, physiological, and anatomical theory; as they change, so must the nature of the bridge laws that link the domains". This idea has great import for understanding the neurobehavioural bases of motor control, since our conceptualization of motor behaviour in terms of what is being controlled and how control is exerted has changed dramatically over the past 50 years. Likewise, the burgeoning information about brain organization and the neural basis of motor control has fundamentally changed our view of the neurophysiological bases of the control of movement (Brooks, 1986). Our discussion of the interface between studies in normality and pathology will take into account these parallels in theories of brain organization and motor control.

The chapter begins with a consideration of the roles played by studies in normality and pathology in advancing our understanding of the processes in motor control. Following this discussion consideration is given to issues important in making comparisons of studies from these two behaviourial states.

The final section is devoted to a discussion of the directions for research necessary in the future to foster a greater interface between findings from normality and pathology.

Roles of Studies in Normality and Pathology

Studies of motor behaviour in normal and pathological states provide somewhat different views as to the mechanisms which may be involved in the control of movement. "As action in a moving film can be elucidated by playing it in slow motion, so motor behaviour and the cognitive processes underlying it become more susceptible to analysis when observed in a pathological condition which reduces the rate at which information is processed" (Roy, 1978, p. 204). Three roles which these studies assume are considered here. First, studies in normality both afford a definition of the nature and extent of pathology and provide a means of focusing the study of pathology on particular mechanisms. Second, studies of pathology, on the other hand, provide a basis for confirming the existence of particular processes or mechanisms derived from studies of normality and third, for identifying mechanisms which might not be observed only from studies of normality.

Defining the Nature and Extent of Pathology

To some extent, studies of motor performance in normality provide a basis for defining the nature and extent of pathology. The usual way of defining pathology is with regard to the product, that is, whether or not the person has achieved the intended goal of the movement. This perspective is exemplified in the area of clinical neuropsychology (Lezak, 1983). A number of perceptual motor tests have been developed examining fine motor control (finger tapping), and visual motor control (pegboard test). These tests have been administered to large numbers of normal people providing a range of performance scores which serve as normative data. The performance scores of persons having or suspected of having neurological impairments are compared to this normative data in order to define the degree of impairment (Lezak, 1983).

Pathology may also be defined with reference to the process, that is, the mechanisms and/or strategies involved in achieving the goal (i.e., the product). Clinical neuropsychology again provides an example of this definition of pathology. In the process-oriented approach to neuropsychological assessment (Milberg, Hebben, & Kaplan, 1986) the focus is more upon the strategies employed by the patient in performing a task rather than simply on whether or not he is able to achieve the goal of the task. Drawing the Rey-Osterrieth Complex Figure (Osterrieth, 1944; Visser, 1973) affords one example of this approach. This figure is composed of a number of component parts. The order in which components of this figure are completed in the drawing process has been documented in the studies of normal children (Waber & Holmes, 1985, 1986) and adults (Visser, 1973). In the same way that overall performance scores provide a normative base, these orders in drawing the components provide a basis for defining the normal "strategies" used in drawing this figure. Binder (1982), for example, in studies with adults, developed three scores reflecting the way the figure is drawn: configural units which are the number of elements in the figure drawn as one unit, fragmented units which are the number of elements not drawn as a unit and missing units which are the number of missing or omitted elements. In examining the performance of patients with left or right brain damage and non-brain-damaged patients he found that the non-brain-damaged patients exhibited very low fragmentation and missing unit scores but very high configuration unit scores. These normal patients, then, tended to draw the figure in organized units.

Very different strategies in drawing were observed in the brain-damaged patients. Both brain-damaged groups exhibited significantly lower configuration unit scores suggesting that they were much less organized in the way they drew the figure. The other unit scores revealed somewhat different patterns in the nature of this disorganization, however. The left-damaged patients had a much higher fragmentation unit score but a lower missing unit score than the right-damaged group. With damage to the left hemisphere, then, all the elements were drawn but in a very fragmented, disorganized manner. With right-hemisphere damage, on the other hand, many of the elements of the figure were omitted.

One might argue that these findings do not really reflect strategies involved in drawing but rather provide a more detailed measure of the product. That is, the observation that drawings are fragmented or have elements missing does not reveal how or why they were drawn this way. A more careful analysis of the movements used in drawing may provide a clearer reflection of the processes or strategies involved.

Another example of this process approach to defining pathology comes from studies of limb apraxia. De Renzi (1985), among others, has examined the ability of patients with lateralized brain damage to perform common gestures (e.g., salute, wave good-bye) to verbal command and to imitation of the examiner's performance of the gesture. In many cases patients are able to perform these gestures more accurately to imitation than to verbal command. De Renzi suggested that performance to verbal command requires the patient to access the movement from memory. It is this process of memory retrieval, he argues, which is impaired, particularly in patients with left-hemisphere damage. The role of memory in the process of response selection and programming will be considered in more detail in the next section of the chapter.

A Focus for studies in Pathology

While studies of normal function provide a basis for defining pathology both in terms of the product and the processes involved, models derived from these studies also form a basis for focusing studies in pathology on particular processes or mechanisms.

Work by Mather (1986) on eye movements in schizophrenics, by Webster (1985, 1986) on movement sequencing in stutterers and by Roy on movement sequencing in patients with lateralized brain damage all provide examples of this role of models derived from studies in normality. Looking more closely at deficits in praxis and sequencing Roy's work (Roy, 1981, 1983, 1985; Roy & Square, 1985) adapted the idea of conceptual and production systems (Newell & Simon, 1972) to the study of disruptions in praxis and sequencing. One example here relates to the role of memory in movement sequencing. Work by Sternberg, Monsell, Knoll, and Wright (1978) indicates that in normals, performing sequences requires the retrieval of elements in the sequence from a memory buffer. This idea, derived from studies of normals, that memory may play a role in praxis and movement sequencing has also been addressed in studies of patients with lateralized brain damage by Roy (1981, 1983) and Jason (1983).

Roy (1981) examined the ability of patients with left-hemisphere and right-hemisphere damage to learn a sequence of four gestures. Each trial involved two phases. In the first phase, the patient was required to perform the sequence indicated by a series of four pictures depicting the actions to be performed at each location on the sequencing board. If patients were successful in performing the sequence on this phase of the trial, the pictures were removed and they were required to perform the sequence from memory. Learning to a criterion of five consecutive correct trials was examined in each phase. The results indicated that, on the first phase where memory demands were minimal, the left and right-hemisphere groups took the same number of trials to reach criterion. On the second phase, however, where the sequence was generated from memory the left-hemisphere patients took significantly more trials. In fact, many of these patients never reached criterion performance within the maximum of 24 trials.

More recent work by Jason (1983) confirmed these findings. Using a somewhat different methodology, Jason compared sequencing performance under two conditions. In both these conditions, the patients were required to imitate a series of four hand postures. In the first condition, the four hand postures were demonstrated to patients and they were required to perform the sequence from their memory of the demonstration. On this task, learning was reflected as the number of trials to reach the criterion of three consecutive correct sequences. On the other task, memory was not required. In this case, the patient imitated each gesture following its demonstration by the examiner. The performance of the sequence was paced by a metronome and the time interval between successive demonstrations was systematically reduced by increasing the pace set by the metronome. Performance on this task was reflected as the metronome pace achieved when the first error appeared in the patient's performance. Results of this study demonstrated no differences between the left and right-hemisphere patients on the metronome-paced sequencing task. On the task requiring the patient to generate the sequence from memory, the left-hemisphere patients took significantly more trials to reach criterion.

More recent work by Roy, Square-Storer, Adams & Friesen (1987) further examined the role of memory in the performance of sequences. In this study, sequences of limb, oral, and verbal gestures were performed under three conditions. In two conditions, the patient was required to perform the sequence from memory. In one of these two conditions the sequence was presented as a series of verbal commands (e.g., pull, push), while in the second, the sequence was demonstrated by the examiner and the patient was then required to imitate it from memory of the examiner's demonstration. The third condition placed no demands on memory. In this case, pictures depicting the actions to be performed at each position remained in place during the patient's performance of each trial. The results from this study again indicated that the left-hemisphere patients performed more poorly than the right-hemisphere patients only under the conditions in which the sequence was generated from memory. The findings of this study extend the previous work by demonstrating that this role of memory in movement sequencing is observed in all three types of movements, limb, oral, and verbal.

Another example of how studies in normality provide a focus for studies in pathology is seen in Stelmach's work with Parkinson's patients (Stelmach, Worringham, & Strand 1986). The question addressed in this work concerns the degree to which Parkinson's patients are able to use advance information in the initiation of motor responses. Stelmach et al. (1986) adopted the movement precueing technique developed by Rosenbaum (1980, 1983) to study processes of movement preparation. Using this technique, subjects were required to make movements of two extents (long or short) with either hand in one of two directions (up or down). Several conditions were involved corresponding to the amount of advance information afforded by the warning signal (i.e., the precue) about the exact nature of the upcoming movement in terms of the underlying dimensions of limb, direction, and extent. This technique permits specific inferences about the processes involved in response selection. For example, the time taken to specify values on each of the dimensions of movement can be estimated, allowing comparisons of their absolute and relative magnitude between groups of patients. The results from this experiment demonstrated that Parkinson patients exhibited longer reaction times than a comparable group of age-matched controls. These elevated reaction times, however, were not primarily caused by delays in response selection. Rather the slowness in movement initiation was thought to be due to processes which are unaffected by advance information such as excessive delays in the motor as opposed to the pre-motor component of reaction time.

Defining Mechanisms to Consider in Normality

While studies of normality may provide insight into the nature and extent of pathology, studies of patients with various types of neurobehavioural deficits afford a means of confirming the role of processes derived from studies of normals. Further, studies of patients may provide insight into mechanisms involved in perceptual and motor tasks which might not be considered through studies of normal people alone. One example of this role of studies of pathology is provided in work examining visual agnosia, the inability to recognize and/or name objects presented visually (Bauer & Rubens, 1985). One type of disorder is termed optic aphasia and represents the inability of a patient to name or point to objects named with a preserved ability to discriminate among visual objects presented. A second disorder, termed associative agnosia, involves the inability of the patient to name an object presented, while still being able to point to the same object if it is named by the examiner. The patient remains able to discriminate among objects presented visually. In a third type of disorder, termed apperceptive agnosia, the patient is unable to name objects presented or to point to objects named by the examiner, as well as being unable to discriminate among objects presented visually. These three disorders suggest that recognition of objects presented visually incorporates a number of processes involving perception and memory. Apperceptive agnosia might be thought of as a failure of processing information at a perceptual stage, while optic aphasia represents a failure at a stage involving access to the name for the object.

A recent study by Jeannerod, Michel, & Prablanc (1984) affords another example of this role of studies in pathology. In this study, they describe a patient who suffered a lesion in the post-central gyrus of the left hemisphere involving areas SI, SII, 5 and 40. As a result of this lesion the patient suffered a relatively selective loss to somatosensory function on the right side without significant involvement to motor control itself. They examined this patient's performance in rapid finger tapping, manual force generation and reaching and grasping movements. These tasks were performed with the aid of vision and with vision of the hands occluded. Comparisons between the hands revealed a marked impairment with the affected right hand, particularly when vision was prevented. Tapping performance and force generation deteriorated markedly when the patient was unable to visually monitor her performance. On the reaching task, performance was particularly impaired as the hand reached the target. This impairment in the grasp was markedly accentuated when vision of the hand was not possible. These findings substantiate the work with normals indicating the important role played by somatosensory information in the control of movement. Further, however, they indicate the important role vision may play in controlling movement when somatosensory information is lost. This substitutive role of vision may have been difficult to observe in studies of normals alone.

Another example of this role of studies in pathology comes from work by Perenin and Vighetto (1982) examining pointing accuracy in patients with lateralized brain damage. Earlier work by Prablanc, Echallier, Komilis & Jeannerod (1979) had indicated the importance of vision in directing the hand to locations in space in normal visuomotor control. Accuracy decreased and variability increased dramatically when vision of the hand was prevented, particularly near the target. In comparing the patients' performance to that of normals under the two visual conditions (i.e., vision of the hand available or not) Perenin and Vighetto observed an effect of no visual feedback in the patients which was much greater than that observed for the normals, with pointing accuracy in particular being affected. Again, these studies in pathology confirm the importance of vision in the control of movement derived from studies in normality.

Taken together these observations suggest that studies in normality and pathology each play a role in developing descriptions of the organization and control of movement. Studies of normality both define the extent of pathology in terms of whether the product or goal of the movement has been achieved and the process or means used in achieving the product or goal of the movement. As well, studies of normality provide a basis for focusing studies in pathology on particular mechanisms. Studies in pathology, on the other hand, afford a means of confirming the existence of mechanisms involved in the control of movement derived from studies in normality as well as providing an opportunity to identify mechanisms which might not be apparent in studies of motor control in normality.

Developing the Normality-Pathology Interface

Clearly, studies in normality and pathology together play an important role in advancing our understanding of mechanisms involved in motor control. However, comparisons of findings from these two populations, particularly as they pertain to the larger issue of brain-behaviour relationships, require a careful consideration of a number of issues which influence the interpretation of these comparisons. These issues centre around models of brain organization, the potential for recovery of function following brain damage, and models of the organization and control of movement. These issues are addressed in this section of the chapter.

Principles of Brain Organization

Advances in understanding brain-behaviour relationships have come through a better understanding of the organization and function of the brain. One of the most widely used methods for interpreting brain organization has come from examining the effects of damage to the brain on behaviour. In interpreting the effects of brain damage Hughlings-Jackson (1958), almost a century ago, made the important distinction between a symptom which is associated with damage to some brain region and a function. This distinction is important since we frequently ascribe as the function of a given brain area that which is lost (i.e., a symptom) when that area is damaged. Weiskrantz (1968) questioned this logic using the analogy of a radio tube's inferred function being to stop the radio from "squeaking". When the tube was in place, the radio performed well. Upon removing the tube the radio commenced a boisterous squeaking sound, hence, the inference that the tube prevents such an unpleasant sound. Wiezkrantz went on to argue that removing the tube resulted in changing the operation of the remaining tubes and, thus, what was heard (squeaking) arose from the operation of the remaining tubes in the absence of the one removed. This observation suggests that the function of any given brain region must be viewed in terms of its relationship to other brain regions.

Another point raised by Hughlings-Jackson was that damage to the brain may lead to two types of effects: loss of function, or negative symptoms, and release of function, or positive symptoms. The negative symptoms were those behaviours which were absent after brain damage and were, he reasoned, presumably generated by the now damaged area. The positive symptoms were those that emerged or became apparent after the brain damage. He reasoned that these symptoms revealed the function of remaining structures in the absence of the contribution from the damaged area. Denny-Brown (1958) has provided an example of these types of symptoms in patients who have suffered damage to the frontal lobe. The loss of control over behaviour reflected in poor judgement and impulsivity, often observed in these patients, represents the negative symptoms. The reappearance of rooting and sucking reflexes represent the positive symptoms. These positive symptoms, to some extent, are thought to reflect the loss of inhibition by the frontal lobes over lower levels that control reflexive behaviour. Again, this proposal with regard to the effects of brain damage on behaviour suggests that the brain must be organized as an integrated system.

The most recent work in functional neuroanatomy indicates that brain organization indeed involves this type of integrated system (Brooks, 1986; Kandel & Schwartz, 1985; Szentagothai & Arbib, 1975). The brain is organized into columns or modules which form the basic units. These units interact through inhibitory pathways such that they influence each other's activity. Despite anatomical and morphological boundaries, it appears that there is no one part of the brain which is in constant control of another. Rather there is a constant interplay. It appears that these modules are organized into networks which afford self organization. This principle reflects that there are properties which emerge out of the network relationship which one could not predict based upon knowledge of the function of a single component of the network. Reciprocal inhibition and lateral inhibition are examples of these emergent properties.

This view of brain organization has been accompanied by a re-evaluation of the concept of a behaviourial function. One of the earliest definitions of function was that it relates to the activity or process carried out by a single organ in the body. For example, the function of the heart is to pump blood, while the function of the kidney is to remove impurities from the blood. This definition of function pervaded the early work on the relationship between brain and behaviour and supported the notion of strict localization as a principle of brain organization reflected most notably in the movement termed phrenology (Olin, 1910).

The definition of function which more readily incorporates the principles of brain organization described above suggests that a behaviourial function relates more to the operation of a system which is dependent upon a number of subprocesses or operations. For example, breathing involves a complex functional system which incorporates the operation of a number of components. The act of breathing is largely controlled by the diaphragm. However, in the event that this muscle is damaged, breathing is controlled through the operation of the intercostal muscles. If these are damaged, breathing is made possible by swallowing air. The act of breathing, then, does not involve the operation of a single "organ" but rather involves the action of a number of components organized into a functional system.

This notion of a functional system was presented initially by Luria (1966) and was termed pleuri-potentialism. He argued that when considering complex behaviours like speech, writing, or praxis one needs to view these as involving a system of functions which are not represented in a single brain region but rather involve a number of brain regions operating in concert. Thus, in the case of speech, when the brain is damaged, the afflicted person does not lose the ability to communicate completely. Rather, depending on the area of the brain damaged, speech and language functions are disrupted in a characteristic way. Disruptions to the anterior regions of the brain in Broca's area leads to what has been termed an expressive disorder, while damage to more posterior regions in Wernicke's area leads to a receptive disorder. More recently this notion of a functional system has been applied to the study of disorders of attention (Mesulam, 1981) and praxis (Roy, 1978).

This concept of a functional system is also exemplified in Hughlings-Jackson's notion of hierarchical levels of control. The implication is that control of the system may be exerted at a number of levels. This notion of levels of control was alluded to in our discussion above of the positive effects of brain damage and has been developed in regard to the study of motor impairments by Grimm & Nashner (Grimm & Nashner, 1978; Grimm, 1983) and Roy (1978, 1983; Roy & Square, 1985). Grimm (1983) argues that motor disorders can be divided into two categories, program or non-program. Program disorders (e.g., Parkinson's Disease, Huntington's Chorea) are those in which "structural alterations occur above the level of motor units and beyond the central termination of primary afferents" (p. 1). Non-program disorders (e.g., peripheral neuropathies) are those in which the problem lies in the neuromuscular system controlling movement. In his study of disorders to praxis and sequencing Roy (1983) argues that apraxia and sequencing disorders may arise from disruptions at a number of levels in a system controlling movement.

This organizational network involving levels of control provides a rich internal environment for movement. This internal environment is afforded through the network of interconnections within levels and across spinal, brainstem, subcortical and cortical levels of control. Given this integrated network movement is preceded by complex supraspinal and spinal tuning of the neuromuscular system which sets constraints on the nature of the ensuing movement (Bernstein, 1967).

While there appears to be an internal environment important in the control of movement, the external environment also plays a role apparent in the rather direct influence cues in the environment have on movement. The nervous system is very sensitive to changes in the environment such that motor responses to these changes are very rapid and seem not to require conscious control. For example, unexpected changes in the terrain elicit rapid corrections through muscle spindle mechanisms to prevent falling. Arbib (1972, 1981) has suggested that these linkages between the environment and the motor system play an important role in the control of movements. The influence of the external environment on the brain is also seen in the affects of early experience in the development of brain structures and their interconnections. Work by Wiesel and Hubel (1985) with kittens demonstrated that deprivation from vision led to selective degeneration of cells in the visual cortex responsive to the form of a visual stimulus.

The implications of these observations on brain organization for understanding the interface between normality and pathology are numerous. One of the most important is that impairments associated with brain damage in different areas may appear to be similar. A closer examination, however, may reveal that they are quite different. Given the notion that behaviour may be organized in the brain in terms of a functional system, it is not particularly surprising that such a difference may exist. For example, following right hemisphere damage, patients may exhibit a disorder termed left neglect. In this disorder the patient tends to miss information in left hemi-space. In their work with these patients, Heilman, Watson and Valenstein (1985) found that the impairment was somewhat different in patients with frontal as opposed to parietal lesions. Frontal patients tended to have a difficulty in making movements in left hemi-space, while patients with parietal damage were unable to attend to stimuli presented in that side of hemi-space. In this case, patients with lesions in either brain area were unable to respond to information in left hemi-space, although for quite different reasons.

The other implication of these principles of brain organization concerns motor equivalence. That is, a movement goal may be achieved by a number of means. In a broader sense, this concept refers to the dissociation between the product (i.e., the movement goal) and the process (i.e., the means by which the product is achieved), alluded to above. Given that there may be a number of control centres and levels of control, it would seem that the movement goal might be achieved in a number of ways and using a number of different strategies and sources of information. For example, in the past few years it has become apparent that Parkinson patients have difficulty in using kinaesthetic information in the control of movement (Marsden, 1982). Some evidence for this finding comes from observations that performance in these patients is facilitated with augmented visual cues. The difficulty with initiating and controlling gait, for example, is greatly reduced if visual markers which act as targets for the foot are placed on the floor along the course the patient is asked to walk. This product-process dichotomy implies that damage to the central nervous system will likely not prevent the achievement of particular movement goals (i.e., the product) but rather will change the means by which these goals are achieved (i.e., process). The implication here for understanding brain-behaviour relationships is clear. We need to be concerned as much about measurement of the movements and strategies used to achieve the movement goal as we are about measuring the movement goal itself. This issue will be considered in more detail in the next section.

The Potential for Recovery of Function

The principles of brain organization discussed above provide the potential for neural plasticity and recovery of function following brain damage (Bach-y-Rita, Lazarus, Boyeson, Balliet, & Myers, 1989). This potential for recovery in itself has profound implications for understanding the normality-pathology interface. In order to clearly understand the implications of recovery of function for this interface between normality and pathology, it is important to consider some factors which seem to be important in recovery.

The potential for recovery of function lies in the neural plasticity of the brain. While a number of mechanisms have been used to explain recovery of function (e.g., Finger & Stein, 1982; Scheff, 1984), recovery seems to arise out of some type of re-organization of neural control centres in the brain. Recent work by Bach-y-Rita et al. (1989) has been focusing on recovery of motor function in the hemi-paretic arm of young head-injured patients. Normally, the control of limb movements is exerted largely by the contralateral hemisphere through the crossed lateral corticospinal tract. Through the ventral corticospinal tract, however, there are projections to each limb from the ipsilateral hemisphere, but it is not clear that the contribution from this hemisphere is significant in the control of movement. In his work, however, Bach-y-Rita has discovered that recovery in the control of the hemi-parietic limb may be due to an increasing contribution in control of the limb from the ipsilateral hemisphere. Recovery of motor control through reorganization may arise from the contribution of brain areas which are close to the damaged area as suggested in this work by Bach-y-Rita. Some of this work suggests that areas which are relatively far removed spatially from the damaged area but which share functional connections with the damaged area may also subserve recovery. Work by Goldberger (1974) examining impairments to upper limb control in monkeys following cerebellar lesioning has found that recovery may be subserved by contributions from the pre-motor and motor areas.

To some extent the basis for this re-organization seems to lie in the reduction of inhibition exerted by damaged brain regions (e.g., Bach-y-Rita et al., 1989; Goldberger, 1974; Kinsbourne, 1971a). In the work by Goldberger alluded to above, for example, recovery from pyramidal tract lesions was facilitated by lesions which reduced the inhibition exerted by surrounding brain regions. The administration of drugs which tended to reduce the inhibitory influence of these surrounding brain regions also facilitated recovery. The role of inhibition is also suggested in work examining recovery of speech and language function in patients with left hemisphere damage. Kinsbourne (1971b) observed that procedures which reduced the inhibitory influence of the damaged left hemisphere over the intact right hemisphere tended to facilitate recovery from speech impairments in these patients.

While reduction of inhibition seems to play a role in the re-organization of control centres in the brain, it also appears that the functional maturity of the undamaged brain areas in a given region may be important implicating the role of age in recovery. The effect of age on recovery is exemplified most clearly in work with animals (e.g., Goldman, 1972; Kolb & Tomie, 1988; Kolb & Whishaw, 1985). Some of this work suggested that areas which mature early and so are "committed" to a functional role may not be able to compensate for damage to another region. On the other hand, areas which mature later and are relatively "uncommitted" functionally at an early stage of development may be able to assume the role of the damaged areas. This notion is exemplified in Goldman's (1972) studies of the effects of lesioning different regions in the frontal lobes on monkeys at different stages of development on subsequent adult behaviour. She found, for example, that lesions in the dorsolateral pre-frontal area of infant and juvenile monkeys have little or no affect on behaviour at this early stage in development when compared to normal adults. On maturing to adulthood, these early lesioned monkeys do show the expected deficits. Lesions early in development in the orbito-frontal region, however, are associated with deficits at this point in development, but the deficits dissipate over development. Goldman reasoned that the dorsolateral area may mature later than the orbito-frontal area. The decreasing deficit with orbito-frontal lesions over development, she thought, reflected the relative uncommitted dorsolateral area assuming the function of this region. The increasing deficit seen with dorsolateral lesions, she suggested, indicated that this area was functionally immature early in development and that the early maturing orbito-frontal region, being functionally committed, was unable to assume the function of the dorsolateral region.

This potential for recovery of function suggests that the interface between normality and pathology is a dynamic one. That is, inferences from pathology as to the mechanisms involved in motor control in the normal state may potentially change depending upon the state of recovery of the brain-damaged person. Further the re-organization of control centres in the brain which seem to subserve recovery of function raises the question of whether the control of performance in this recovered state is the same as that observed in normality. In compensatory approaches to recovery and rehabilitation the aim is to teach the patient to carry out tasks using other muscle groups. In this case there is no question that control is different. In so-called non-compensatory approaches discussed by Bach-y-Rita et al. (1989) the question of control is less clear. The product-process dimension alluded to above in several places is important here. If we focus primarily on the product, whether or not the goal of the movement is achieved, for example moving their arm, we may observe that the patients are able to re-acquire this performance in their recovered state. If, however, we look more closely at the way in which they perform (i.e., the process) we may observe that the basis of control is not like that observed in normality. Isaacson (1975) in his work with brain-damaged children has talked about the myth of recovery of function arguing that while the child is able to achieve the movement goal, the way in which they move to that goal is fundamentally different than that observed in normal children (cf., Kolb & Tomie, 1988). These observations suggest again that it is extremely important to develop measures of the control processes involved in movement in order to clearly understand the interface between normality and pathology.

Models of the Organization and Control of Movement

At the outset of the chapter we noted that the link between brain and behaviour involves an awareness of the principles of organization of each of the components in this relationship. To this point we have discussed principles pertaining to brain organization. We now move our focus to the other component in this relationship, motor behaviour. Models of the organization and control of movement have changed substantially over the past two decades. The view that the system is organized as a strict hierarchy in which control is largely exerted by some central executor in a top-down fashion is no longer strongly held. Various models (e.g., Gallistel, 1980; Kelso & Tuller, 1981; Reed, 1982; Roy, 1983) now suggest that the system is organized more as a heterarchy in which control may be exerted at one of a number of levels. A coalitional style of control is also proposed where movements are seen to occur in an environmental context in which the environment may play a role in directing movement.

These current views of the organization and control of movement relate well to the principles of brain organization we discussed. The concept of a functional system with multiple control centres and levels of control and the importance placed on internal and external environmental contexts are all seen as key features in these models. Movement, then, may be seen as controlled both neurologically and behaviourially using common principles. The implication of this congruence is that we might ask similar questions about the control of movement observed in performance in normal and pathological states. These types of investigations particularly amplify two of the roles played by studies in normality and pathology discussed in the first section of the chapter: studies in normality provide a focus for studies in pathology and studies in pathology afford a means of confirming the role of processes derived from studies in normality. Moreover, it may be possible to better understand behaviourial impairments by simulating them in normals (cf., Kinsbourne, 1971a). Finally, impairments associated with pathology may be somewhat demystified in that these disorders, to some extent, may be viewed as aberrations of mechanisms involved in the control of movement in the normal state. For example, in comparing errors observed in apraxia and normality Roy (1982, p. 282) suggests that the "errors which are common to both the normal and pathological states ... reflect a disruption in the cognitive and/or perceptual-motor processes concerned with intention, planning and response organization".

Considerations For Future Research

These observations with regard to principles of brain organization, the accompanying potential for recovery of function and models of the control of movement have important implications for the direction of future research on the interface between normality and pathology in motor control. The development of more adequate measures of motor performance and the precise and accurate measurement of neuropathology are two implications which will be considered below.

Developing Descriptions of Motor Performance

In describing motor performance it is important to consider both the product and the process involved. As we discussed at several points in the chapter this dissociation affords an opportunity to examine more precisely the relationship between performance in normality and pathology. The measures we use, then, should enable one to examine both of these dimensions of performance, although our discussion at this point will focus mainly on the process.

The process dimension of performance is revealed through the use of two methods, descriptive or manipulative. The former aspect describes the movements, strategies or subcomponents involved in the performance of a task, while the latter refers to the manipulation of task demands so as to uncover the mechanisms involved in task performance. Both of these means of studying the process dimension may afford important insights into how a particular movement goal is achieved. A closer examination of each of these aspects suggests how these insights might be revealed.

Considering first the descriptive method it is apparent that the dissociation between product and process is not always clear. Where the movement goal or product may be achieved using any one of a number of movements or strategies, in what have been referred to as open skills (Poulton, 1957), the dissociation is quite easily made. The distinction becomes much less obvious in situations where the movement goal requires the performer to employ a particular strategy or movement pattern. Such is the case in closed skills like movement in gymnastics (Poulton, 1957). Although this product-process distinction may not always be clear, it remains important to provide as detailed a description of performance as possible in order to reflect both whether and how the movement goal was achieved.

This descriptive aspect of performance has been addressed in several ways. One approach has focused on describing the strategies employed in performance. The work by Waber and Holmes (1985, 1986) alluded to earlier examining strategies in drawing the Rey-Osterrieth Figure is an example of this approach. A second approach involves describing the movements involved in performance. One example here is the work by Roy, Square, Adams and Friesen (1985) on apraxia indicating that gestural movements may be examined at several levels of analysis which provide increasingly detailed descriptions of performance. The analysis which has most often been used simply reflects whether the gesture (e.g., salute) has been achieved or not. A somewhat more fine-grained analysis involves describing the types of errors observed in the patients' performance (e.g., Charlton, Roy, MacKenzie, & Square, 1986; Haaland & Flaherty, 1984; Rothi, Heilman, Mack, Verfaellie, & Brown, 1988; Roy, Clark, Aigbogun & Square-Storer, 1987; Roy, Square-Storer; Patla, MacKenzie & Charlton, 1987). The most detailed level of analysis employs the notation of movements (e.g., Fentress, 1984; Golani, 1973) and the description of the kinematic details (e.g., velocity, acceleration) of movements involved in performance (e.g., Marteniuk, MacKenzie, Jeannerod, Athenes, & Dugas, 1987).

This approach to describing movements has proven very useful in more clearly understanding the normal control processes involved in limb (e.g., Atkeson & Hollerbach, 1985; Jeannerod, 1984; Marteniuk et al., 1987; Soechting, 1984) and oral (e.g., Abbs, Gracco, & Cole, 1984) movements and the disruptions to control of limb (e.g., Roy et al., 1985) and oral/verbal (e.g., Itoh, Sasanuma, Hirose, Yosioka, & Ushijima, 1980) movements.

A third approach involves describing the components of a task. The reaction time paradigm provides a particularly fruitful example. Reaction time can be fractionated into two components, premotor time and motor time (Botwinick & Thompson, 1966). A number of studies in normality have indicated that different variables influence each component. Studies of brain-damaged patients have also provided some insight into the neurobehavioural mechanisms involved. For example, damage to the motor area of cortex and the underlying white matter leads to lengthening of reaction time which appears largely due to elevations in the motor component.

The other method for studying the process dimension of performance involves manipulating the perceptual, decision or effector demands of a task so as to infer the mechanisms underlying performance. This method has its root in the limiting principle from information processing and has proven useful in delineating mechanisms involved in a wide range of cognitive and motor tasks (e.g., Schmidt, 1982). In work with normals Sternberg et al. (1978) and Rosenbaum (1985) have revealed several mechanisms involved in the organization and production of movement sequences. Likewise, Posner (1980; Posner & Presti, 1987) has identified a number of mechanisms involved in shifting attention through space. Using somewhat similar methodologies work with patients with various types of neurological deficits has provided some insights into the neurological substrates underlying mechanisms identified in these investigations with normals.

The study of movement sequencing with stroke patients by Roy (1981, 1983; Roy et al., 1987) and others (e.g., Jason, 1983; Kimura, 1977, 1982) has pointed to the importance of the left hemisphere in movement sequencing. Work by Marsden (Benecke, Rothwell, Dick, Day, & Marsden, 1987) with Parkinson's patients has revealed the role of the basal ganglia in sequencing tasks. Studies of attentional deficits in patients with cortical as opposed to basal ganglia disorders by Posner (Posner, Choate, Rafal, & Vaughan, 1985; Posner, Cohen, & Rafal, 1982; Posner, Walker, Friedrich, & Rafal, 1984) has revealed that damage to the right hemisphere disrupts the disengaging of attention while basal ganglia disorders impair the efficient movement of attention through space.

These observations clearly evidence the importance of examining both the product and process dimensions of performance in order to comprehend the interface between normality and pathology. Future research will need to pay even closer attention to these two dimensions. Considering our discussion of the organization of the nervous system and the potential for recovery of function, damage to the brain precipitates a number of changes in the function of and relationship among remaining brain regions. Depending on the functional integrity of these remaining brain regions one may see tremendous interindividual variation in the process dimension of performance at any given point in time. Moreover, as these remaining brain regions undergo reorganization during the recovery period one may see enormous changes in the movement patterns and strategies used to achieve any given movement goal (e.g., Golani, Wolgin, & Teitelbaum, 1979; Whishaw, O'Connor & Dunnett, 1986). In both cases only careful studies of the process dimension will afford clear comparisons between performance in normality and pathology.

Measures of the Location and Extent of Neuropathology

Another important consideration in developing links between normality and pathology in motor control relates to the use of appropriate measures of neuropathology. Just as one needs to carefully describe the behaviourial manifestations of neurological impairments through analyses of the product and process dimensions of performance so one must accurately identify the location and extent of neuropathology. Over the past two decades many new neuroradiological and electrophysiological techniques have been developed which permit much more precise localization of brain lesions. Of the neuroradiological techniques available one of the most widely used is computerized axial tomography (CAT). The CAT scan images of the brain are generated from the degree of absorption of x-rays by various brain structures (e.g., Plets, Baert, Nijs, & Wilms, 1987). This technique has been used to identify the location and extent of neuropathology in many deficits (see Kertesz, 1983) including movement disorders such as apraxia (e.g., Basso, Faglioni, Luzzatti, 1985). A more recent technique which provides images similar to CAT scans although with somewhat greater resolution is called magnetic resonance imaging (MRI, see Daniels, Haughton & Naidich, 1987). This technique has also been used to relate observed neuropsychological deficits with the location of brain lesions, including movement disorders such as apraxia (e.g., Watson, Heilman, & Bowers, 1985). A third procedure, positron emission tomography (PET, see Heiss, Beil, Herholz, Pawlik, Wagner, & Weinhard, 1985; Phelps, 1977; Phelps, Hoffman, Huang, & Kuhl, 1978) involves a completely different method of generating the brain scan images. In the CAT and MRI techniques the image reflects the structural integrity of the brain. The PET scan, however, reflects the functional integrity of the brain in terms of its metabolic activity as measured by the rate of glucose utilization. This procedure has also been used in neuropsychological research (see Benson,

Metter, Kuhl, & Phelps, 1983) although to a lesser extent to date than CAT and MRI scanning.

While each of these techniques offers a view of the localization of brain lesions, each has their limitations (see Kertesz, 1983, Chapter 1). The important point here relates to which of these techniques reflects the location and extent of the lesion most effectively. From the standpoint of precision in localization CAT and MRI scans provide much better resolution than do PET scans. Both the CAT and MRI procedures reflect only the structural integrity of brain tissue, however. This fact may lead to considerable errors in describing the full extent of a lesion since brain tissue which is metabolically underactive and, therefore, not exhibiting complete functional integrity may appear structurally intact. The PET scan image which is sensitive to the functional integrity of brain tissue may, then, provide the most valid measure of the extent of a lesion.

The incongruence between PET scan and CAT/MRI scan images of the brain is revealed by Benson et al. (1983). They describe the case of a 48 year old male who experienced sudden onset of a mild right hemiparesis and aphasia. The PET scan image revealed marked hypometabolism of the temporo-parietal regions of the left subcortical nuclear areas and a somewhat lesser degree of hypometabolism of the left hemisphere. The CAT scan, however, appeared largely normal. This potential for incongruity among these neuroradiological measures leads, of course, to the question of which measure do we use to relate to observed behaviourial deficits. The only solution at this point would seem to be to use all these measures of neuropathology where feasible and attempt to interrelate findings from each technique to observed impairments of function. These types of comparative studies (e.g., Benson et al., 1983; Lee & Rao, 1987) have begun in the past few years.

These types of comparative studies in pathology may lead to insights into the normality-pathology interface. An even more fruitful approach, however, may be to compare brain activity in normals associated with the performance of various tasks as reflected by metabolic or electrophysiological (e.g., Phelps, Kuhl, & Mazziotti, 1980) measures to the location of brain lesions in patients who show deficits in these same tasks.

While an understanding of the interface between normality and pathology will be facilitated through the use of effective measures of neuropathology, this approach by itself has several limitations. First, several types of neuropathology such as Parkinson's disease cannot be well imaged using the neuroradiological procedures discussed. These diseases reflect disruptions to neurotransmitter systems rather than structural or metabolic disorders (but see Nahmias, Garnett, Firnau, & Lang, 1985). Secondly, due to individual differences in brain organization related to such factors as sex, handedness and age, persons with similar lesions may manifest somewhat different behaviourial deficits. Finally, knowledge of the precise location and extent of a brain lesion reveals nothing of the functional integrity of the apparently undamaged tissue. For these reasons it is necessary to augment information about neuropathology gleaned from neuroradiological techniques with complete neurological and neuropsychological assessments to measure the degree of deficits behaviourially and to identify areas of preserved function. For example, the degree of motor impairment in Parkinson's disease can be quantified (Fahn, 1982; Hoehn & Yahr, 1967). This measure rather than any neuroradiological measure would reflect the degree of neuropathologic deficit. It is this measure, then, which would be correlated with other behaviourial measures. Work by Saint-Cyr and his colleagues (Saint-Cyr, Taylor & Lang, 1988; Taylor, Saint-Cyr & Lang, 1986) which attempts to identify cognitive impairments in Parkinson's disease affords an example of this approach. In this research they use various measures of tremor and bradykinesia to reflect the severity of the motor deficit in the patients and relate these measures to their measures of cognitive deficits.

Summary

The processes involved in motor learning and control have been largely studied in normal individuals. Patients with a variety of motor impairments due to various types of pathology have been reported for over 100 years in the neurology literature. It is only in the last two decades that more systematic and sophisticated investigations of these motor impairments have been initiated. The focus of this chapter has been on discussing how comparisons between studies in these two states, normality and pathology, may lead to insights into the nature of the learning and control of movement.

At the outset the role of studies in normality and pathology was considered. Studies in normality were seen to afford a view of the nature and extent of pathology as well as to provide a focus on particular mechanisms in studies in pathology. Studies in pathology, on the other hand, were thought to enable confirmation of mechanisms identified from studies in normality. The second section was devoted to factors important in making these comparisons in normality and pathology. The principles of brain organization and the accompanying potential for recovery of function as well as models of the organization and control of movement were considered. Given these observations directions for future research were presented. The need to measure both the product and the process involved in movement as well as to use appropriate measures of neuropathology was discussed.

Author Notes

1. This chapter is partially based on a reaction paper presented in a symposium entitled Human Pathology in Motor Behavior at the annual meeting of the North American Society for the Psychology of Sport and Physical Activity, Vancouver, B.C., June, 1987.

2. Preparation of this manuscript was partially funded by a grant from NSERC.

3. Send requests for reprints to Eric A. Roy, Department of Kinesiology, University of Waterloo, Waterloo, Ontario, Canada, N2L 3G1.

References

Abbs, J. H., Gracco, V. L., & Cole, K. J. (1984). Control of multimovement coordination: Sensorimotor mechanisms in speech motor programming. *Journal of Motor Behavior, 16*, 195-231.

Arbib, M. A. (1972). *The metaphorical brain: An introduction to cybernetics as artificial intelligence and brain theory.* New York, NY: Interscience.

Arbib, M. A. (1981). Perceptual structures and distributed motor control. In J. M. Brookhart & V. B. Mountcastle (Eds.), *Handbook of physiology*, Volume II:2 (pp. 1499-1480). Bethesda, MD: American Psychological Society.

Atkeson, C. G., & Hollerbach, J. M. (1985). Kinematic features of unrestrained vertical arm movements. *Journal of Neuroscience, 5*, 2318-2330.

Bach-y-Rita, P., Lazarus, J. C., Boyeson, M. G., Balliet, R., & Myers, T. (1989). Neural aspects of motor function as a basis of early and post-acute rehabilitation. In J. A. Delisa, D. Currie, B. Gans, P. Gatens, J. A. Leonard, & M. McPhee (Eds.), *Principles and practice of rehabilitation medicine.* Philadelphia, PA: J.B. Lippincott.

Basso, A., Faglioni, P., & Luzzatti, C. (1985). Methods in neuroanatomical research and an experimental study of limb apraxia. In E. A. Roy (Ed.) *Advances in psychology: Vol. 23. Neuropsychological studies of apraxia and related disorders* (pp. 179-202). Amsterdam: North-Holland.

Bauer, R. M. & Rubens, A. B. (1985). Agnosia. In K. M. Heilman & E. Valenstein (Eds.), *Clinical neuropsychology*. (pp. 187-241). New York, NY: Academic Press.

Benecke, R., Rothwell, J. C., Dick, J. P. R., Day, B. L., & Marsden, C. D. (1987). Disturbance of sequential movements in patients with Parkinson's disease. *Brain, 110,* 361-379.

Benson, F., Metter, E. J., Kuhl, D. E., & Phelps, M. E. (1983). Position computed tomography in neurobehavioural problems. In A. Kertesz (Ed.) *Localization in neuropsychology* (pp. 121-139). New York, NY: Academic Press.

Bernstein, N. A. (1967). *The coordination and regulation of movements.* London: Pergamon Press.

Binder, L. M. (1982). Constructional strategies on complex figure drawings after unilateral brain damage. *Journal of Clinical Neuropsychology, 4,* 51-58.

Botwinick, J. & Thompson, L. W. (1966). Pre-motor and motor components of reaction time. *Journal of Experimental Psychology, 71,* 9-15.

Brooks, V. B. (1986). *The neural basis of motor control.* New York, NY: Oxford University Press.

Charlton, J., Roy, E. A., MacKenzie, C., & Square, P. (1986) Impairments to sequencing and motor control in apraxia. *Canadian Psychology, 27,* 432.

Daniels, D. L., Haughton, V. M., & Naidich, T. P. (1987). *Cranial and spinal magnetic resonance imaging.* New York, NY: Raven Press.

Denny-Brown, D. (1958). The nature of apraxia. *Journal of Nervous and Mental Disease, 126,* 9-32.

De Renzi, E. (1985). Methods of limb apraxia examination and their bearing on the interpretation of the disorder. In E. A. Roy (Ed.), *Advances in psychology: Vol. 23. Neuropsychological studies of apraxia and related disorders* (pp. 45-64). Amsterdam: North Holland Co.

Fahn, S. (1982). Fluctuations of disability in Parkinson's disease: Pathophysiology. In C. D. Marsden & S. Fahn (Eds.), *Movement disorders* (pp. 123-145). London: Butterworths.

Fentress, J. C. (1984). The development of coordination. *Journal of Motor Behavior, 16* (2), 99-134.

Finger, S. & Stein, A. G. (1982). *Brain damage and recovery: Research and clinical perspective.* New York, NY: Academic Press.

Gallistel, C. R. (1980). *The organization of action.* Hillsdale, NJ: Lawrence Erlbaum.

Golani, I. (1973). Homeostatic motor processes in mammalian interactions: A choreography of display. In P. P. G. Bateson & P. H. Klopfer (Eds.), *Perspectives in ethology* (Vol. 2, pp. 69-134). New York, NY: Plenum Press.

Golani, I., Wolgin, D. L., & Teitelbaum, P. (1979). A proposed natural geometry of recovery of function from akinesia in the lateral hypothalamic rat. *Brain Research, 164,* 237-267.

Goldberger, M. E. (1974). Recovery of movement after CNS lesions in monkeys. In D. G. Stein, J. J. Rosen, & N. Butters (Eds.), *Plasticity and recovery of function in the central nervous system* (pp. 265-337). New York, NY: Academic Press.

Goldman, P. S. (1972). Developmental determinants of cortical plasticity. *Acta Neurobiologica Experimentalis, 32,* 495-511.

Grimm, R. J. (1983). Program disorders of movement. In J. E. Desmedt (Ed.), *Motor control mechanisms in health and disease* (pp. 1-11). New York NY: Raven Press.

Grimm, R. J., & Nashner, L. M. (1978). Long loop dyscontrol. In J. E. Desmedt (Ed.), *Cerebral motor control in man: Long loop mechanisms, Progress in clinical neurophysiology* (Vol. 4, pp. 70-84) Basel, Switzerland: S. Karger.

Haaland, K. & Flaherty, D. (1984). The different types of limb apraxia errors made by patients with left vs. right hemisphere damage. *Brain and Cognition, 3,* 370-384.

Heilman, K. M., Watson, R. T., & Valenstein, E. (1985). Neglect and related disorders. In K. M. Heilman & E. Valenstein (Eds.), *Clinical neuropsychology* (pp. 243-293). New York, NY: Oxford University Press.

Heiss, W. D., Beil, C., Herholz, K., Pawlik, G., Wagner, R., & Weinhard, K. (1985). *Atlas of position emission tomography of the brain.* Heidelberg: Springer-Verlag.

Hoehn, M. M. & Yahr, M. D. (1967). Parkinsonism: Onset, progression and mortality. *Neurology, 17,* 427-442.

Hughlings-Jackson, J. (1958). *Selected writings of John Hughlings-Jackson.* New York, NY: Basic Books.

Isaacson, R. L. (1975). The myth of recovery from early brain damage. In N. R. Ellis (Ed.), *Aberrant development in infancy* (pp. 1-25), Hillsdale, NJ: Lawrence Erlbaum.

Itoh, M., Sasanuma, S., Hirose, H., Yosioka, H., & Ushijima, T. (1980). Abnormal articulatory dynamics in a patient with apraxia of speech. *Brain and Language, 7,* 227-239.

Jason, G. (1983). Hemispheric asymmetries in motor function: I. Left hemisphere specialization for memory but not performance. *Neuropsychologia, 21,* 35-46.

Jeannerod, M. (1984). The timing of natural prehension movements. *Journal of Motor Behavior, 16,* 235-254.

Jeannerod, M., Michel, F., & Prablanc, C. (1984). The control of hand movements in a case of hemianesthesia following a parietal lesion. *Brain, 107,* 899-920.

Kandel, E. R. & Schwartz, J. H. (1985). *Principles of neural science* (2nd ed.). New York, NY: Elsevier Science Publishing.

Kelso, J. A. S., & Tuller, B. (1981). Towards a theory of apractic syndromes. *Brain and Language, 12,* 224-245.

Kertesz, A. (Ed.) (1983). *Localization in neuropsychology.* New York, NY: Academic Press.

Kimura, D. (1977). Acquisition of a motor skill after left hemisphere damage. *Brain, 100,* 527-542.

Kimura, D. (1982). Left-hemisphere control of oral and brachial movements and their relation to communication. *Philosophical Transactions of the Royal Society of London, B298,* 135-149.

Kinsbourne, M. (1971a). Cognitive deficit: An experimental analysis. In J. L. McGaugh (Ed.), *Psychobiology* (pp. 285-348). New York, NY: Academic Press.

Kinsbourne, M. (1971b). The minor cerebral hemisphere as a source of aphasic speech. *Archives of Neurology, 25,* 302-306.

Kolb, B., & Tomie, J. (1988). Recovery from early cortical damage in rats. IV. Effects of hemidecortication at 1, 5, or 10 days of age on cerebral anatomy and behaviour. *Behavioral Brain Research, 28,* 259-274.

Kolb, B., & Whishaw, I. Q. (1985). Earlier is not always better: Behavioral dysfunction and abnormal cerebral morphogenesis following neonatal cortical lesions in the rat. *Behavioral Brain Research, 17,* 25-43.

Lee, S. H., & Rao, K. C. V. G. (1987). *Cranial computed tomography and MRI.* New York, NY: McGraw-Hill.

Lezak, M. (1983). *Neuropsychological assessment* (2nd ed.). New York, NY: Oxford University Press.

Luria, A. R. (1966). *Higher cortical functions in man.* New York, NY: Basic Books.

Marsden, C. D. (1982). The mysterious function of the basal ganglia: The Robert Wartenburg Lecture. *Neurology, 32,* 514-539.

Marshall, J. C. (1982). Models of the mind in health and diseases. In A. W. Ellis (Ed.) *Normality and pathology in cognitive functions* (pp. 1-18). New York, NY: Academic Press.

Marteniuk, R. G., MacKenzie, C., Jeannerod, M., Athenes, S., & Dugas, C. (1987). Constraints on human arm movement trajectories. *Canadian Journal of Psychology, 41,* 365-378.

Mather, J. A. (1986). Saccadic eye movements to seen and unseen targets: Occilomotor errors in normal subjects resembling those of schizophrenics. *Journal of Psychiatric Research, 20,* 1-8.

Mesulam, M. M. (1981). A cortical network for directed attention and unilateral neglect. *Annals of Neurology, 10,* 309-325.

Milberg, W. P., Hebben, N., & Kaplan, E. (1986). The Boston process approach to neuropsychological assessment. In I. Grant & K. M. Adams (Eds.), *Neuropsychological assessment of neuropsychiatric disorders* (pp. 65-86). New York, NY: Oxford University Press.

Nahmias, C., Garnett, C.E., Firnau, G. & Lang, A. Striatal dopamine distribution in parkinsonian patients in life. *Journal of Neurological Sciences*, 69, 223-230.

Newell, A. & Simon, H. A. (1972). *Human problem solving.* Englewood Cliffs, NJ: Prentice-Hall.

Olin, C. H. (1910). *Phrenology.* Philadelphia, PA: The Penn Publishing Co.

Osterrieth, P. A. (1944). Le test de copie d'une figure complex. *Archives de Psychologie, 30,* 206-356.

Perenin, M. T., & Vighetto, A. (1983). Optic ataxia: A specific disorder in visuomotor coordination. In A. Hein & M. Jeannerod (Eds.), *Spatially oriented behavior* (pp. 305-326). New York, NY: Springer-Verlag.

Phelps, M. E. (1977). Emission computed tomography. *Seminars in Nuclear Medicine, 7,* 337-365.

Phelps, M. E., Hoffman, E. J., Huang, S. C., & Kuhl, D. E. (1978). ECAT: A new computerized tomographic imaging system for positron-emitting radiopharmaceuticals. *Journal of Nuclear Medicine, 19,* 635-647.

Phelps, M. E., Kuhl, D. E., & Mazziotti, J. C. (1980). Tomographic mapping of the metabolic changes in the visual cortex during visual stimulation of volunteers and patients with visual defects. *Journal of Nuclear Medicine, 21,* 21.

Plets, C., Baert, A. L., Nijs, G. L., & Wilms, G. (1987). *Computed tomographic injury and anatómic correlation of the human brain.* Boston, MA: Martinus Nijhoff.

Posner, M. I. (1980). Orienting of attention. *Quarterly Journal of Experimental Psychology, 32,* 3-25.

Posner, M. I., Choate, L., Rafal, R. D., & Vaughan, J. (1985). Inhibition of return: Neural mechanisms and function. *Cognitive Neuropsychology, 2,* 211-228.

Posner, M. I., Cohen, Y., & Rafal, R. D. (1982). Neural systems control of spatial orienting. *Proceedings of the Royal Society of London, B298,* 187-198.

Posner, M. I., & Presti, D. E. (1987). Selective attention and cognitive control. *Trends in Neurosciences, 10,* 13-17.

Posner, M. I., Walker, J. A., Friedrich, F. J., & Rafal, R. D. (1984). Effects of parietal lobe injury on covert orienting of visual attention. *Journal of Neuroscience, 4,* 1863-1874.

Poulton, E. C. (1957). On prediction in skilled movement. *Psychological Bulletin, 54,* 467-478.

Prablanc, E., Echallier, J. F., Komilis, E., & Jeannerod, M. (1979). Optimal response of eye and hand motor systems in pointing at a visual target. I. Spatio-temporal characteristics of eye and hand movements and their relationships when varying the amount of visual information. *Biological Cybernetics, 35,* 113-24.

Reed, E. S. (1982). An outline of a theory of action systems. *Journal of Motor Behavior, 14,* 98-134.

Rosenbaum, D. A. (1980). Human movement imitation specification of arm, direction, and extent. *Journal of Experimental Psychology: General, 109,* 444-474.

Rosenbaum, D. A. (1983). The movement precuing technique: Assumptions, applications and extensions. In R. A. Magill (Ed.), *Advances in psychology: Vol. 12. Memory and control of action* (pp. 231-274). Amsterdam: North-Holland.

Rosenbaum, D. A. (1985). Motor programming: A review and scheduling theory. In H. Heuer, U. Kleinbeck & K. M. Schmidt (Eds.), *Motor behavior: Programming, control and acquisition* (pp. 1-33). Berlin: Springer-Verlag.

Rothi, L. J. G., Heilman, K. M., Mack, L., Verfaellie, M., & Brown, P., (1988, in press). Ideomotor apraxia error pattern analysis. *Aphasiology.*

Roy, E. A. (1978). Apraxia: A new look at an old syndrome. *Journal of Human Movement Studies, 4,* 191-210.

Roy, E. A. (1981). Action sequencing and lateralized cerebral damage: Evidence for asymmetries in control. In J. Long & A. Baddeley (Eds.), *Attention and performance IX* (pp. 265-298). Hillsdale, NJ: Lawrence Erlbaum.

Roy, E. A. (1982). Action and performance. In A. Ellis (Ed.), *Normality and pathology in cognitive functions* (pp. 265-298). London: Academic Press.

Roy, E. A. (1983). Neuropsychological perspectives on apraxia and related action sequencing disorders. In R. Magill (Ed.) *Advances in psychology: Vol. 12. Memory and motor control* (pp. 293-320) Amsterdam: North-Holland Co.

Roy, E. A. (Ed.) (1985). *Advances in psychology, Volume, 23, Neuropsychological studies of apraxia and related disorders.* Amsterdam: North Holland Co.

Roy, E. A., Clark, P., Aigbogun, S., & Square-Storer, P. (1987). Evidence for bimanual impairments in fine motor control with left hemisphere damage. *Journal of Clinical and Experimental Neuropsychology, 9,* 78.

Roy, E. A,. & Square, P. A. (1985). Common considerations in the study of disruptions to limb, oral and verbal praxis. In E. A. Roy (Ed.), *Advances in psychology: Vol. 23. Neuropsychological studies of apraxia and related disorders* (pp. 111-161). Amsterdam: North Holland Co.

Roy, E. A., Square, P. A., Adams, S,. & Friesen, H. (1985), Error/movement notation systems in apraxia. *Semiotic Inquiry, 4,* 402-412.

Roy, E. A., Square-Storer, P. A., Patla, A., MacKenzie, C., & Charlton, J. (1987). Developing systems for describing apraxic performance: Comparisons between normal and brain-damaged adults. *Canadian Psychology, 28,* 522.

Roy, E.A., Square-Storer, P.A., Adams, S. & Friesen, H. (1987) Disruptions to sequencing of limb, oral and verbal movements: Effects of sequence length and presentation at annual meeting of the North American Society for the Psychology of Sport and Physical Activity, Vancouver, B.C., June, 1987.

Saint-Cyr, J. A., Taylor, A. E., & Lang, A. E. (1988). Procedural learning and neostratal function in man. *Brain, 111,* 941-959.

Scheff, S. W. (Ed.) (1984). *Aging and recovery of function in the central nervous system.* New York, NY: Plenum Press.

Schmidt, R. A. (1982). *Motor control and learning: A behavioral analysis.* Champaign, IL: Human Kinetics Publisher.

Soechting, J. E. (1984). Effect of target size on spatial and temporal characteristics of a pointing movement in man. *Experimental Brain Research, 54,* 121-132.

Stelmach, G. E., Worringham, C. J., & Strand, E. A. (1986). Movement preparation in Parkinson's disease: The use of advance information. *Brain, 109,* 1179-1194.

Sternberg, S., Monsell, S., Knoll, R., & Wright, C. (1978). The latency and duration of rapid movement sequences: Comparisons of speech and typewriting. In G. E. Stelmach (Ed.), *Information processing in motor control and learning* (pp. 118-152). New York, NY: Academic Press.

Szentagothai, J., & Arbib, M. A. (1975). The module concept in cerebral cortex architecture. *Brain Research, 95,* 475-496.

Taylor, A. E., Saint-Cyr, J. A., & Lang, A. Z. (1986). Frontal lobe dysfunction in Parkinson's disease: The cortical focus on neostriatal outflow. *Brain, 109,* 845-853.

Visser, R. S. H. (1973). *Manual of the complex figure test.* Amsterdam: Swets Zeitlinger B.V.

Waber, D. P., & Holmes, J. M. (1985). Assessing children's copy productions of the Rey-Osterrieth Complex Figure. *Journal of Clinical and Experimental Neuropsychology, 7,* 264-280.

Waber, D. P., & Holmes, J. M. (1986). Assessing children's memory of the Rey-Osterrieth Complex Figure. *Journal of Clinical and Experimental Neuropsychology, 8,* 563-580.

Watson, R. T., Heilman, K., & Bowers, D. (1985). Magnetic resonance imaging scan in a case of callosal apraxia and pseudoneglect. *Brain, 108,* 535-536.

Webster, W. G. (1985). Neuropsychological models of stuttering. I. Representation of sequential response mechanisms. *Neuropsychologia, 23,* 263-267.

Webster, W. G. (1986). Neuropsychological models of stuttering. II. Interhemispheric interference. *Neuropsychologia, 24,* 737-741.

Weiskrantz, L. (1968). *Analysis of behavioral change.* New York, NY: Harper & Row Co.

Whishaw, I. Q., O'Connor, W. T., & Dunnett, S. B. (1986). The contributions of motor cortex, nigrostiatal dopamine and caudate-pritanmen to skilled forelimb use in the rat. *Brain, 109,* 805-843.

Wiesel, T. N., & Hubel, D. H. (1985). Comparison of the effects of unilateral and bilateral eye closure on cortical unit responses in kittens. *Journal of Neurophysiology, 28,* 1029-1040.

Problems in Movement Control
G. Reid (editor)

SKILL ACQUISITION RESEARCH WITH PERSONS WITH DEVELOPMENTAL DISABILITIES: RESEARCH DESIGN CONSIDERATIONS

A.E. Wall
Department of Physical Education
McGill University

For our purposes, developmental-disabilities research will refer to psychological, educational, and motor learning investigations into the characteristics, needs, and learning processes of children and youth who have been categorized as learning disabled or mentally handicapped. Space constraints allow for only a brief discussion of some of the major issues in the field of developmental disabilities research; however, they will provide a background from which to examine current and future directions in adapted physical activity research.

A Holistic View of Developmental Disabilities

Concerns with Reductionism

In his opening address to the Alpbach Symposium in 1968 entitled: Beyond reductionism, Paul Weiss a famous developmental neurobiologist, stated:

> "Just like the painter, who steps back from his canvas to gain perspective, so the laboratory scientist emerges above ground occasionally from the deep shaft of his specialized preoccupation to survey the cohesive, meaningful fabric developing from innumerable component tributary threads, spun underground much like his own. Only by such shuttling back and forth between the worm's eye view of detail and the bird's eye view of the total scenery of science can the scientist gain and retain a sense of perspective and proportions." (p. 3)

His recognition for the need to temper reductioninst science with a holistic perspective was applauded by other distinguished scientists at that time and it has been reinforced by important statements on the need to take a broader view in psychology by other researchers (Maslow, 1969).

In recent years, developmental and educational psychologists working with persons with developmental disabilities have also stressed the importance of taking a broader theoretical perspective. Recently, Poplin (1988) categorized psychological research in learning disabilities under four major models and time periods: the medical (1950's), psychological process (1960's), behaviourial (1970's), and cognitive-learning strategy (1980's). She examined how each of these models addressed the major questions of etiology, diagnosis, assessment, instruction, treatment and goals of the program. Her analysis and discussion of each of the models is worth careful consideration, but we will simply relate the general conclusions she makes about them.

Poplin's main premise is that the field of research in learning disabilities has made little progress because of the reductionist nature of science that underlies the above four models. She contends that the scientific method used in both psychological and educational research is based on reductionist principles. By using reductionist methods, these fields base their research on the fallacious belief that a complex whole can simply be explained by studying its parts. All of the models are "examples of erroneously believing that a complex whole such as human learning problems can be broken down into component parts . . . in order to design more effective practice in assessment and instruction" (p. 394). Thus, learning is usually segmented into parts which results in tasks that are "tedious and disconnected from students' lives" (p. 395).

Poplin takes special exception to the fact that instruction in each model is deficit driven and that much of the school day is spent on finding what is wrong with the student or what the student has not learned. She "wonders if our students' trouble with self-concept is not exacerbated by our deficit-driven methodologies" (p. 395). Finally, Poplin notes that each of the models almost exclusively promotes school goals rather than life goals, a point that is of central importance to those who wish to promote physically active lifestyles for all individuals.

The above brief analysis of the models used in the field of learning disabilities research has identified concerns with reducationism that merit our consideration as we examine theoretical frameworks in the adapted physical activity field.

Concerns with IQ and Developmental Level

A recent examination of research in mental retardation by Baumeister (1987) may also prove instructive. Baumeister, a well-known researcher in the field of mental retardation, begins by noting that "mental retardation is primarily a behaviourial concept, defined in relation to standards for different ages and cultures" (p. 796). He notes that the current American Association on Mental Deficiency definition is multidimensional: "Mental retardation refers to significantly subaverage intellectual functioning existing concurrently with deficits in adaptive behaviour and manifested during the developmental period" (Grossman, 1983).

Baumeister (1987) identifies a number of problems with the above definition, not the least of which is a major problem with the concept of intelligence itself. As he notes, the "intense and sometimes acrimonious debate over the nature of intelligence has profound implications for defining mental retardation, but these have yet to influence the committee process by which 'mental retardation' has been defined" (p. 796). The recent work of Gardner (1983) on broader conceptions of intelligence, underscores the major changes taking place in this field. The notion that one has a number of "frames of mind" or intelligences, including bodily-kinesthetic intelligence, is of special interest to those working in the fields of adapted physical activity and motor learning (Gardner, 1983).

Baumeister goes on to ask what clinically useful information is obtained from IQ scores. He contends that "beyond predicting academic performance within the relatively fixed school system; intelligence tests have dubious validity for differential diagnosis of mental retardation" (p. 96). Baumeister notes that correlations between measures of achievement outside of school and IQ are relatively low; furthermore, "different environments contribute to identifying adaptive behaviour or intellectual incompetence by different criteria or with varying degrees of sensitivity" (p. 796). He concludes his analysis of the usefulness of IQ scores as follows:

> The most compelling position against the use of IQ scores is that a single composite score yields little information about either cause or corrective action. To improve cognitive competence, an IQ score is not needed. The purpose of schooling is to help children learn and develop skills needed in adjusting to their environments (p. 797).

In addition to the above comments on the definition of mental retardation, Baumeister makes a number of important observations on research that is based on traditional IQ classification methods. First, he notes that homogeneous groups of mentally handicapped subjects "exhibit significantly more between-individual differences on various tasks than do similarly grouped non-retarded subjects" (p. 797). Furthermore, mentally handicapped individuals "show greater within-subject variability than non-handicapped individuals" (p. 797). He recommends that classification schemes need to include focused behaviourial measures and not simply general behaviourial attributes if they are to be of any value in developmental disability research. Certainly, the issues raised by Baumeister must be considered when we examine the appropriateness of our research designs.

Concerns with Motor Learning Research

A complete review of the literature in the field of adapted physical activity and motor learning is beyond the scope of this chapter; however, a short summary and discussion of an important review paper by Hoover and Wade (1985) on motor learning research with mentally handicapped individuals will provide a helpful background for our discussions. From the outset, Hoover and Wade acknowledge that the broad field of motor learning and especially the areas of motor development and special education have not had strong theoretical underpinnings. They divide their historical review into three periods: the pre-information processing period (1900-1950), the information processing period (1947-present), and the post-information processing period (1975-to date).

The pre-information processing period was influenced by stimulus-response psychology and Hoover and Wade report that most of the mental retardation research on motor skills during that period was relatively atheoretical in nature. The information processing period from 1947 to the present was marked by the emergence of models based on a cybernetic view of performance in which comparative research on skill acquisition looked for information - capacity limitations to explain the generally lower motor performance capabilities of mentally handicapped individuals (Wade, Hoover & Newell, 1983). The focus of comparative research during that period was to identify and describe the information processing differences between mentally handicapped and non-handicapped individuals.

The authors carefully review comparative studies that examined differences in stimulus input and coding, (Baumeister & Kellas, 1968; Nettelbeck & Brewer, 1976; Nettelbeck & Kirby, 1980), stimulus - response integration (Brewer & Nettelbeck 1977; Brewer, 1978; Wade, Newell & Wallace, 1978; Bankhead & Mackay, 1982) and response parameters (Berkson, 1960; Wade, Newell & Wallace, 1978; Hoover, Wade & Newell, 1981). They conclude their review of research in this period by reinforcing Newell's (1985) observation that "the information processing approach has been no more than another description of the motor performance of mentally retarded persons" (p.242).

Hoover and Wade report that the major research thrust in recent years has focused on the effects of strategic behaviour and metacognition on the motor performance of mentally handicapped individuals. Brewer and Nettelbeck (1979) experienced difficulties trying to ensure that the subjects in their target aiming studies appropriately followed their verbal instructions. Subjects with IQ's below 70 clearly favoured being accurate rather than fast even though instructions to "go as fast as you can" were given. Hoover and Wade (1985) point out that the way subjects interpret instructions is an important factor to consider in research studies with persons with mental handicaps.

More recent studies of motor memory with mildly mentally handicapped individuals using the linear positioning task show large performance decrements as retention intervals increase apparently due to a lack of strategic processing (Horgan, 1983; Kelso, Goodman, Stamm & Hayes, 1979). Reid (1980) was one of the first to show the beneficial effects of strategic training on the retention of target positions in a motor memory task. Recent research has shown that training in strategic behaviours can positively affect motor performance; however, some difficulties have been found in the maintenance and generalization of such strategies (Brown, 1974; Borkowski & Cavanaugh, 1979).

Hoover and Wade's article reflects the state of the art in the field of mental retardation and motor performance up until fairly recently. It shows that a considerable amount of comparative research has been based on chronological-age and mental-age match designs using laboratory type tasks to explain performance and information processing differences largely on the basis of IQ and MA. Given the concerns that Baumeister (1987) raises about the validity of the intelligent quotient, the usefulness of MA and CA matches, and the lack of attention to socio-cultural factors, and coupling them with those of Poplin (1988), who stresses the need to take a more contextualist approach, and it is clear that research in our field certainly needs a more inclusive framework with which to guide itself.

If we wish to understand the motor performance and skill acquisition of developmentally-delayed individuals so that we can help them participate more fully in physical activity, then it seems evident that our research should be at a behavioural level of analysis and focus on ecologically-valid tasks. Furthermore, it will be extremely important to consider the knowledge base of the person; a subject to which we know turn.

A Knowledge-based Approach to Skill Acquisition

In 1985, Wall and his colleagues criticized the atheoretical nature of much of the research done with physically awkward children (Wall, McClements, Bouffard, Findlay & Taylor, 1985). In response to the types of concerns and issues outlined by Poplin and Baumeister and recognizing the relevance of the expert novice studies that showed the importance of domain-specific knowledge, they developed a knowledge-based approach to motor development that emphasized the emergence of five types of knowledge about action and discussed how they apply to the developmental problems faced by physically awkward children. They suggested that such a model might be a valuable heuristic device that could help generate new ways of viewing and enhancing skill acquisition and performance among developmentally-disabled individuals.

This section reviews some expert-novice studies that provide the background for a brief outline of the model and a brief description of studies that provide evidence to support the validity of some of its underlying principles.

Domain-Specific Expertise

In an early study of expertise in chess, de Groot (1965) tried to understand why chess masters played better than less-experienced players. He initially thought that masters could think further ahead during a game which would enable them to accurately assess the value of different moves. He presented actual game situations to masters and less experienced players and asked them to think aloud as they selected their next move. In contrast to his initial expectation, de Groot found that the masters did not think further ahead; rather their moves were simply qualitatively better than the less skilled players. In a subsequent study, de Groot examined whether chess masters had developed a greater knowledge base that allowed them to appreciate the significance of different game positions which, in turn, allowed them to select better chess moves. He allowed masters and less experienced players to view an actual chess game board for five seconds and asked them to recall the placement of the different pieces as accurately as possible. de Groot's results showed that the experts were much better on this short term memory task than their less-skilled colleagues. de Groot's study was a pioneering one that demonstrated the importance of a person's knowledge base in skilled performance.
Chase and Simon (1973) followed up on de Groot's work to demonstrate that the above differences were not simply due to differences in short-term memory capacity. In an expert-novice study that has become a classic in the field, they presented masters, intermediates and novices actual game and random chess situations for five seconds and asked them to reproduce them as accurately as possible. In the actual game situation, recall performance was directly related to skill in chess; however, there were no differences in the recall of the random presentations. Thus, when meaningful chess situations were presented the experts could perceive relevant patterns and remember them very well but their much more extensive domain-specific knowledge did not help them encode randomly placed pieces. In such expert-novice studies, it is essential that this skill level by recall condition interaction be demonstrated so that initial group differences in short-term memory capacity can be ruled out as an explanation of the differences in recall.

In an early demonstration of the influence of domain-specific knowledge and expertise during childhood, Chi (1978) presented 10 year old chess players and college students digit span and memory for chess position tasks. The adults remembered more numbers on the short term memory test but the expert children were able to remember far more chess positions than the less-skilled adult subjects. Chi's study was one of the first to show the developmental importance of domain-specific knowledge; more importantly, it brought into question some of the fundamental axioms of stage theories of development, as it highlighted the role of a person's knowledge base rather than their chronological or developmental age.

In another developmental study, Gobbo and Chi (1986) examined the effects of knowledge about dinosaurs on 7 year old children who were very knowledgeable or less experienced in this domain. When presenting the children a series of dinosaur pictures, the authors asked them to tell all they knew about each of the dinosaurs. The less experienced children described only the explicitly presented features of each dinosaur; in contrast, the expert children described those features but also gave detailed descriptions about the diet, habitat and behaviour of the dinosaurs. Even when they were unfamiliar with a specific species, the expert children were able to logically infer about the characteristics of these dinosaurs demonstrating the influence of domain-specific knowledge on thinking and reasoning skills.

Chi and Ceci (1987) report a study by Ceci, Bronfenbrenner & Bober (1987) that demonstrates the effect of domain-specific knowledge on children's ability to reason. Elementary school children were seated in front of a video monitor and asked to predict the direction and distance that a target dot would travel. The children used a joystick to indicate where the target would terminate on the screen. To make this prediction, the children would have to consider the interactive effects of three variables: namely, the size, speed and colour of the target. Results show that the children were completely unsuccessful in doing this task. However, when the same task was presented in a video-game format in which the children were asked to "fire a missile" at where the spaceship (target dot) would stop, the children could do so easily. Chi and Ceci (1987) contend that context in this problem solving task was crucial. Quite simply, when the children could use their extensive video-game knowledge base they were able to do much more complex reasoning than when the task was separated from their content knowledge.

A recent study by Ceci and Liker (1986) has special relevance for our discussion as it underlines the importance that domain-specific knowledge plays in complex reasoning and problem solving in individuals with relatively low intelligence. The study examined the ability of men with intelligence scores between 80-90 "to engage in multiple-regression type thinking when they attempted to select winners at a racetrack" (p. 166). A strong correlation between their subjects' low IQ's and their lack of formal schooling was found; however, their ability to use complex reasoning as they tried to predict winners showed the influence that their extensive knowledge base about horse racing had on the generation and use of complex reasoning skills.

The above studies provide evidence to support the important role that domain-specific knowledge plays in expert performance. They also show that such knowledge influences attentional and memory control processes that directly affect learning and performance. A knowledge-based approach to motor development emphasizes the role of domain-specific knowledge in the action domain and contends that such knowledge can be categorized into five types, namely, declarative, procedural, affective, metacognitive and metacognitive skills. A brief discussion of each type of knowledge about action follows along with a description of studies related to them.

Declarative Knowledge

Factual information stored in memory that can influence the development and execution of skilled action has been called declarative knowledge about action (Wall et al., 1985). Such factual information is thought to be of considerable importance in skill development as it allows one to assess the context, variables, and strategies that affect learning and performance (Anderson, 1982; Wall, 1986).

Declarative knowledge consists of numerous schemata that are organized into structures of knowledge within specific domains (Bartlett, 1932; Rumelhart, 1980). In the action domain, an individual's declarative knowledge base includes information about the body and its morphological and biomechanical constraints, the physical environment and objects in it, and the interaction between the person, moving objects, and the environment. The development of language is central to the emergence of such general declarative knowledge about action (Bruner, 1983). The use of words to define and label specific skills, describe and categorize skilled actions and ultimately to control learning, are a crucial part of this general declarative knowledge base about action.

Recently, considerable information has been generated on declarative knowledge within specific domains and the effect that differences in skill level have on the structure and use of such factual knowledge.

As early as 1980, Allard and her colleagues demonstrated the effect of expertise in specific sport skills on the perceptual and memory skills of their subjects. They found that expert players "recall a greater amount of information about player positions in game structured stimuli" in both basketball (Allard, Graham & Paarsalu, 1980) and field hockey (Starkes and Deakin, 1984, p. 123). In another study of expertise in basketball, Allard and Burnett (1985) presented expert women basketball players and non-playing controls, 30 pictures depicting various aspects of the game of basketball. They were asked to sort the pictures into appropriate categories in any way that they wished. The expert players used more categories than the non-players and a hierarchial cluster analysis showed that the categories used by the experts discriminated much better than those that were used by the non-players. The experts categorized the pictures according to the use or significance of each skill while the non-players used more surface features such as what the players were actually doing in each picture. Allard and Burnett (1985) conclude that "at very least, sport expertise has a declarative component and may be described at some level as a semantically rich domain" (p. 302). Further evidence for the development of a domain-specific declarative knowledge base emerges from recent developmental studies.

In their introduction to a study of the relation of declarative knowledge development to children's basketball performance, French and Thomas (1987) make a number of observations about the structure of declarative knowledge. Using evidence from recent cognitive science studies, they note that declarative knowledge is usually conceptualized as a propositional network of interconnected nodes and links (Anderson, 1982; Chi & Rees, 1983; Chi & Ceci, 1987). The different nodes represent associations between concepts. Within a specific domain, more experienced individuals have larger semantic networks with more nodes, and more defining features on each node or concept. Thus, a person with expertise in a domain "has the distinct advantage of access to more and better organized information, which aids in the retrieval of information" (French & Thomas, 1987, p. 16).

With the above ideas as a conceptual framework, French and Thomas (1987) constructed a 50-item multiple choice test to assess declarative knowledge in the sport of basketball. The test measured a player's knowledge of the rules, playing positions and terminology used in basketball. Dribbling and shooting tests, ratings by coaches, and an open-ended basketball interview on appropriate actions to take in five playing situations were used to measure basketball skill.

As was expected, players rated as experts in both the 8-10 and 11-12 year old groups were more conceptually knowledgeable about basketball and were more physically skilled in the game than their less-skilled peers. On all measures of skill and declarative knowledge, an age related developmental trend did not appear, rather, as Chi (1978) found, the order of performance on the measures within the study was older experts, younger experts, older child novices, and younger child novices showing the importance of knowledge base differences rather than chronological age.

More importantly, canonical correlations between dribbling and shooting skills showed a significant relationship with the use of basketball knowledge supporting a strong relationship between declarative and procedural knowledge within this domain. In fact, French and Thomas (1987) conclude that two functions underlie children's basketball performance, namely,

> a cognitive decision-making component related to knowledge of basketball, and . . . a motor skill component involving execution and control related to dribbling and shooting skill. Thus, skilled performance of children in basketball involves a basic foundation in motor skills and specific sport knowledge (p. 29).

Procedural Knowledge

As discussed above, declarative knowledge refers to the storage of information about something, whereas procedural knowledge refers to how to do something (Anderson, 1982; Norman & Shallice, 1980). From a knowledge-based perspective, procedural knowledge about action is viewed as underlying all aspects of an action sequence including the perceptual, cognitive, response initiation and execution phases (Wall, 1986; Singer, 1980; Stelmach & Diggles, 1982).

Action sequences are under the control of sets of schemas that are activated when an appropriate set of conditions are met. Norman and Shallice (1980) provide a theory of how such schemas can be activated to flexibly control actions. From their perspective, well learned actions are controlled by a source schema that organizes a set of related component schemas; furthermore, with sufficient practice and familiarity with stimulus conditions such action sequences can be run off relatively automatically. They contend that deliberate attentional control is needed only in novel, technically difficult or dangerous situations. Recent advances in neuroscience are congruent with such thinking. Explanations of the development and control of action sequences from a Darwinian view of the operation of neural networks provides evidence from a lower level of analysis for the validity of such ideas and underlines the importance of experience and practice in the emergence of skilled action. For an excellent introduction to the application of neural Darwinian principles in the action domain readers are encouraged to read William Calvin's (1990) book, *The Cerebral Symphony*. Calvin's use of committee analogies to explain the role of "cerebral committees of neurons" is especially helpful and demonstrates the value of metaphor when explaining neuroscientific concepts that underly skilled action (p. 216).

As noted above procedural knowledge can be viewed from a process perspective; that is, it can represent the information processing processes that underlie skilled action as outlined above. At the same time, it can be viewed from a product, or developmental, perspective that reflects the quantity and quality of skilled actions that a person has acquired through experience and learning. Procedural knowledge about action will be examined from both of these perspectives in this chapter.

Recent evidence from a number of studies of expertise in sport demonstrate the enhanced performance of skilled athletes in certain components of the information processing sequence that underlies skilled action. The following section reviews some of these studies.

As early as 1978, Jones and Miles found that advanced tennis players were able to predict the landing position of the ball faster than were beginners. In a similar way, Salmela and Fiorito (1979) showed that skilled hockey goaltenders used pre-shot visual cues to predict wrist shots better than slap shots. Furthermore, the goaltenders could identify the side of the net that a puck was aimed at better than the intended height. Using a corneal-reflection eye movement apparatus, Bard and Fleury (1981) showed that expert hockey goaltenders fixated on the stick and puck while beginners used a greater number of ocular fixations on the puck. They suggest that the experts used stick cues including position and speed whereas beginners waited until contact was made with the puck before deciding how to block the shot.

In a multi-task examination of expertise in field hockey, Starkes (1987) measured simple reaction time, dynamic visual acuity, coincident anticipation, ball detection and accuracy, complex decision speed and accuracy, shot prediction accuracy when the ball was in sight and occluded, and the recall accuracy of structured and unstructured information about the game. In keeping with the findings of past studies of sport expertise, none of the hard-wired factors figured significantly in the prediction of "skilled performance" (Cockerill, 1981; Sanderson, 1981; Starkes & Deakin, 1984). However, national field hockey team members could predict the placement of shots more accurately than the varsity players and controls. Furthermore, Starkes provided brief visual exposure (1/60 sec.) to 24 slides depicting game situations and required her subjects to decide whether the optimal offensive play was to shoot, dribble, or dodge with the ball. Data on the accuracy of the decision confirmed that national players made the most accurate decisions; however, no group differences in voice reaction times were found. Starkes (1987) concludes that "for expert field hockey players the determining factors appear to be how well they are able to encode and use information regarding game structure and how well they can predict placement of a shot following view of ball impact" (p. 158). In terms of a knowledge based approach, such findings suggest that the important differences in sport skill may well not be found in "hard-wire" structural differences between skilled and less-skilled athletes but rather in the acquired procedural knowledge about action that has been termed "software" (Starkes & Deakin, 1984; Wall, 1986).

The above expert-novice studies of perceptual skill in sport settings clearly demonstrate the effects of procedural knowledge base differences in adult groups. In a recent developmental study, Abernethy (1988) asked the more fundamental question of how such differences in perceptual skill emerge. Using matched samples of expert and novice badminton players at ages 12, 15, 18, and the adult years, the subjects were shown film clips of opponents hitting the badminton shuttle and asked to predict where the shuttle would land. However, the subjects were presented varying amounts of temporal information leading up to and following the contact point. Radial error in metres was used to evaluate the discrepancy between the actual landing position of the shuttle and the subject's prediction.

Expert players in the 12 year old group did not improve their prediction accuracy across the five temporal occlusion conditions prior to and following contact. However, the 15 year old experts increased their prediction accuracy after the point of contact and the two time frames following it. The 18 year-old experts showed improved prediction accuracy even earlier as they extracted anticipatory information at frame 2 prior to contact and at the 3 other frames following it. As Abernethy and Russell (1987) had shown in an earlier study, adult experts were able to improve their prediction accuracy by extracting anticipatory information at all five time frames. In contrast to the systematic effect of increasing age on the prediction accuracy of the experts, the novice players demonstrated no increase in anticipatory skill with age. Abernethy (1988) concludes that the above data makes it clear that expert badminton players show a developmental improvement in their capability to extract information at earlier times in the stroke sequence. In fact, he contends "that task - specific practice, and not maturation per se, is the principal avenue through which improvements in anticipatory performance takes place" (p.215).

Marchiori, Wall and Bedingfield (1987) used a kinematic analysis of the stationary slap shot to assess procedural knowledge differences between two physically awkward children and two age-matched non-awkward children. The filmed performances of the non-awkward subjects showed relatively accurate and precise slap shots as measured by the angular velocity curves and peak stick velocity times in relation to contact time with the puck. In contrast, the movement patterns of the physically awkward boys were very inconsistent and showed a lack of both skill and power. Even after 1200 practice trials, 40 trials per day for 5 days for 6 weeks, under the supervision of their parents, their performances were still very inaccurate and inconsistent. The authors caution that their findings need replication; however, the results are congruent with observations made in gymnasium and clinical situations that underline the minimal procedural skill of physically awkward children.

Affective Knowledge About Action

Affective knowledge about action refers to the subjective feelings that individuals have about themselves in action situations. Such feelings are developed through countless movement experiences in play, physical activity, and sport settings. Unfortunately, not all children develop positive feelings about physical activity. Griffin and Keogh (1982) suggest that positive attitudes to physical activity depend on the development of movement confidence. They contend that movement confidence depends on the degree to which an individual develops movement competence within physical activity settings. Children who can handle the culturally-normative demands of their socio-cultural environment enjoy many more positive experiences than those who are less skilled. Positive experiences generate feelings of confidence and motivate children to participate more fully in physical activity settings. Furthermore, they result in the development of a positive self-concept that can influence learning and performance (Harter, 1978, 1981, 1982).

In contrast, the less-skilled performer receives considerably less positive reinforcement simply because they do not have a sufficient repetoire of physical skills, that is, procedural knowledge, to handle the task demands that they meet in physical activity settings. The mentally handicapped or physically awkward youngster who cannot run well, ride a bike, catch a ball, or swim across a pool, encounters hundreds of negative reinforcements during a given week. The ethnographic studies of physical activity settings by Griffin (1985) documents the negative verbal and social consequences that these youngsters receive in culturally-normative play and sport environments. It is not surprising that less-skilled children attempt to withdraw from as many physical activity settings as possible.

In addition to attempting to avoid physical activity, children and adolescents who are mentally handicapped or physically awkward often exhibit a syndrome of learned helplessness that is characterized by a lack of motivation, minimal persistence in the face of difficulties, and a general apathy to involvement in challenging situations (Dweck, 1980; Gibson, 1980). Clearly, such motivational tendencies will adversely affect skill acquisition and the development of sufficient domain-specific knowledge to participate effectively and enjoyably in physical activities.

A knowledge-based approach to skill acquisition underscores the importance of the above observations. The negative self-concepts, inappropriate attributions, and the lack of effort and persistence in difficult situations are powerful determinants of performance and development.

Vallerand and Reid (current volume) provide further evidence of this fact and make a number of helpful suggestions to ameliorate these problems. Unfortunately, all too often our research studies forget the powerful influence of affective knowledge. Perhaps, the use of a more holistic theoretical framework will encourage researchers and professionals to at least recognize, if not account for, this extremely powerful aspect of development.

Metacognitive Knowledge

The concept of metacognition refers to the executive control of a person's cognitive information processing capabilities. It has been categorized in a number of ways; however, for the purposes of this chapter, a distinction between metacognitive knowledge and metacognitive skills will be made. Metacognitive knowledge is declarative knowledge about what one knows or does not know. Wellman (1984) contends that such higher-level knowledge develops as children grow older; in fact, he suggests that children develop an extensive set of concepts related to how their minds operate. For example, they begin to realize that they can retrieve material to be remembered, and organize it into meaningful chunks or units that will facilitate the recall of it. In the motor domain, they begin to appreciate the value of remembering locations through the use of verbal cues such as a clock face or the directions on a compass. As they grow older, children begin to appreciate the factors that influence their cognitive processing (Flavell, Friedricks & Hoyt, 1970; Brown, 1978; Kopp, 1982; Bransford, Sherwood, Vye & Rieser, 1986; Glaser & Bassok, 1989).

Furthermore, they begin to realize what skills they have acquired and when and where it is appropriate to use them. Unfortunately, very little empirical research has been done on the development of metacognitive knowledge in the motor domain. Anecdotal evidence from personal interviews with skilled athletes suggests that they become very aware of the skills that they can do well, and, in fact, one of the marks of true expertise is that they are able to "stay within themselves", that is, they are able to predict when they are ready to try more difficult actions, take a sensible chance in a game, or employ a novel strategy to fool their opponents. The in-depth interviews Orlick and Partington (1985) conducted with Canadian Olympic athletes shows that many of them keep extensive notes on their performances as well as specific details on the progress that they are making while training. Clearly, the assessment and awareness of one's metacognitive knowledge base is an important aspect of skill development that requires further empirical and experimental research.

Metacognitive Skills

Metacognitive skills are responsible for the executive control of cognitive activity including the planning, monitoring and evaluation of learning and performance. Extensive research in the verbal-cognitive domain shows that such higher-level self-regulation skills emerge with increasing age and experience (Brown, 1975;1977; Chi, 1978; Flavell, 1976; Wellman, 1977;1984). Reid (1980) was one of the first to show the beneficial effect of instruction on the use of rehearsal strategies by mentally handicapped children performing a linear positioning task. Winther and Thomas (1981) and Weiss (1983) demonstrated the positive effects of using labelling strategies to enhance memory for movements.

In an excellent developmental study, Gallagher and Thomas (1986) examined the effects of grouping and recoding strategies on the learning of a series of movements. Grouping refers to the encoding strategy of combining new information into larger units. Recoding is the combining of several groups of information into long term memory within a given unit or chunk. The use of such strategies enables the learner to recall more information with less effort. Subjects in the study were 5, 7, 11 and 19 years of age.

The authors found that strategically organizing a series of movements for 5 year old children does not aid their recall. Such organization helps the 7 year olds in an immediate recall situation but not in transfer conditions. The 11 year old children could use and transfer the imposed organizational strategy; however, they could not develop a suitable strategy to enhance the recall of instructional input. Adults demonstrated that they could use and transfer imposed strategies and employ suitable strategies to also improve their recall of an unorganized series of movements.

Gallagher and Thomas (1986) stress the importance of the knowledge base of their subjects in the generation and use of cognitive strategies. They note that "the implementation of a deliberate organizational strategy is not content free, but depends upon the nature of the to-be-remembered information to which the strategy is applied" (p.124). They recommend that future studies examine the relationship between the knowledge base and the use of strategies.

Starkes, Deakin , Lindley and Crisp (1987) were the first to actually report on the effects of knowledge base differences on the use of strategies with ecologically-valid tasks in the motor skills domain. They recruited skilled young dancers from the National Ballet School of Canada as their expert subjects. Six girls and 2 boys with an average age of 11.3 years and with an average of 5.1 years ballet experience were categorized as the expert group while the novice ability group came from two local ballet schools. They had an average age of 10.9 years and had an average of 4.7 years experience in ballet. The subjects were presented with two conditions, a structured choreographed sequence and an unstructured sequence, both consisting of eight elements with which the dancers in both skill groups were familiar. Recall of the sequences was assessed motorically by performing the steps as well as verbally.

The results clearly supported the expected skill by recall condition interaction; the expert dancers showed enhanced recall over their age-matched novice peers in both the motor-structured and verbal-structured sequences. As expected, the motor-unstructured sequences were recalled significantly less accurately and there were no differences between the expert and novice dancers. The most interesting aspect of the study was the differences in metacognitive strategies used by the dancers. After viewing each sequence,

> novices rushed to perform or verbalize what they had seen. The experts inevitably asked if they could think about the sequence before performing it. During this very brief consolidation or rehearsal time they used small hand and foot movements to represent elements, and on rare occasions verbally labelled different steps. This consolidation seemed critical to the expert children (p. 227).

The above strategies are clearly metacognitive in nature. They are executive control strategies that experts use to enhance their overall learning and performance. Starkes and her colleagues reinforce the distinction made earlier in this chapter between declarative and procedural knowledge in the motor domain and the importance of domain-specific knowledge in the generation and use of metacognitive strategies.

Vickers (1988) examined the effect of expertise in gymnastics in a multi-phased study. Her 12 - 13 year old subjects were elite female gymnasts who were nationally ranked and intermediate gymnasts who were regionally ranked. The novice subjects were highly skilled soccer players with limited or no gymnastic experience. The 10 elite gymnasts had competed for an average 5.8 years while the 10 intermediates had 3.5 years of competitive experience.

An initial eye movement study in which eye fixations and body parts were analyzed during slide presentations of six sequences of gymnastics showed that the intermediate gymnasts observed the head more often than the elites who clearly attended to the hips more frequently in three of the six sequences. More importantly, the novice gymnasts attended to much more off body information such as fixating on equipment and the surrounding environment. The second phase was a resequencing study of selected slides from the initial eye movement phase to examine Carrol and Bandura's (1985) finding that the value of physical practice was more beneficial than visual practice in the development of a "cognitive representation" of a complex movement sequence. Vickers hypothesized "that the more highly skilled the gymnast the better able to reconstruct a photographic representation of each sequence" (p.61). As expected, the mean time to resequence the photographs and the number of error scores were inversely related to expertise in gymnastics. The third phase of the study examined the level of agreement between verbal description of the important parts of key photographs in the gymnastic sequences and the eye fixation data. The percent match between eye fixations and verbal reports were 68.3%, 76.3% and 66.6% for the experts intermediates and novices respectively.

Vickers (1988) discusses the above results from both a cognitive and ecological perspective. However, her conclusion is clear: the knowledge base of the gymnasts plays a very important role in what is attended to and how well it is cognitively represented. In terms of this discussion, she underscores the importance of procedural knowledge in studies of motor skill by stating that "physical skill level therefore should be considered as an independent variable in choosing subject groups for future research in teaching, coaching and judging behaviour" (p. 71).

The above observations are congruent with the results from recent expert performance studies in developmental psychology. Glaser and Bassok (1989) state that:

> The experience of experts enables them to develop executive skills for monitoring performance; they rapidly check their work on a problem, accurately judge its difficulty, apportion their time, assess their progress, and predict the outcomes of their performance... These self-regulatory skills vary in individuals and appear to be less developed in those with performance difficulties. Superior monitoring skills both reflect the efficient representational skills of experts in their domains and contribute to the utility of their knowledge. Because knowledge of a rule or procedure is enhanced when one can oversee its applicability and monitor its use, self-regulatory skills are important outcomes of learning.

The more general point that must be made is that the knowledge base of the person plays a significant role in problem solving situations. Consider the mentally handicapped or physically awkward youngster who has developed very few skills; that is, they have minimal procedural knowledge within the domain-specific area of ball catching. Also assume that they have a relatively meagre conceptual or declarative knowledge background about catching and its uses. Such a situation is especially true of mentally handicapped individuals who clearly are less proficient, by definition, within the verbal-cognitive domain in addition to having less experience in ball catching. Contrast the effects of such undeveloped knowledge bases with that of a young expert who plays little league baseball on a regular basis, and reflect on the effects of such knowledge base differences in terms of the following description of the importance of knowledge in problem solving by experts:

> As competence is attained, elements of knowledge become increasingly interconnected so that proficient individuals access coherent chunks of information. Beginners' knowledge of a domain is spotty, consisting of isolated definitions and superficial understandings of central terms and concepts. As proficiency develops, these items become structured and are integrated with past organizations of knowledge so that they are retrieved from memory rapidly and in larger units (cf Rumelhart & Norman, 1978). The exceptional memory retrieval of experts in a domain is based on the structured content of stored information (Ericsson & Staszewski, 1988). These organized structures of knowledge are referred to as schemata (Bartlett, 1932; Rumelhart, 1980). Such structures evolve and are modified and elaborated to

> facilitate more advanced thinking, and they enable forms of representation that are correlated with the ability to solve problems. (Glaser & Bassok, 1989, p. 647).

Clearly, developmentally-delayed youngsters are at a considerable disadvantage when faced with motor problems to solve.

Bouffard (1986) in a doctoral dissertation, based on a knowledge-based perspective, examined the ability of mildly and moderately handicapped adolescents to problem solve in a simulated table tennis situation. The rationale for the study stemmed from evidence documenting the difficulties mentally handicapped individuals face trying to access and use knowledge to solve problems in the cognitive domain (Borkowski & Büchel, 1983; Brown & Barclay, 1976; Brown, 1982; Campione & Brown, 1978; Campione, Brown & Ferrara, 1982) as well as studies that show similar difficulties in the solution of movement problems (Sugden, 1978; Reid, 1980).

In an initial study, eight males and eight females with IQ's between 45 and 70 were asked to return a table tennis ball projected at them under a control condition and an instructional condition in which they were told the future landing position of the ball. Analysis of video-taped data showed that subjects in the instructional condition used the declarative information to move closer to the future path of the ball prior to attempting a return hit. However, the strokes used by the subjects to return the ball were quite variable and only the high IQ group ($60<IQ<70$) actually hit more balls during the experimental condition. Bouffard (1986) suggests that:

> ...it is only when a rather consistent kinematic motor pattern is developed that knowledge about the future landing location of the ball is beneficial; otherwise the players frequently miss the ball even if they are close to it. Hence, a priori knowledge does not insure better performance unless a minimal level of movement consistency has been developed (p.104).

This observation underscores the strong interaction that exists between procedural skill level and the ability to use declarative knowledge effectively. In other words, conceptual knowledge alone will not necessarily improve motor performance unless the response aspects of an action are sufficiently proceduralized.

In a second experiment, another eight males and females with similar IQ's were provided information on the future landing position of the ball through the placement of a barbie-doll type figure on the ball projection machine. A control condition was also used. As in the initial study, the subjects in the experimental group moved closer to the landing position of the ball showing that "the positioning strategy used by the players is a function of knowledge (p.149). However, no differences in the number of balls hit were found. An analysis of the mover-environment relationships (Keogh & Sugden, 1985) clearly places Bouffard's task in the open-skill (Gentile, 1975) category. During the flight of the ball, Bouffard (1986) notes that the subjects "had to perceive as well as anticipate the spatio-temporal characteristics of the flight of the ball, decide where to move their body and what type of stroke to use and, finally; initiate the selected response in due time" (p.88).

Bouffard reports that the majority of his subjects had minimal experience with table tennis. However, "being forced to look at Barbie, guess where the ball will land, and hit the ball was, most likely, a new movement situation for the players." Thus, they were in the cognitive phase of skill acquisition that is characterized by inaccuracy of movement, high performance variability, and concern with "getting the idea of the movement" (Fitts & Posner, 1967; Gentile, 1972). Bouffard contends that the subjects were in an information overload situation in which most of their attentional capacity was used to predict where the ball was going rather than on tracking the ball to effectively return it. Kinematic studies of sport skills in both skilled and unskilled individuals reflect the differences in accuracy and precision that comes with the proceduralization of movement skill (Marchiori, Wall & Bedingfield 1986; Tyldesley & Whiting, 1977; Whiting, 1988). It seems that the lack of procedural knowledge in table tennis directly affected the ability of the subjects to use the declarative information provided in this study.

The above examination of studies related to the five types of knowledge about action underlines the importance of a person's knowledge base and indicates the interactive effects that differences in each of them plays in learning and performance. The next section of this chapter examines some of the research design considerations that stem from such a holistic view of motor development with persons with developmental disabilities.

Skill Acquisition Research Design Considerations

Planning motor skill acquisition studies in the area of developmental disabilities requires that an investigator consider a host of factors. As mentioned earlier in this paper, a number of research design difficulties stem from the limited view of what actually develops in motor development. These concerns are not new; in fact, they are congruent with recent observations made by developmental psychologists studying the acquisition of cognitive skills (Glaser, 1984; Glaser & Bassok, 1989; Siegler, 1983). In this section, the importance of evaluating a learner's knowledge base, carefully selecting and analyzing the task-to-be learned in relation to that knowledge-base, and the need to plan intervention strategies that are appropriate for the developmental level of the learner will be emphasized.

Developmental Level and Knowledge About Action

Comparative researchers have long been concerned with the question of developmental level. For over thirty years the questionable merits of chronological and mental age matches have been debated. One might even argue that the central design question of all research with developmentally-delayed individuals, if not all developmental research, revolves around the issue of developmental level. As mentioned above, an appreciation of the importance of the notion of developmental level led to the development of a more holistic approach to skill acquisition that emphasizes the importance of the learner's knowledge base.

As outlined earlier, a knowledge based approach to skill acquisition stresses the interactive influence of five types of knowledge about action. Studies from the cognitive science, sport expertise, and developmental psychology literature provide considerable support for this knowledge based approach. Further research is needed to develop means to effectively assess a person's knowledge base; however, it is clear that it is no longer sufficient to use only chronological age or mental age indices to assess developmental level. It is particularly important with developmentally-delayed individuals that we examine the effects of increased knowledge within specific domains since one of the major characteristics of the motor performance of such individuals is the unevenness of their development.

Using the above knowledge based principles, one would expect that the physical proficiency of persons with developmental disabilities would diminish as one examines their repertoire of simple, reactive, and complex skills. A culturally-normative skills framework might prove to be helpful in assessing the general developmental level of an individual (Smith, 1987). More careful analysis of domain-specific strengths and weaknesses would also be needed depending on the purpose of the research study. In developing such evaluation instruments, it will be particularly important to assess all five types of knowledge about action.

The Importance of Domain-specific Knowledge

A knowledge-based approach also emphasizes the importance of domain-specific knowledge in the learning process. As outlined above, studies of expert novice differences demonstrate the effect that domain-specific knowledge has on the learning process. Experts in a given domain have access to more extensive knowledge bases, acquire additional knowledge more readily, and generate much more sophisticated problem solving strategies than novices do. The domain-specific knowledge of the learner directly influences such metacognitive skills as planning, monitoring, and evaluating (Glaser, 1984; Siegler, 1983). Therefore, it is necessary to evaluate the person's knowledge base prior to the implementation of any intervention strategy. This is particularly true in the motor domain where the skills that are acquired often vary greatly.

The Learner-Task Match

It is a given to call for the analysis of the task-to-be learned in developmental skill acquisition research. However, beyond the analysis of the event, temporal, and spatial uncertainty, or the degree to which it is a simple, reactive or complex skill, it is essential that the demands of a task be evaluated in relation to the developmental level or knowledge base of the person.

Research with mentally handicapped and physically awkward adolescents suggests that many of them show symptoms of learned helplessness; that is, when they are asked why they succeed or fail on a motor task they usually attribute their success to the relatively stable factor of the task being too easy whereas they attribute their failures to the stable internal factor of their lack of ability (Gibson, 1980). The important point for the design of learning studies is that individuals with such negative motivational tendencies often do not try to use effective problem solving or self-control strategies when they are faced with tasks that are beyond their capabilities. Hence, the degree of difficulty of the task must be evaluated in relation to the general and domain-specific knowledge of the learner. Smith (1978) contends that learners are optimally motivated when their subjective expectancy of success or failure is about 50/50. He stresses the importance of ensuring that the task-to-be learned is appropriate for a given learner. By doing so, the learner is more likely to view it as a skill task that is subject to learner control rather than a chance task that generates feelings of learned helplessness. Clearly, the learner-task match must be a crucial consideration in our research design deliberations.

Phase of Skill Acquisition

In addition to determining the match between the knowledge base of the learner and the task-to-be learned, it is important to consider the phase of skill acquisition at which a given learner is operating. Again, it is the knowledge base of the learner that will determine this matter. For example, a person with considerable expertise in juggling will be at a relatively proceduralized level of performance when juggling two or three balls while a novice would be at the initial cognitive phase of simply trying to get the idea of the task (Gentile, 1972; Magill, 1985). Such considerations are especially important when we design comparative or developmental studies in which wide individual differences in developmental level are present.

The question of the phase of skill acquisition also influences the selection of the number of trials to be presented in a learning study. Clearly, the effect of a given intervention strategy can be dramatically affected by the learner's phase of skill acquisition.

Matching the Intervention Strategy to the Learner

The perennial problem with task selection in developmental research has been floor and ceiling effects. Most researchers are aware of this problem in relation to the selection of the dependent variable for a given task. It is equally important that the independent variable, whether it be verbal instruction, the use of physical prompts, or covert rehearsal strategies, be suitably matched to the knowledge base of the learner. It is especially important to consider this matter when verbal instructions, contextual information, or problem solving methods are the intervention strategies being used. Developmentally delayed children are by definition often deficient in these knowledge domains, hence, attention to this design issue would seem to be sensible. The plethora of non-significant treatment x aptitude interactions might well be due to insufficient attention to this research design factor.

A consideration of the above factors that impinge on sound developmental research designs would surely make even the most experienced researcher nervous. Clearly, the day of using large groups of uncategorized learners who receive some form of undifferentiated treatment is past. The complexity of the developmental skill acquisition process requires the use of more sophisticated factorial designs in which we, at least, block on the relevant factors or move towards the use of single-subject designs. In a short but most informative article, Cole (1988) discusses the value of using analysis of covariance procedures when analysing treatment-control group differences especially when small sample sizes are a problem. Small group sizes are a very real problem to those investigating the effects of skill acquisition treatment programs on the motor performance of persons with developmental disabilities. Cole discusses the factors that influence the relative power of statistical tests with the posttest-only approach, the change-score approach, and an analysis of covariance approach. In almost all cases, the analysis of covariance approach provides the most statisical power and Cole highly recommends its use. If factorial designs are to be used, it seems appropriate that analysis of covariance techniques be used with them.

A number of effective single subject research designs have been generated which have been successfully used with a variety of disabled populations.

Excellent reviews of such methods are available for those who are not familiar with them (Watkinson & Wasson, 1984).

Space does not permit a discussion of the merit or procedures related to the above two design approaches; however, if we are to understand developmental skill acquisition, especially in developmentally-delayed populations where wide individual and intra-individual differences are the norm, then we will have to study smaller groups of subjects or individuals where we can observe the interaction of the person's knowledge base, with specific task, environment and intervention factors.

Program Development Research Considerations

The program development research process may benefit from a consideration of the ideas that underly a knowledge-based approach to motor development. The following suggestions are designed to encourage a more holistic view of our attempts to help developmentally-disabled individuals to enjoy the benefits of physical activity.

Situational Analysis

Careful thought needs to be given to the demands that different physical activity environments place on participants. Smith (1986) defined five physical activity opportunity options: unstructured participation, structured participation, recreational competition, low intensity competition and high intensity competition and identified the types of skills and abilities needed for success in them. Program development researchers need to understand this continuum of programs and focus their work on particular physical activities or sports within them, according to the interests, needs, and capabilities of the developmentally-disabled individuals with whom they are working.

The key physical, social, and life skills required for participation need to be identified so that an effective person-activity match can be made. Special attention should be given to the physical skills required and the bandwidth of proficiency that is acceptable within each environment. The role of support persons and strategies to facilitate participation should also be noted. Such a situational analysis can help ensure that programs are designed to meet the interests, needs, and capabilities of the participant.

Developmental Evaluation

A knowledge-based approach to developmental evaluation could be of considerable help in program development research. Evaluation checklists and scales will certainly vary in complexity and detail; however, they should attempt to provide information on all five types of knowledge about action. In the past, developmental evaluations in the motor domain focused mainly on the physical skills of participants. Clearly, a careful assessment of a participant's physical skill repertoire should be made and the accuracy, precision, and automaticity of each skill noted; however, it is also important to consider the declarative knowledge base of the person. Conceptual knowledge of the key terms, rules, playing patterns, strategies, and etiquette of an activity or sport should be assessed. Special care should be given to the identification of words and phrases used in the teaching, learning, and control of skill within practice and game situations. As noted earlier, developmentally-disabled individuals may lack such domain-specific knowledge which, in turn, can greatly affect their learning and performance.

The attitudes, feelings, and motivations of the participant should also be assessed. In doing so, it is important to consider not only the feelings of the person in relation to physical activity in general but to record differences in attitude and motivation within different activity areas. Observations on the positive effects of competence, and the negative effects of a lack of it require that such attitudinal information be domain-specific.

The development of expertise requires that a person acquire executive control skills. Care should be taken to ensure that information is recorded on the growth of metacognitive knowledge in the procedural, declarative, and affective areas. At the present time, such information is rarely recorded; however, more research into the assessment, evaluation, and use of metacognitive knowledge about action is sorely needed.

A developmental evaluation would not be complete without an assessment of the metacognitive skills of the person. Information on the planning, monitoring, evaluating, and problem solving skills of the participant could be of immense help when facilitating learning and performance. Again depending on the purpose of the program, information should be noted on the development of verbal comprehension and listening skills, observational modelling and attentional control skills, and intelligent practice strategies. Such executive control strategies are essential for the growth of skill mastery and further research on the identification, documentation, and evaluation of them is clearly needed.

Activity Prescription

Much more attention needs to be given to research into the prescription of activities. Given the limited time available for instruction and the enormous amount of practice, both physical and mental, that is required for skill mastery, it is essential that we develop better means by which to prescribe skills for instruction. Clearly, the learner's interest and knowledge base will be central to this process; however, the availability of proper instruction, practice opportunities, and supportive environments must also be considered. Careful thought should also be directed to the selection of skills-to-be-learned that will have the broadest possible use in the community. Opportunities for ongoing participation should be identified so that the skills and domain-specific knowledge that are learned will result in as much enjoyable participation as possible. Further research is clearly needed to investigate means to enhance the activity-prescription process.

Effective strategies to enhance skill acquisition with developmentally-disabled individuals have been developed; the use of task analysis, progressive learning principles, response prompting continuums, and skill maintenance techniques have significantly helped the physical skill acquisition process (Watkinson & Wall, 1982). However, more research needs to be devoted to the development and use of declarative knowledge about action. Key concepts and descriptors related to the skill acquisition process generally, and, in specific sports and activities, must be identified and taught. Special efforts must be made to develop metacognitive awareness in the developmentally-disabled once they have acquired sufficient knowledge within a given domain.

Research into the development of goal setting procedures that lead to an emphasis on learning goals rather than performance goals need to be completed. Research on the use of modelling, observational skills, attentional control, response organization and feedback strategies to control and enhance learning is also needed. The development of such metacognitive skills must be closely related to domain-specific knowledge. In sum, a much broader view of skill acquisition must be taken in order to meet the wide individual differences and needs of the developmentally-disabled.

Author Notes

1. Send request for reprints to A.E. Wall, Department of Physical Education, McGill University, Montreal, Quebec, Canada, H2W 1S4.

References

Abernethy, B. (1988). The effects of age and expertise upon perceptual skill development in a racquet sport. *Research Quarterly, 59*(3), 210-221.

Abernethy, B. & Russell, D.G. (1987). Expert-novice differences in an applied selective attentional task. *Journal of Sport Psychology, 9*, 326-343.

Allard, F. & Burnett, N. (1985). Skill in sport. *Canadian Journal of Psychology, 39*(2), 294-312.

Allard, F., Graham, S. & Paarsalu, M.E. (1980). Perception in sport: Basketball. *Journal of Sport Psychology, 2*, 14-21.

Anderson, J.R. (1982). Acquisition of cognitive skill. *Psychological Review, 89*, 396-406.

Bankhead, I. & Mackay, D.N. (1982). Fine motor performance in subjects of subnormal, normal, and superior intelligence. I. Reaction time and task complexity. *Journal of Mental Deficiency Research, 26*, 73-89, 98-106.

Bard, C. & Fleury, M. (1981). Considering eye movement as a predictor of attainment. In I.M. Cocherill & W.W. MacGilvary (Eds.), *Vision and Sport* (pp. 28-41). Cheltenham, England: Stanley Thomas.

Bartlett, F.C. (1932). *Remembering*. Cambridge: Cambridge University Press.

Baumeister, A.A. (1987). Mental retardation: Some concepts and dilemmas. *American Psychologist*, 796-800.

Baumeister, A.A. & Kellas G. (1968). Reaction time and mental retardation. In N.R. Ellis (Ed.), *International Review of Research in Mental Retardation, 3*, New York: Academic Press, 163-192.

Berkson, G. (1960). An analysis of reaction time in normal and mentally deficient young men, I. Duration threshold experiment. *Journal of Mental Deficiency Research, 4*, 51-58.

Borkowski, J. & Cavanaugh, J (1979). Maintenance and generalization of skills and strategies by the retarded. In N.R. Ellis (Ed.), *The Handbook of Mental Deficiency, 2*, Hillsdale, NJ: Erlbaum, 569-617.

Borkowski, J.G. & Buchel, F.P. (1983). Learning and memory strategies in the mentally retarded. In M. Pressley & J.R. Levin (Eds.), *Cognitive strategy research* (pp. 103-128). New York: Springer-Verlag.

Bouffard, M. (1986). *Knowledge, Anticipation and the Solution of Movement Problems by Mentally Retarded Adolescents.* Unpublished doctoral dissertation, University of Alberta, Edmonton, Alberta.

Bransford, J., Sherwood, R., Vye, N. & Rieser, J. (1986). Teaching thinking and problem solving: Research foundations. *American Psychologist, 41*(10), 1078-1089.

Brewer, N. (1978). Motor components in the choice reaction time of mildly retarded adults. *American Journal of Mental Deficiency, 82*, 37-43.

Brewer, N. & Nettelbeck, T. (1977). Influence of contextual cues on the choice reaction time of mildly retarded adults, *American Journal of Mental Deficiency, 82*, 37-43.

Brown, A.L. (1974). The role of strategic behavior in retardate memory. In N.R. Ellis (Ed.), *International Review of Research in Mental Retardation, 7.* New York: Academic Press, 55-111.

Brown, A.L. (1975). The development of memory: Knowing, knowing about knowing, and knowing how to know. In H.W. Reese (Ed.), *Advances in child development, 10*, 103-152, New York: Academic Press.

Brown, A.L. (1977). Development, schooling, and the acquisition of knowledge. In R.C. Anderson, R.J. Spiro & W.E. Montague (Eds.), *Schooling and the acquisition of knowledge* (pp. 241-253). Hillsdale, NJ: Erlbaum.

Brown, A.L. (1982). Learning and development: The problems of compatibility, access and induction. *Human Development, 25*, 89-115.

Brown, A.L., & Barclay, C.R. (1976). The effects of training specific mnemonics on the metamnemonic efficiency of retarded children. *Child Development, 47*, 71-80.

Bruner, J.S. (1983). *Child's Talk.* New York: Norton.

Calvin, W. (1990). *The Cerebral Symphony.* Toronto: Bantam Books.

Campione, J.C., & Brown, A.L. (1978). Toward a theory of intelligence: Contributions from research with retarded children. *Intelligence, 2*, 279-304.

Carroll, W.R., & Bandura, A. (1985). The role of visual monitoring and motor rehearsal in observational learning of action patterns. *Journal of Motor Behaviour, 17*, 269-282.

Ceci, S.J., & Liker, J. (1986). A day at the races: The study of IQ, expertise, and cognitive complexity. *Journal of Experimental Psychology, General, 118*, 164-169.

Ceci, S.J., Bronfenbrenner, V., & Baber, J.G. (1987). Memory development and ecological complexity: The case of prospective memory. In M. Perlmutter & F. Weinert (Eds.) *Future Trends in Memory Development Research*, New York: Springer-Verlager.

Chase, W.G., & Simon, H.A. (1973). The mind's eye in chess. In W.G. Chase (Ed.), *Visual information processing* (pp. 215-281). New York: Academic Press.

Chi, M.T.H. (1978). Knowledge structures and memory development. In R.S. Siegler (Ed.), *Children's thinking: What develops?* (pp. 73-96). Hillsdale, NJ:Erlbaum.

Chi, M.T.H. & Rees, E.T. (1983). A learning framework for development. In M.T.G. Chi (Ed.), *Trends in memory development research*, New York: Karger.

Chi, M.T.H., & Ceci, S.J (1987). Content knowledge: Its role, representation, and restructuring in memory development. *Advances in Child Development and Behaviour, 20*, 91-142.

Cockerill, I.M. (1981). Peripheral vision and hockey. In I.M. Cockerill & W.W. McGillvary (Eds.), *Vision and Sport* (pp. 54-63). Cheltenham, England: Stanley Thomas.

Cole, D.A. (1988). Statistics for small groups: The power of the pretest. *Journal of the Association for Persons with Severe Handicaps, 13*(3), 142-146.

de Groot, A. (1965). *Thought and choice in chess.* The Hague: Mouton.

Dweck, C.S. (1980). Learned helplessness in sport. In C.H. Nadeau, W.R. Halliwell, K.M. Newell and G.C. Roberts (Eds.), *Psychology of motor behaviour and sport - 1979.* Champaign, IL: Human Kinetics.

Fitts, P.M. & Posner, M.I. (1967). *Human performance.* Belmont, CA: Brooks/Cole.

Flavell, J.H. (1976). Metacognitive aspects of problem solving. In L.B. Resnick (Ed.), *The nature of intelligence* (pp. 231-235). Hillsdale, NJ: Erlbaum.

Flavell, J.H., Fredricks, A.G., & Hoyt, J.D. (1970). Developmental changes in the memorization process. *Cognitive Psychology, 1*, 324-340.

French, K.E., & Thomas, J.R. (1987). The relation of knowledge development in children's basketball performance, *Journal of Sport Psychology, 9*, 15-32.

Gallagher, J.D., & Thomas, J.R. (1986). Developmental effects of grouping and recoding on learning a movement series. *Research Quarterly for Exercise and Sport, 57*(2), 117-127.

Gardner, H. (1983). *Frames of mind: The theory of multiple intelligence*. New York: Basic Books.

Gentile, A.M. (1972). A working model of skill acquisition with application to teaching. *Quest, 17*, 3-23.

Gibson, B.J. (1980). An attributional analysis of performance outcome and alleviation of learned helplessness on motor performance tasks: A comparative study of educable mentally retarded and non-retarded boys. Unpublished doctoral dissertation, University of Alberta.

Glaser, R. (1984). Education and thinking: The role of knowledge. *American Psychologist, 39*, 93-104.

Glaser, R., & Bassok, M. (1989). Learning theory and the study of instruction. *Annual Review of Psychology, 40*, 631-666.

Gobbo, C., & Chi, M.T.H. (1986). How knowledge is structured and used by expert and novice children. *Cognitive Development, 1*, 221-237.

Griffin, P.S. (1985). Boys' participation styles in a middle school physical education team sports unit. *Journal of Teaching Physical Education, 4*, 111-122.

Griffin, N.S., & Keogh, J.F. (1982). A model for movement confidence. In J.A.S. Kelso & J.E. Clark (Eds.), *The development of movement control and co-ordination* (pp. 213-236). New York: Wiley.

Grossman, H.J. (Ed.) (1983). Classification in mental retardation. Washington, D.C.: American Association of Mental Deficiency.

Harter, S. (1978). Effectance motivation reconsidered: Toward a developmental model. *Human Development, 21*, 34-64.

Harter, S. (1981). The development of competence motivation in the mastery of cognitive and physical skills: Is there still a place for joy? In G.C. Roberts and D.M. Landers (Eds.), *Psychology of motor behaviour and sport -1980*. Champaign, IL: Human Kinetics.

Harter, S. (1982). The perceived competence scale for children. *Child Development, 53*, 87-97.

Hoover, J.H., Wade, M.G., & Newell, K.M. (1981). The trainability of reaction time and movement time in moderately mentally handicapped workers. *American Journal of Mental Deficiency, 85*, 389-395.

Hoover, J.H., & Wade, M.G. (1985). Motor learning theory and mentally retarded individuals: A historical review. *Adapted Physical Activity Quarterly, 2*, 228-252.

Horgan, J.S. (1983). Mnemonic strategy instruction in coding, processing, and recall of movement-related cues by mentally retarded children. *Perceptual and Motor Skills, 57*, 547-557.

Jones, C.M., & Miles, T.R. (1978). Use of advance cues in predicting the flight of a lawn tennis ball. *Journal of Human Movement Studies, 4*, 231-235.

Kelso, J.A.S., Goodman, D., Stamm, C.L., & Hayes, C. (1979). Movement coding and memory in retarded children. *American Journal of Mental Deficiency, 82*, 601-611.

Keogh, J., & Sugden, D. (1985). *Movement skill development*. New York: Macmillan.

Kopp, C.B. (1982). Antecedents of self-regulation: A developmental perspective. *Developmental Psychology, 18*, 199-214.

Magill, R.A. (1985). *Motor learning: Concepts and applications* (2nd ed.). Dubuque, IA: Wm. C. Brown.

Marchioi, G.E., Wall, A.E., & Bedingfield, E.W. (1987). Kinematic analysis of skill acquisition in physically awkward boys. *Adapted Physical Activity Quarterly, 4*, 306-315.

Maslow, A.H. (1969). *The Psychology of Science*. Chicago: Henry Regency.

Nettelbeck, T., & Brewer, N. (1976). Effects of stimulus-response variables on the choice reaction time of mildly retarded adults. *American Journal of Mental Deficiency, 81*, 85-92.

Nettelbeck, T., & Kirby, N.H. (1980). Measures of timed performance and intelligence. *Intelligence, 7*, 39-52.

Newell, K.M. (1985). Motor skill acquisition and mental retardation. Overview of traditional and current orientations. In J.E. Clark & J.H. Humphries (Eds.), *Motor development: Current selected research, 1.* Princeton, NJ: Princeton Books Co., 183-191.

Norman, D.A., & Shallice, T. (1980). *Attention to action: Willed and automatic control of behaviour.* (Tech. Rep.). San Diego: University of California, Center for Human Information Processing.

Orlick, T., & Partington, J. (1985). *Psyched: Inner views of winning.* Ottawa: Coaching Association of Canada.

Poplin, M.S. (1988). The reductionistic fallacy in learning disabilities: Replicating the past by reducing the present. *Journal of Learning Disabilities, 21*(7), 389-400.

Reid, G. (1980). The effect of memory strategy instruction in the short-term motor memory of the mentally retarded. *Journal of Motor Behaviour, 12*, 221-227.

Rumelhart, D.E. (1980). Schemata: The building blocks of cognition. In R. Spiro, B. Bruce & W. Brewer (Eds.), *Theoretical issues in reading comprehension* (pp. 38-58). Hillsdale, NJ: Erlbaum.

Rumelhart, D.E., & Norman, D.A. (1978). Accretion, tuning, and restructuring: Three modes of learning. In J.W. Cotton, R.L. Klatzky (Eds.), *Semantic Factors in Cognition*. Hillsdale, NJ: Erlbaum.

Salmela, J.H., & Fiorito, P. (1979). Visual cues in ice hockey goaltending. *Canadian Journal of Applied Sport Sciences, 4*, 56-59.

Sanderson, F.H. (1981). Visual acuity and sports performance. In I.M. Cocherill & W.W. MacGillvary (Eds.). *Vision in Sports* (pp. 64-79). Cheltenham, England: Stanley Thomas.

Siegler, R.S. (1983). How knowledge influences learning. *American Scientist*, 631-640.

Singer, R.N. (1980). Motor behaviour and the role of cognitive processes and learner strategies. In G.E. Stelmach and J. Requin (Eds.), *Tutorials in motor behaviour.* New York: Holland Publishing Company.

Smith, M.F.R. (1978). Attribution, achievement motivation, and task difficulty in physical education. Paper presented at the B.C. Conference on the Teaching of Physical Education, Victoria, B.C.

Smith, M.F.R. (1987). Understanding and changing physical activity delivery systems, *CAHPER Journal, 53*(5), 39-44.

Starkes. J.L. (1987). Skill in field hockey: Nature of the cognitive advantage. *Journal of Sport Psychology, 9*, 146-160.

Starkes, J.L., & Deakin, J. (1984). Perception in sport: A cognitive approach to skilled performance. In W.F. Straub & J.M Williams (Eds.), *Cognitive Sport Psychology* (pp. 115-128). Lansing, N.Y.: Sport Science Associates.

Starkes, J.L., Deakin, J.M., Lindley, S., & Crisp, F. (1987). Motor versus verbal recall of ballet sequencing by young expert dancers. *Journal of Sport Psychology, 9*, 222-230.

Stelmach, G.E., & Diggles, V.A. (1982). Control theories in motor behaviour. *Acta Psychologica, 50*, 83-105.

Sugden, D.A. (1978). Visual motor short term memory in educationally subnormal boys. *British Journal of Educational Psychology, 48*, 330-339.

Tyldesley, D.A., & Whiting, H.T.A. (1977). Operational timing. *Journal of Human Movement Studies, 1*, 172-177.

Vickers, J.N. (1988). Knowledge structures of expert-novice gymnasts. *Human Movement Science, 7*, 47-72.

Wade, M.G., Hoover, J.H., & Newell, K.M. (1983). Training and trainability in motor skills performance of mentally retarded persons. In J. Hogg & P. Mittler (Eds.), *Advances in mental handicap research* (vol. 2, pp. 175-200). New York: Wiley & Sons.

Wade, M.G., Newell, K.M., & Wallace, S.A. (1978). Decision time and movement time as a function of response complexity in retarded persons. *American Journal of Mental Deficiency, 83*, 135-144.

Wall, A.E. (1986). A Knowledge-based approach to motor skill acquisition. In *Motor development in children: Aspects of coordination and control*, M.G. Wade & H.T.A. Whiting (Eds.) Dordrecht: Martinus Nyhoff Publishers.

Wall, A.E., McClements, J., Bouffard, M., Findlay, H., & Taylor, M.J. (1985). A knowledge-based approach to motor development: Implications for the physically awkward. *Adapted Physical Activity Quarterly, 2*, 21-42.

Watkinson, E.J. & Wasson, D.L. (1984). The use of single-subject time series designs in adapted physical activity. *Adapted Physical Activity Quarterly, 1*, 19-29.

Weiss, M (1983). Modeling and motor performance: A developmental perspective. *Research Quarterly for Exercise and Sport, 54*, 190-197.

Weiss, P.A. (1968). The living system: Determinism stratified (3-55). In A. Koestler & J.R. Smythies (Eds.), *Beyond Reductionism*. New York: Macmillan.

Wellman, H.M. (1977). The early development of intentional memory behaviour. *Human Development, 20*, 86-101.

Wellman, H.M. (1984). The development of concepts of the mental world. *Behavioral and Brain Sciences, 7*(4), 651-652.

Whiting, H.T.A. (1982). Skill in sport: A descriptive and prescriptive appraisal. In *New Paths to Sport Learning and Excellence*, J.H. Salmela, J.T. Partington & T. Orlick (Eds.), Ottawa: Sport in Perspective.

Whiting, H.T.A. (1988). Mediation in learning complex cyclical actions, In *Cognitive and Neuropsychological Approaches to Mental Imagery* (pp. 269-277), M. Denis (Ed.), Martinus Nijhoff.

Winther, K.T. & Thomas J.R. (1981). Developmental differences in children's labelling of movement. *Journal of Motor Behaviour, 13*, 77-90.

SECTION II:

PERSPECTIVES

Problems in Movement Control
G. Reid (editor)

NORMAL AND ABNORMAL RHYTHMS IN NEUROMOTOR CONTROL: ANALYSIS, MODELLING AND IMPLICATIONS

A. Beuter
Departement de Kinanthropologie
Université du Québec à Montréal

and

Center for Nonlinear Dynamics in Physiology and Medicine
McGill University

When observing the behaviour of an individual performing a repetitive task such as walking it is relatively easy to detect whether the limb segments involved in the motion are controlled "normally" or "abnormally". Our eyes act as a reliable, intuitive pattern recognition tool to distinguish "normal" and "abnormal" gait rhythms. These rhythmical motions are found in all domains of human behaviour from life support activities such as chewing, walking, breathing, etc., to leisure activities such as running, swimming, rowing, cycling, or riding. These activities are usually performed smoothly by athletes and healthy individuals or may appear incoordinated because of lack of training, exhaustion or pathology. Recently, the control mechanisms responsible for these rhythmicities have become the focus of a number of experimental and theoretical studies reviewed in Rensing, an der Heiden and Mackey (1987).

Since motion is a fundamental property of most animal life, its disturbance can be used as a neurodiagnosis (Chusid, 1973). Changes in *motor power* (i.e., weakness, paresis and paralysis) may result from lesions of peripheric nerves (i.e., neuropathy) and/or of the muscles themselves (i.e., myopathy). *Increased movement* (i.e., hyperkinesia) is often combined with disturbances in tonus (i.e., hypertonia and hypotonia) and may involve the extrapyramidal system, the spinal cord and reflex arc, and/or muscular activity. Signs of disturbed tonus and increased movements include, for example, rigidity, tremor, spasms, dystonia or myoclonus. *Disturbances in synergy* are generally due to lesions of the cerebellum or its pathways and lead to a lack of integrated, coordinated action between muscle groups. Typical symptoms and signs include ataxia, adiadochokinesia and dysmetria (see definitions below). *Gait problems* may arise from a variety of causes such as drug poisoning, brain tumours, multiple sclerosis, muscular dystrophy or poliomyelitis and may include disturbances in the programming of movement, or disturbances in the afferent and/or efferent pathways (Grimm, 1984). These disturbances are grouped in specific syndromes and semiologies (e.g., the pyramidal syndrome or the extrapyramidal, cerebellar, and ataxic semiologies) which can affect all levels of the nervous system from the neuromuscular junction to the motor cortex. As noted some of the disturbances directly affect the rhythms of motion. They correspond to a disorder in the temporal organization of motion, however the exact role of the nervous system in the production of these disorders is unclear. Tremor, for example, is one prominent and striking oscillatory feature of normal and abnormal motor control (Desmedt, 1978; Freund, 1987; Koller, 1984; Marsden, 1984) which may involve various levels of the nervous system but the exact mechanisms producing this behaviour are not fully understood yet.

Researchers are trying to understand how the mechanisms responsible for normal rhythms can change and produce abnormal behaviours. Are the mechanisms involved basically intact with control parameters operating in an unusual range or are they different? In a Guillain-Barré syndrome, for example, the demyelinization of the peripheral nerves lead to a pathological process of impulse conduction, while after stroke, a structure may be destroyed and the whole system must reorganize itself. It is clear that the development of new therapeutic strategies depends on this information. Indeed, if the mechanisms are intact and the control parameters operate in different regions, the therapeutic strategies should attempt to move the system from regions of parameter space in which they exhibit pathological behaviour into a region in which they are again classified as healthy (Glass & Mackey, 1979; Mackey & Glass, 1977). The re-adjustment of these control parameters mechanically, electrically, or pharmacologically could reposition the control system in a range of parameter space associated with "healthy" dynamical behaviour (Mackey & Milton, 1987; Stein, Gordon, Oguztöreli & Lee, 1981).

In this chapter, I show that some of the abnormal manifestations of motor control may be the result of temporal disorders in the oscillatory processes underlying movement behaviours. First, oscillatory processes observed in human movement behaviour are described. Second, the mechanisms underlying normal and abnormal neuromotor control in tremor are examined. Third, basic concepts used in modelling neuromotor control are introduced and finally, the implications of this approach for the development of intervention strategies in motor control are outlined.

Oscillatory Processes in Neuromotor Control

Neurophysiological control systems are characterized by processes which occur at regular intervals under the control of the nervous system (i.e., breathing, masticating, speech, etc.). Far from being static, the functions of the nervous system are dynamic and produce complex biological oscillations (Keidel, Keidel, Tirsch & Poppl, 1987; Kopell & Ermentrout, 1986). Rhythmical movements are presumably controlled by neural networks located at the spinal level. However, little is known about the coupling between the neural oscillators (i.e., central pattern generators) or about the descending supraspinal influences they receive (Bassler, 1986).

Hildebrandt (1987) noted that oscillations have a great variety of period length ranging from a fraction of a second (e.g., neural action) to one day (e.g., circadian rhythm). The genesis of the electrical signals associated with physiological oscillations is not fully understood. However, these signals are widely used in medical diagnosis to provide useful information about the structure and function of the brain (EEG), heart (ECG) and muscles (EMG).

Abnormalities in physiological rhythms are of major clinical importance (Glass & Mackey, 1979; Mackey & Glass, 1977; Mackey & Milton, 1987). In neuromotor control, examples of rhythm abnormalities include myoclonus (sudden isolated muscle contractions), fibrillation (denervated muscle), ataxic gait (unsteady gait), spasms (involuntary contractions of large muscle groups), bradykinesia (slow movements), athetoid movements (oscillation between flexion and extension), dystonia (undulant and sinuous movements of the body and trunk), choreiform movements (coarse, quick and jerky movements with no rhythmicity), hemiballism (continuous coordinated activity of the axial and proximal extremity musculature), adiadochokinesia (inability to execute quickly opposite movements), asterixis or flapping tremor (absence of fixed position), dysarthria (explosive and irregular speech), and, titubation (rhythmical oscillations of head and sometimes trunk in cerebellar disease). Although abnormal motor rhythms are well described in clinical neurophysiology, the implications of the oscillatory basis of movement, which is a fundamental aspect of motor control, has been left relatively unexplored in humans until recently (Delcomyn, 1980; Delong, 1978; Kelso, 1981; Stein, 1977). General examples of physiological systems in health and disease in which both regular and irregular rhythms have been observed are presented in Mackey and Milton (1987).

Qualitative description of neuromotor rhythms

To understand the mechanisms of these rhythms requires an integration of neurophysiology and a branch of mathematics called nonlinear dynamics

(Poincaré, 1954). Developments in nonlinear dynamics during the last 25 years have made it possible to reconstruct the dynamical processes of complex physiological systems from analysis of their time series. These normal and abnormal oscillatory behaviours contain a rich variety of dynamics (i.e., distinct qualitative behaviours). Abnormalities may correspond to three types of qualitative changes including the appearance of a regular/irregular rhythm, the transition from one rhythm to another with a different periodicity, or the disappearance of a rhythm. These qualitative changes are called bifurcations and occur when one or more parameters are varied. In this perspective, the concept of dynamical disease has been proposed by Mackey and Glass (1977). A dynamical disease is "a disease that occurs in a intact physiological control system operating in a range of control parameters that leads to abnormal dynamics" (Rensing et al., 1987, p. 1). The difficulty, of course, is to work backwards from observing the oscillations to inferring the appropriate underlying dynamics.

Modelling oscillatory processes

Most physiological systems contain significant nonlinearities and time delays in their feedback mechanisms. Rensing et al. (1987) indicated that "These time delays may arise because, for example, of the time required for a cell to mature, of the time for the nerve impulse to travel along the axon and across the synapse, or the time for hormonal signals to travel from their site of production to target organs by diffusion and/or passage through the circulation" (p. 3). Some of the qualitative behaviours of the oscillatory processes can be reproduced by relatively simple non-linear mathematical models which suggests that "dynamic complexity may be the norm rather than the exception in nonlinear systems" (Rensing et al., 1987, p. 3).

Mathematical models provide a simple and concise way to explore the dynamics involved in normal and abnormal oscillatory behaviours and to predict the occurrence of qualitative changes as the system parameters are varied. Detailed description of the mathematical models used cannot be further discussed in the context of this chapter but can be found elsewhere (Edelstein-Keshet, 1988; Glass & Mackey, 1988). Modelling human oscillatory systems has been applied to cardiac (Goldberger, 1987), respiratory (Raschke, 1987), and circadian rhythms (Hildebrandt, 1987). Recently, this approach has been applied to neural control (Longtin & Milton, 1988) and to neuromotor control (Akamatsu, Hannaford & Stark, 1986; Bunz, & Haken 1987; Freund, 1987; Kraus, Bittner, Klotz & Przuntek, 1987). As a physiological system, the neuromotor system contains a number of feedback loops with latencies and gains whose values are crucial in the determination of complex dynamical behaviour in motor control. In general, the latency of a reflex (i.e., the time delay around the reflex arc) influences its frequency while the gain influences its stability. Stein and Oguztöreli (1978) indicated that "as the gain is increased so that the oscillation changes from a damped oscillation to a maintained oscillation, to an oscillation which grows to some large amplitude, the frequency may increase by less than 1 Hz" (p. 37). It is known that negative feedback systems may oscillate when the time delay becomes large (Grodins, 1963; Guyton, Crowell & Moore, 1956). In neuromotor control, oscillations in the stretch reflex and tremor have been described by Lippold (1981) and Merton, Morton and Rashbass (1967) respectively.

As mentioned above tremor is a prominent and striking feature of motor control which has been extensively studied in animal and human models. It contains rich dynamics and can also be reset or modulated through sensory actions (Beuter, Larocque & Glass, 1989; Glass, Beuter & Larocque, 1988). Thus, tremor is examined below as a typical example or normal and abnormal motor control.

Description of Tremor

Physiological tremor

Physiological tremor can be defined as a more or less regular oscillation of a body part around a fixed point in space that typically occurs between 8 to 12 Hz (Elble, 1986; Elble & Randall, 1976; Lippold, 1970; Shahani & Young, 1978; Stiles, 1980). This oscillation has a period of 80 to 330 ms and may grow, decay or be maintained (Stein & Oguztöreli, 1978). Although research regarding its cause and a reason for its existence began several hundred years ago, it has failed to fully explain why tremor occurs and what role it may play in the human motor system. Tremor appears to result from several factors which interact in varying proportions depending on the amplitude and nature of the tremor. These factors include the limb natural resonance, the inherent firing properties of motoneurons combined with low-pass filter properties of the muscle system, an instability in the stretch reflex arc associated with synchronization of motoneuron discharge at 8-12 Hz, the size principle of motor unit activation, the ballistocardiac impulse, circulating catecholamines and supraspinal rhythmic input to motoneurons (Marsden, 1984). In other words, tremor can arise from mechanical, reflex or central oscillations and may be considered as a property of the system rather than as any single element comprising it (Allum, 1984; Stein & Oguztöreli, 1978). In fact, Elble (1986) recently concluded that several factors continuously force the mechanical and reflex properties of the body to produce tremor.

Supraspinal influences on physiological tremor

Interest in supraspinal influences started in the 1940's when Lindqvist (1941) suggested that there was a correspondence between alpha rhythms and physiological tremor. This led to the hypothesis that physiological tremor was due to some cerebral pacemaker driving motoneurons to fire synchronously at about 8 Hz. This hypothesis was later abandoned after Marsden, Meadows, Lange and Watson (1969) found no correspondence between finger tremor of the two hands.

Oscillations such as breathing, walking, etc., are produced by the central nervous system and other oscillations can be induced when damage or chemical modification of structures of the CNS occur. Working on animal models of tremor, Lamarre (1984) has shown that under the effect of harmaline, the olivo-cerebellar system can generate tremors at 8-12 Hz or 6-8 Hz which show some similarity with normal and essential tremor respectively. The role of these higher centres in the absence of the drug is unknown but Holmes (1922) observed that physiological tremor in the extended hand disappeared after unilateral damage of the cerebellum. Recently, Keidel et al. (1987) recorded simultaneously electroencephalogram, vibromyogram and tremor and found a "striking temporal order of cyclic change in the degree of coupling between cortical and spinal neuronal populations" (p. 76). Keidel et al. (1987) suggested that the CNS "periodically alters the level of activity and degree of 'synergy' between different (parallel processing) structures and systems rather than maintaining a steady state" (p.77). They also suggest that a common central oscillating mechanism (i.e., a clock) is responsible for the well organized temporal pattern that they observed. As detailed aspects of oscillatory processes such as tremor are studied, it becomes apparent that we lack both a global and a local understanding of their neurofunctional organization and interaction. As suggested by Marsden (1984), it is important to examine the involvement of spindle feedback and stretch reflex in tremor, the interaction of long-latency stretch reflex (perhaps transcortical) with enhanced physiological tremor, and the involvement of the inferior olive rhythmic activity in physiological tremor. A better understanding of these neurophysiological aspects of tremor could contribute to the development of intervention strategies in abnormal motor control.

Pathological tremor

In general, tremor is a symptom used in clinical neurology to differentiate the structure affected in the central nervous system. Examples of pathological tremor include Parkinsonian, essential, chronic alcohol intoxication, cerebellar, and neuropathic tremor (Marsden, 1984; Shahani & Young, 1978; Struppler, Erbel & Velho, 1978). Classification of pathological tremor is based on the preferential appearance of tremor at rest (complete relaxation), postural tremor (anti-gravity innervation), action tremor (volitional innervation) and/or intention tremor (goal-directed movement). Larger amplitude and lower frequency are some of the consistent differences between physiological and pathological tremor. The origin of these differences is still partly unknown.

Changes in the characteristics of physiological tremor are not necessarily a sign of pathology. For example, Enhanced Physiological Tremor (EPT), can be induced by beta-adrenergic overactivity caused by anxiety, fright, hypoglycaemia, or bronchodilators which alter the muscle spindles output (Ia bursts). EPT can also be induced by exercise or fatigue and may correspond to a change in synchronization of motor unit firing (Lippold, 1981; Stiles, 1976). EPT is absent at rest, appears in posture and is present but not intensified during movement (Marsden, 1984). It is distinguished from physiological tremor by a greater tendency for synchronization of single motor discharges. Surface recordings of the EMG from the active muscle show discrete bursts (Hagbarth & Young, 1979; Young & Hagbarth, 1980). The cause of this change is unclear.

Parkinsonian tremor is associated with a lesion in the basal ganglia and is mainly found in muscles of the distal extremities. It is predominantly a resting tremor characterized by reciprocal alternating innervation (i.e., alternating contraction of agonists and antagonists), sometimes accompanied by a postural tremor, and rarely by an action tremor. If it can be easily suppressed by voluntary innervation, then it is said to be a true Parkinsonian syndrome. It has a low peak frequency, a strong motor unit synchronization, and a reflex loop oscillation with a high gain. Comparisons between normal and Parkinsonian tremor are illustrated in Figure 1. As suggested by Marsden (1984) further research should examine if action tremor is distinct from rest tremor, what lesions (in addition to damage to the nigrostriatal system) are essential for the appearance of Parkinsonian rest tremor, and if Parkinsonian rest tremor can be reset by peripheral input.

In the conclusion of a comprehensive review on the role played by the basal ganglia in neuromotor control Lee (1984) wrote "The lesioning, stimulating, and recording experiments in animals have provided us with a large number of semi-isolated fragments of information, but we are still lacking the unifying thread required to tie all these pieces together into a meaningful hypothesis of movement." (p. 128). This may well indicate that the study of the basal ganglia should now be regarded as the common ground for research performed by basic investigators, clinical neurologists as well as theoreticians. Thus the formulation of theoretical models may contribute significantly to our understanding of the specific role of the basal ganglia in normal and abnormal neuromotor control.

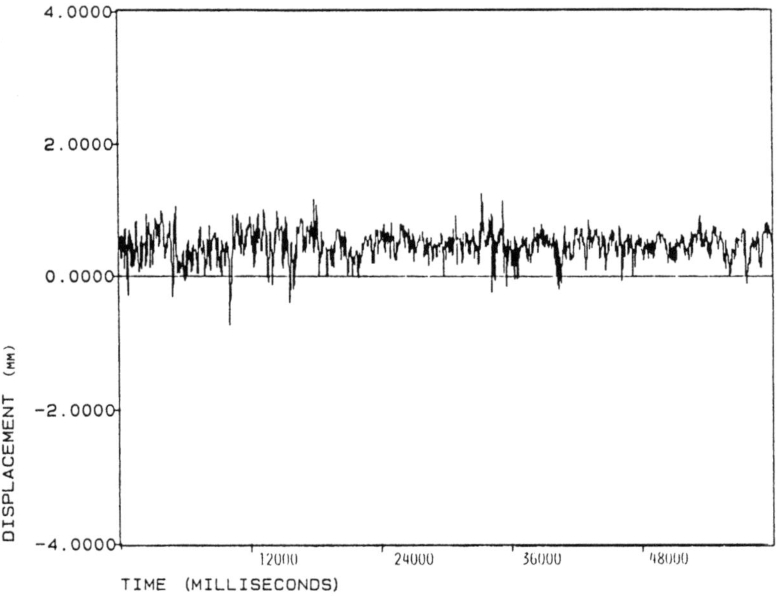

Figure 1 (a): Finger tremor recorded with visual feedback in a normal subject for 60 s. The subject was asked to maintain a constant finger position relative to a stationary baseline displayed on an oscilloscope. The amplitude and frequency of the physiological tremor is relatively consistent across days and trials.

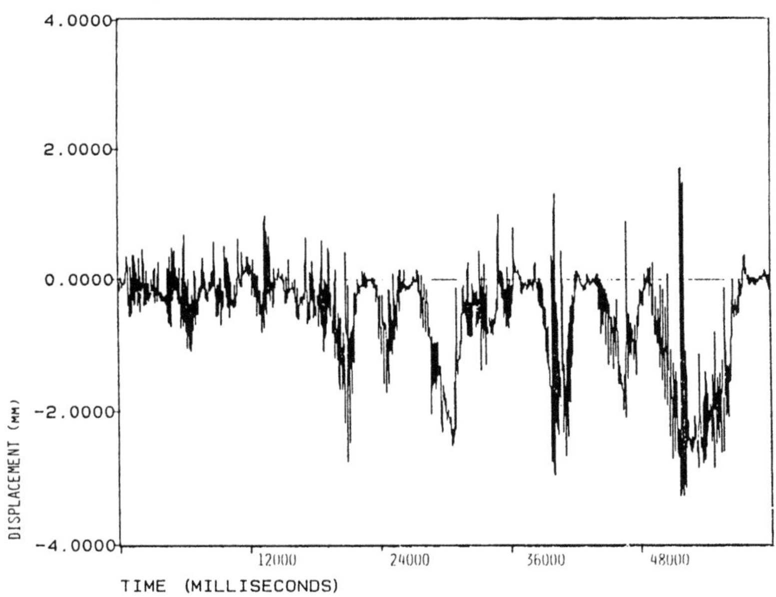

(b): Finger tremor recorded with visual feedback in a Parkinsonian subject for 60 s. The subject was asked to maintain a constant finger position relative to a stationary baseline displayed on an oscilloscope. Note the change in amplitude during the experiment. This phenomenon may correspond to a transition between postural and action tremor induced by a voluntary effort made by the subject to maintain a position close to the baseline.

Tremor and temporal organization of motor control

Freund (1987) noted two relationships between the oscillatory properties of tremor and invariant principles of the temporal organization of motor control. First, movements are limited to frequencies below the peak tremor frequency (i.e., below 6 to 8 Hz). Second, the firing range of motor units is limited between about 8 and 30 Hz for the forearm and hand muscles (i.e., above the peak tremor frequency). Freund (1987) noted that movement and firing range occupy adjacent segments in the frequency domain and that "if extrapyramidal lesions lead to the development of pathological tremor, the range of movements and the range of motor unit firing rates become abnormally low as well as that of rapid alternating movements" (p. 82). The fact that the range of tremor peak frequencies lies exactly between the ranges of movement and motor firing suggests a possible connection between the frequency of voluntary movement control, tremor, and motoneuron firing rate. It also stresses the need for new models of motor rhythms to simulate neuromotor control, and to predict the behaviour of the system in normal and abnormal conditions of operation.

Modelling Neuromotor Control

Current research on modelling, control and simulation of human movement involves such diverse fields as robotics, kinesiology, rehabilitation, and prosthetics. According to Brogan (1985) the scientist must specify the purpose of the model, the boundary of the system, and reduce the actual system to an interconnection of simple idealized elements preserving the mechanisms of storage, dissipation and transfer of energy. Although drastic simplification may be selected to reduce the complexity to a manageable expression, the model must correlate functionally, morphologically, anatomically and physiologically with the real system (Hemami, 1985) and equations must be developed to describe the mathematical relationships between variables.

According to Hemami (1985) the complex nature of the human body in motion often cannot be analyzed with conventional mathematical tools such as the solution of differential and integral equations of motion. The nonlinear functions, complicated relations, and large dimensionality needed to simulate even simple movements has led to the extensive use of digital computer simulations. So far, efforts have been invested more into local rather than global modelling of human movement, that is, the modelling of limbs, muscles or nerves.

Control Theory

Appropriate knowledge from control theory can be applied to simplified local or global models of human motor systems. A movement is simulated and compared with an equivalent movement performed by a human subject. One of the major difficulties in studying the control of human movements is the fact that only the output (i.e., forces, displacements) of the real system are available but the input are not completely understood. A control system is composed of an interconnection of components or functional units so combined as to command, direct or regulate itself or another system to produce the desired result. The interaction between the system input and output will dictate one of two general classes of control systems (i.e., the open-loop and closed-loop or feedback system). In the open-loop control system (i.e., as in a ballistic movement) the control action is independent of the output while in the closed-loop control system (i.e., as in a ramp movement) the control action depends on the output (Figure 2). This last system is commonly called a feedback control system. A simple example of a negative feedback system related to motor control is illustrated in Figure 3.

Feedback

Because of its major role in biological control systems, the characteristics of a feedback system must be briefly mentioned. They include accuracy of response, reduced sensitivity to variations in systems characteristics, reduced effects of nonlinearities and distortion, an increased bandwidth (or range of input frequency over which the system responds satisfactorily), and a tendency toward oscillation or instability (Figure 2b). Feedback mechanisms can be manipulated in terms of gain and/or latency. Physiological systems may involve a combination of positive, negative and mixed feedback mechanisms, and these feedback loops interact in a complex fashion and are not easily manipulated.

The components of the control system can be represented in different forms including input-output mathematical equations and block diagrams which offer a clear representation of the system (Figure 2). The solution of the mathematical equations represent the system behaviour. The techniques for solving linear equations are well developed in the mathematical and engineering literature. However, within the context of dynamical systems the mathematical models used include finite difference equations, ordinary differential equations, partial differential equations, and time delay differential equations whose solutions are sometimes impossible to find because they are nonlinear. Approximation or simplification of these mathematical models using a system of linear ordinary differential equations is usually not acceptable since it does not respect the reality of the system. As mentioned above, except in some special cases, complete analytical solution to systems of non-linear equations is not possible.

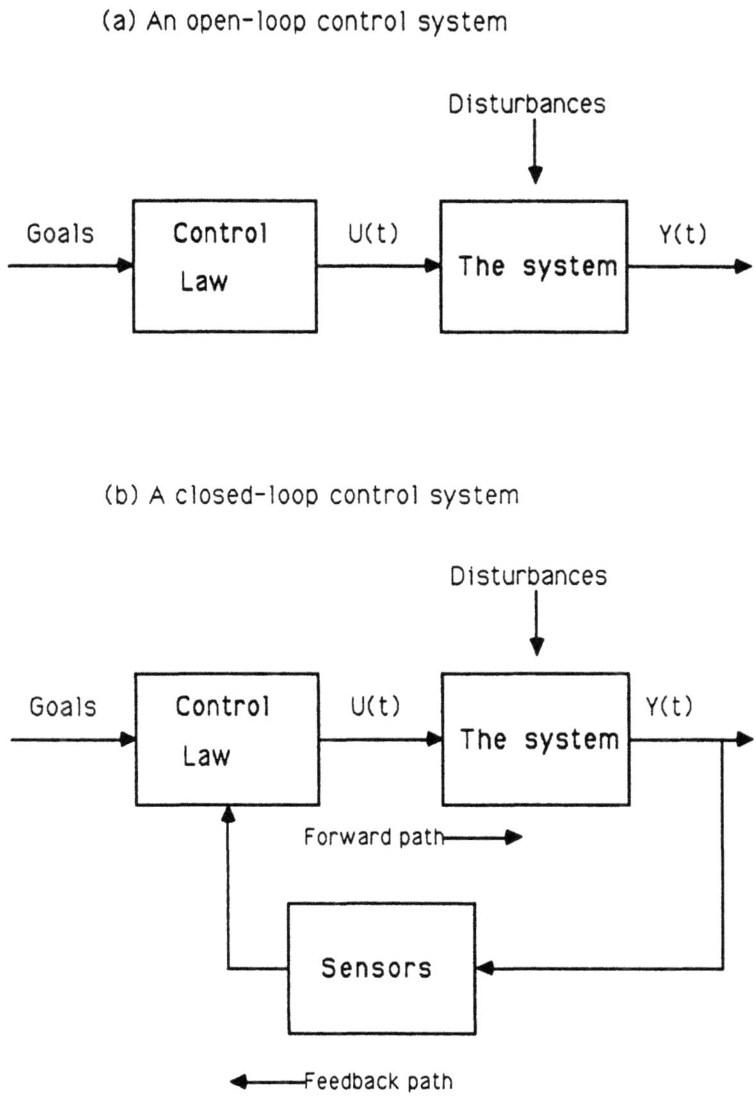

Figure 2: These block diagrams allow a clear representation of the simplest kind of control system which consists of two basic elements, the plant and the controller: (a) is an example of an open-loop control system and (b) is an example of a closed-loop control system. In an open-loop control system the output has no effect on its control, while in a closed-loop system the output affects the control of the system (i.e., measurement errors can be detected and corrected as is illustrated in Figure 3. Figure adapted from Brogan (1985).

(a)

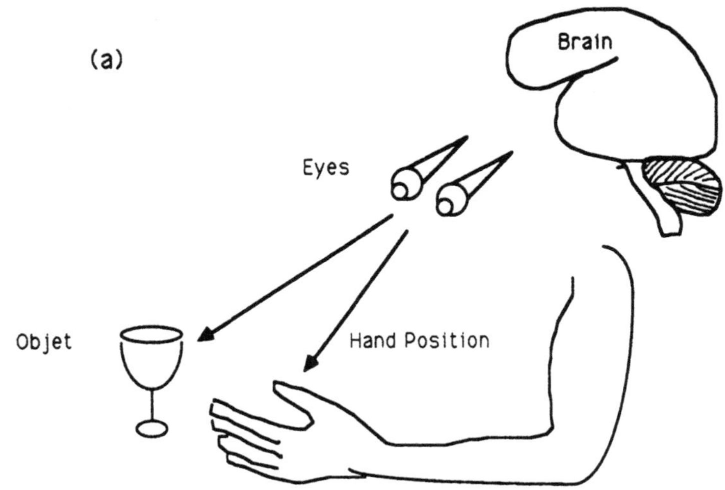

(b)

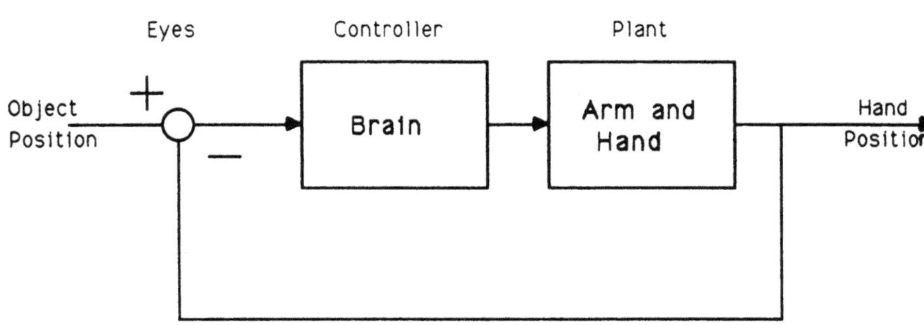

Figure 3: Illustration of a closed-loop control system in which the subject reaches for an object. The object position in 3 dimensional space is determined using vision (a). Commands are sent to the upper limb muscles to contract. In a negative feedback system, information about the *current* trajectory of the hand is fed back into the control action at the comparator and compared with the *desired* hand trajectory (b). The two important characteristics to consider in such a system are the loop time or latency of the feedback pathway and the gain of the system. As explained by Lohr and Wisniewski (1987) if the loop time is short compared to changes in the input, the system will work relatively well. If the loop time is lengthened, oscillations will occur as the comparator attempts to decrease the error signal. Similarly, if the gain is too high, oscillations may also occur. This example represents the simplest possible case. Reaching for an object is a very complex movement involving vision, proprioception and motor control. Information about initiation, execution of the movement follow multiple serial and parallel afferent and efferent neural pathways as well as feedback and feedforward control mechanisms.

Modelling tremor

Despite the number of studies undertaken, the mechanisms of physiological and pathological tremor are still unclear. As mentioned above, tremor is the result of complex interactions between influences (e.g., circulating catecholamines, heart beat, visual feedback, stretch reflex, motoneuron firing rate, natural resonance of the limbs, etc.). The investigation of the dynamics of tremor strictly from an experimental standpoint could become inefficient and limit our global view of tremor since all the pertinent relationships between parameters would have to be measured on a systematic and logical basis. One way to speed up the process is to model tremor using mathematical concepts adequately describing the experimental time series. This model could have some predictive value and provide some estimate of the output for an input for which the model was not originally developed (Agarwal & Gottlieb, 1985). Experimental manipulations could then be used to verify the model predictions.

Experimentally based mathematical models and computer simulations of animal and human tremor generally classify tremogenic influences into mechanical, reflex and central oscillations. Feedback loops involved in this system are illustrated in Figure 4 (Stein & Oguztöreli, 1978). Efforts to model tremor have been slow because of the complex nature of the system and the difficulty to open or manipulate these feedback loops. Existing models consider either the mechanical or neuromuscular oscillators with or without feedback loops. They do not incorporate the nonlinear properties of the spinal cord which is assumed to act as a simple linear summing amplifier (Agarwal & Gottlieb, 1985).

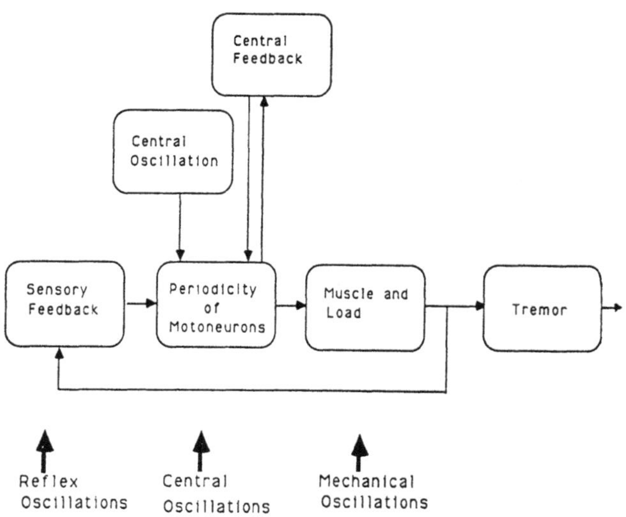

Figure 4: Illustration of the role of mechanical, segmental and central oscillation in tremor. The respective influence of these oscillations in physiological and pathological tremors varies. This figure is modified from a figure presented in Stein and Oguztoreli (1981).

A mechanical type of model is illustrated by Feldman's model (1964) and is in agreement with the work of Dietz, Hillesheimer and Freund (1974), and Elble and Randall (1976). These researchers found that the degree of synchronization of the motor units is correlated with the amplitude of physiological tremor (i.e., stronger tremor correspond to greater synchronization) with a 8-12 Hz peak. Christakos and Lal (1980) used Feldman's model to simulate tremor in muscle force during a moderate contraction. The simulated data showed a 9 Hz peak in the spectral analysis which could correspond to experimental physiological tremor.

A neuromuscular type of model based on oscillations in the stretch reflex loop has been influenced by work from Mathews (1964) and Lippold (1970). Stein and Oguztöreli (1978) modeled tremor using three feedback loops with different latencies and gains. Their simulations revealed that shorter delays produced a 8-12 Hz spectral peak corresponding to physiological tremor while longer time delays produced a 4-6 Hz spectral peak corresponding to pathological tremor. A more detailed description of tremor models are available in Agarwal and Gottlieb (1985).

Modelling tremor requires that a number of simplifications (e.g. linearization of the system) and assumptions (e.g., the mode of operation of short and long delays) be made. When these simplifications and assumptions are made in an appropriate way they allow scientists to represent the phenomenon in a parsimonious and powerful way, and to make predictions about the internal state variables of the system that could be tested experimentally when possible. Although significant progress has been made in modelling the motor system, these models still need improvements with regards to nonlinearities and predictive capabilities.

Future Directions and Concluding Remarks

In this chapter I have attempted to show that oscillatory processes play an important role in motor control disorders and that theoretical analysis of these processes has been left relatively unexplored until recently. Temporal organization and disorders in motor rhythms have been described using physiological and pathological tremors as examples. The need for models of normal and abnormal motor control was demonstrated. The challenge in future research will be to identify the control parameters involved in normal and abnormal neuromotor control. These control parameters will have to be explored experimentally and their dynamics will have to be described and modeled. Today, one of the challenging problems in motor control is to study the dynamics produced by the complex interactions between negative feedback loops having different gain and latencies (Glass et al., 1988). The neural networks involved at the spinal supraspinal and cortical levels are complex and may involve other kinds of control processes such as feedforward or mixed feedback in addition to negative feedback. Sometimes a loop can be "opened" and a control parameter such as the time delay around the loop can be manipulated (Beuter et al., 1989; Longtin & Milton, 1988). However most of the time, loops cannot be opened and the researcher must observe the changes in dynamics corresponding to lesions of specific structures of the CNS found in patients with neurological diseases such as Parkinsonism or cerebellar dysfunction.

In the past, motor control scientists have assumed the existence of motor programs as ready-to-use models creating smooth, fast and skillful motor actions. Sets of commands are sent to the muscles with the proper timing and the movement sequence can, in principle, be carried out with limited peripheral feedback. Changes in the motor output are attributed to adjustments of the motor program parameters through feedback (Brooks, 1986). Thus, a two-way interaction exists between sensory input and motor programs, and ongoing biological oscillations can, to a certain extent, be manipulated (Stein et al., 1981). Based on this observation, Stein et al. (1981) have suggested that 100 ms torque steps (i.e., brief perturbations) could be used to reset neural oscillations between flexion and extension at the wrist in patients with essential and Parkinsonian tremor. They found that essential tremor could be reset to a considerable degree while Parkinsonian tremor could not, indicating a stronger sensory involvement in essential tremor. Sensory actions on biological oscillations have been classified by Stein et al. (1981) and include *modulation* (i.e., change in the amplitude of a phase or the frequency of an oscillation), *resetting* (i.e., change in the timing on a long term basis without modifying the frequency or amplitude in a durable way), *repatterning* (i.e., phase transition between two qualitatively different modes of functioning), and *gating* (i.e., switching on or off of an oscillation). It should be noted that the same sensory input can produce different motor effects depending on other external and internal factors (Stein et al., 1981). I have briefly illustrated the action of sensory input on biological oscillations using pathological tremor as an example. It was suggested that the same approach could be exploited in clinical settings for other manifestations of abnormal motor control in the future. For example, Tatton, Eastman, Bedingham, Verrier, and Bruce (1984) have suggested that a defective utilization of sensory input from the mecanoreceptors may cause bradykinesia, rigidity, and decrease movement repertoire in Parkinsonian patients and in monkeys treated with a substance called MPTP. Animals exposed to MPTP develop a syndrome clinically indistinguishable from Parkinson's disease (Tatton et al., 1984). If this hypothesis is verified, it may be possible to design and test therapeutic strategies adapted to this and other neurological diseases.

An alternative approach to motor control is to assume the existence of self-organizing properties in the motor system (Bunz & Haken, 1987). These properties can produce organized behaviours without the express intervention of the control centres. In this perspective, transitions occur between different modes of functioning when a control parameter reaches a critical value. These modes of operation can change from rest to periodic or aperiodic oscillations, or to more or less complicated oscillations. What is the functional significance of these dynamics in motor control? Goodman and Kelso (1983) observed a clear and systematic relationship between physiological tremor and movement initiation under a variety of experimental conditions. Tremor appears to act as a background facilitation to perform voluntary movements efficiently. The delay sometimes observed in Parkinsonian patients for movement initiation may come from waiting for the correct timing in the cycle to arrive (Hallett, Shahani & Young, 1977). Goodman and Kelso (1983) concluded that tremor plays an important functional role and that the motor control system is sensitive to its own dynamics. This unifying view of motor control could be useful in the development of strategies to reposition the system in a "healthy" range of parameter space.

Future progress will be achieved if an understanding of how a natural system works is developed using sophisticated computers, a theory of systems and an adequate knowledge of physiology (Hemami, 1985). Areas needing immediate attention include the programming of movement variables, neural communication, model parameters and structure, the role of the spinal cord in controlling the amplitude, phase frequency and coupling of oscillators and the identification of feedback loops in the CNS. With these new research efforts, the movement experience of normal and disabled individuals shall be better understood and dealt with.

Author Notes

1. Send request for reprints to Anne Beuter, Departement de Kinanthropologie, Université du Québec à Montréal, Case Postal 8888, Succursale "A", Montréal, Québec, H3C 3P8.

References

Akamatsu, N., Hannaford, B., & Stark, L. (1986). An intrinsic mechanism for the oscillatory contraction of muscle. *Biological Cybernetics, 53,* 219-227.

Allum, J. H. J. (1984). Segmental reflex, muscle mechanical and central mechanisms underlying human physiological tremor. In L. J. Findley & R. Capildeo (Eds.), *Movement disorders: Tremor* (pp. 135-155). London: Macmillan.

Agarwal, G. C., & Gottlieb, G. L. (1985). Mathematical modelling and simulation of the postural control loop: Part I, II, and III. *CRC Critical Reviews in Biomedical Engineering, Vol. 8, Issue 2,* (pp. 93-134), Vol. 11, Issue 2, (pp. 113-154), Vol. 12, Issue 1, (pp. 49-93).

Bassler, U. (1986). On the definition of central pattern generator and its sensory control. *Biological Cybernetics, 54,* 65-69.

Beuter, A., Larocque, D., & Glass, L. (1989). Complex oscillations in a human motor system. *Journal of Motor Behavior, 21,* 277-289.

Brogan, W. L. (1985). *Modern control theory.* Englewood Cliffs, NJ: Prentice Hall.

Brooks, V. B. (1986). *The neural basis of motor control.* New York, NY: Oxford University Press.

Bunz, H., & Haken, H. (1987). Quantitative theory of change in oscillatory hand movements: Application of methods of synergetics. In L. Rensing, U. an der Heiden & M. C. Mackey, (Eds.), *Temporal disorder in human oscillatory systems* (pp. 102-109). Berlin: Springer-Verag.

Christakos, C. N., & Lal, S. (1980). Lumped and population stochastic models of skeletal muscle: Implications and predictions. *Biological Cybernetics, 36,* 73-80.

Chusid, J. G. (1973). *Correlative neuroanatomy and functional neurology* (15th Ed.). Palo Alto, CA: Lange.

Delcomyn F. (1980). Neural basis of rhythmic behavior in animals. *Science, 210,* 492-498.

Delong, M. R. (1978). Possible involvement of central pacemakers in clinical disorders of movement. *Federation Proceedings, 37,* 2171-2175.

Desmedt, J. E. (Ed.). (1978). *Physiological tremor, pathological tremor and clonus: Progress in Clinical Neurophysiology* (Vol. 5). Basel, Switzerland: S. Karger.

Dietz, V., Hillesheimer, W., & Freund, H. J. (1974). Correlation between tremor, voluntary contraction and firing patterns of motor units in Parkinson's disease. *Journal of Neurology, Neurosurgery and Psychiatry, 37,* 927-937.

Edelstein-Keshet, L. (1988). *Mathematical models in biology.* New York, NY: Random House.

Elble, R. J. (1986). Physiological and essential tremor. *Neurology, 36,* 225-31.

Elble, R. J., & Randall, J. E. (1976). Motor unit activity responsible for 8 to 12 Hz component of human physiological finger tremor. *Journal of Neurophysiology, 39,* 370-383.

Feldman, A. G. (1964). Calculation of the spectrum of physiological tremor on the basis of the work of the motor units (trans.) *Biofizika, 9,* 726.

Freund, H. J. (1987). Central rhythmicities in motor control and its perturbations. In L. Rensing, U. an der Heiden & M. C. Mackey (Eds.), *Temporal disorder in human oscillatory systems* (pp. 79-82). Berlin: Springer-Verlag.

Glass, L., & Mackey, M. C. (1979). Pathological conditions resulting from instabilities in physiological control systems. *Annals of the New York Academy of Sciences, 316,* 214-235.

Glass, L., & Mackey, M. C. (1988). *From clocks to chaos: The rhythms of life.* Princeton, NJ: Princeton University Press.

Glass, L., Beuter, A., & Larocque, D. (1988). Time delays, oscillations and chaos in physiological control systems. *Mathematical Biosciences, 89,* 1-15.

Goldberger, A. L. (1987). Nonlinear dynamics, fractals, cardiac physiology and sudden death. In L. Rensing, U. an der Heiden & M. C. Mackey (Eds.), *Temporal disorder in human oscillatory systems* (pp. 118-125). Berlin: Springer-Verlag.

Goodman, D., & Kelso, J. A. S. (1983). Exploring the functional significance of physiological tremor: A biospectroscopic approach. *Experimental Brain Research, 49,* 419-431.

Grodins, F. S. (1963). *Control theory and biological systems.* New York, NY: Columbia University Press.

Grimm, R. J. (1984). Disorderly walks. *Neurologic Clinics, 2,* 615-631.

Guyton, A. C., Crowell, J. W., & Moore, J. W. (1956). Basic oscillating mechanisms of Cheyne-Stokes breathing. *American Journal of Physiology, 187,* 395-398.

Hemami, H. (1985). Modelling, control, and simulation of human movement. *CRC Critical Reviews in Biomedical Engineering, 13*(1), 1-34.

Hagbarth, K. E., & Young, R. R. (1979). Participation of the stretch reflex in human physiological tremor. *Brain,* 102, 509-526.

Hallett, M., Shahani, B. T., & Young, R. R. (1977). Analysis of stereotyped voluntary movements at the elbow in patients with Parkinson's disease. *Journal Neurology, Neurosurgery and Psychiatry, 40,* 1129-1135.

Hildebrandt, G. (1987). The autonomous time structure and its reactive modifications in the human organism. In L. Rensing, U. an der Heiden & M. C. Mackey (Eds.), *Temporal disorder in human oscillatory systems* (pp. 160-175). Berlin: Springer-Verlag.

Holmes, G. (1922). Clinical symptoms of cerebellar diseases. *Lancet, 1,* 1177 1182 1231-1237; *2,* 59-65, 111-15.

Keidel, M., Keidel, W. D. Tirsch, W. S., & Poppl, S. J. (1987). Studying temporal order in human CNS by means of "running" frequency and coherence analysis. In L. Rensing, U. an der Heiden & M. C. Mackey (Eds.), *Temporal disorder in human oscillatory systems* (pp. 69-78). Berlin: Springer-Verlag.

Kelso, J. A. S. (1981). On the oscillatory basis of movement. *Bulletin of the Psychonomic Society, 18,* 63.

Koller, W. C. (1984). Diagnosis and treatment of tremors. *Neurologic Clinics, 2,* 499-514.

Kopell, N., & Ermentrout, G. B. (1986). Subcellular oscillations and bursting. *Mathematical Biosciences, 78,* 265-291.

Kraus, P. H., Bittner, H. R., Klotz, P., & Przuntek, H. (1987). Investigation of agonist/antagonistic movement in Parkinson's disease from an ergotic point of view. In L. Rensing, U. an der Heiden & M. C. Mackey (Eds.), *Temporal disorder in human oscillatory systems* (pp. 110-115). Berlin: Springer-Verlag.

Lamarre, Y. (1984). Animal models of physiological, essential and Parkinsonian-like tremor. In L. J. Findley & R. Capildeo (Eds.), *Movement disorders: Tremor* (pp. 183-194). London: Macmillan.

Lee, R. G. (1984). Physiology of the basal ganglia: An overview. *Canadian Journal of Neurological Sciences, 11,* 124-128.

Lindqvist, T. (1941). Finger tremor and the alpha waves of the electro-encephalogram. *Acta Medica Scandinavia, 108,* 580-585.

Lippold, O. C. J. (1970). Oscillation in the stretch reflex arc and the origin of the rhythmical 8-12 c/s component of physiological tremor. *Journal of Physiology, 206*, 359-382.

Lippold, O. C. J. (1981). The tremor in fatigue. In R. Poater & J. Whelen (Eds.), Human muscle fatigue: Physiological mechanisms. *Ciba Foundation Symposium, 82*, 234-248.

Longtin, A., & Milton J. G. (1988). Complex oscillations in the pupil light reflex with 'mixed' and delayed feedback. *Mathematical Biosciences, 90*, 183-199.

Mackey, M. C., & Glass, L. (1977). Oscillation and chaos in physiological control systems. *Science, 197*, 287-289.

Mackey, M. C., & Milton, J. G. (1987). Dynamical diseases. *Annals of the New York Academy of Sciences, 504*, 16-32.

Marsden, C. D. (1984). Origin of normal and pathological tremor. In L. J. Findley & R. Capildeo (Eds.), *Movement disorders: Tremor* (pp. 37-84). London: Macmillan.

Marsden, C. D., Meadows, J. C., Lange, G. W., & Watson, R. S. (1969). Variations in human physiological finger tremor with particular reference to changes with age. *Electroencephalography and Clinical Neurophysiology, 27*, 169-178.

Mathews, P. B. C. (1964). Muscle spindles and their motor control. *Physiological Reviews, 44*, 219.

Merton, P. A., Morton, R. A., & Rashbass, C. (1967). Visual feedback in hand tremor. *Nature, 216*, 583-584.

Poincaré, H. (1954). *Oeuvres.* Paris: Gauthier-Villar.

Rensing, L., U. an der Heiden & Mackey, M. C. (1987). *Temporal disorder in human oscillatory systems.* Berlin: Springer-Verlag.

Raschke, F. (1987). Coordination in the circulatory and respiratory systems. In L. Rensing, U. an Der Heiden & M. C. Mackey (Eds.), *Temporal disorder in human oscillatory systems* (pp. 152-158). Berlin: Springer-Verlag.

Shahani, B. T., & Young, R. R. (1978). Action tremors: A clinical neurophysiological review. In J. E. Desmedt (Ed.). *Physiological tremor, pathological tremors and clonus: Progress in clinical neurophysiology,* (Vol. 5, pp. 129-137). Basel, Switzerland: S. Karger.

Stein, P. S. G. (1977). Application of the mathematics of coupled oscillator systems to the analysis of the neural control of locomotion. *Federation Proceedings, 36,* 2056-2059.

Stein, R. B., Gordon, T., Oguztöreli, M. N., & Lee, R. G. (1981). Classifying sensory patterns and their effects on locomotion and tremor. *Canadian Journal of Physiological Pharmacology, 59,* 645-655.

Stein, R. B., & Oguztöreli, M. N. (1978). Reflex involvement in the generation and control of tremor and clonus. In J. E. Desmedt (Ed.), *Physiological tremor, pathological tremor and clonus: Progress in clinical neurophysiology,* (Vol. 5, pp. 8-50). Basel, Switzerland: S. Karger.

Stiles, R. N. (1976). Frequency and displacement amplitude relations for normal hand tremor. *Journal of Applied Physiology, 40,* 44-54.

Stiles, R. N. (1980). Mechanical and neural feedback factors in postural hand tremor of normal subjects. *Journal of Neurophysiology, 44,* 40-59.

Struppler, A., Erbel, F., & Velho, F. (1978). An overview on the pathophysiology of Parkinsonian and other pathological tremors. In J. E. Desmedt (Ed.), *Physiological tremor, pathological tremor and clonus: Progress in clinical neurophysiology,* (Vol. 5, pp. 114-128). Basel, Switzerland: S. Karger.

Tatton, W. G., Eastman, M. J., Bedingham, W., Verrier, M. C., & Bruce, I. C. (1984). Defective utilization of sensory input as the basis for bradykinesia, rigidity and decreased movement repertoire in Parkinson's disease: A hypothesis. *Canadian Journal of Neurological sciences, 11,* 136-143.

Young, R. R., & Hagbarth, K. E. (1980). Physiological tremor enhanced by manoeuvres affecting the segmental stretch reflex. *Journal Neurology, Neurosurgery and Psychiatry, 43,* 248-256.

Problems in Movement Control
G. Reid (editor)

PHYSICAL CONSTRAINTS ON THE MOVEMENT OF DISABLED PERFORMERS

Allen W. Burton
Michael G. Wade
School of Physical Education and Recreation
University of Minnesota

The term "constraints" is not new, but recently the term has become increasingly more popular with movement scientists when discussing the development of motor skills. In 1973, Connolly contributed a chapter on the learning of manual skills in young children in a volume entitled *Constraints on Learning* (Connolly, 1973). Nine years later, a chapter by Kugler, Kelso, and Turvey (1982), focused on the implications of a scaling up of morphological characteristics on the development of movement coordination and control. This brought a new awareness of the importance of physical constraints to researchers in the field. In a volume entitled *Motor Development in Children: Aspects of Coordination and Control,* Newell (1986) discussed the effect of organismic, environmental, and task constraints on the development of coordination. Recently, some of the ideas spawned by these authors have been the focus of new research and have generated some new solutions to old problems (e.g., Thelen, Fisher, & Ridley-Johnson, 1984). However, the effect of physical constraints on the movement performance of handicapped individuals has not been included in this recent work; thus, it is not surprising that a chapter on constraints should appear in the present volume.

The term "constraints" is not the only newcomer to the movement science vernacular. As suggested above, "coordination" and "control" are both terms used with increasing frequency to describe skill development in much the same way that the terms "learning" and "performance" have been used when dissecting a motor learning curve. The term "coordination" refers to the elements of skill expression that permit more than one limb segment to act in unison with others. Central to this component of skill is the timing relationship between the limb segments. The term "control" refers to the individual's capacity to modulate the timing or the forces produced in the particular muscles acting on the limb segments involved in the skilled activity. The distinction drawn between coordination and control perhaps is best described by the early proponents of the term, Kugler, Kelso, and Turvey (1980): "A constraint 'coordinates' in the sense that it enforces (automatically) a relationship among several variables; the partitioning into essential and nonessential variables 'controls' in the sense that it identifies the means by which the relationship can be systematically modified--qualitatively and quantitatively" (p. 14).

One chapter does not do justice to this subject matter, thus we limit ourselves here by: (a) discussing the most common disabilities, (b) describing the nature of the physical constraints found in those disabilities, and (c) suggesting how they impact on movement skill and performance. As a first step, we will examine historically the idea of physical constraints as a means of discussing motor skill development. As noted above, it is only recently that a constraints perspective--especially a physical constraint perspective--has gained popularity among researchers in the area.

Theoretical discussions in the 1970s rarely made reference to the physical parameters of the individual. That is not to say that reference to physical constraints in relation to movement development cannot be found in the literature; it just did not receive the attention that it deserved. In the late 1960s and through the 1970s, the common view of motor development cast the developing child in the style of a rather simple computer. The literature published in the 1970s often referred to the child as an immature processor of information, with the so-called "building blocks" of motor skill--sub-routines--gradually increasing in complexity (Bruner & Bruner, 1968; Connolly, 1970). [For a review of the theoretical development during this period, the reader is referred to Wade (1976).] While the computer metaphor held sway in experimental psychology in general and in the area of motor development in particular during this period, there was at least one dissenting voice. Wickstrom (1970) promoted the view that kinematics (the displacement, velocity, and acceleration of the various body segments) was the critical factor in understanding the development of skill and performance in children.

Over 40 years ago, data were available that demonstrated the principle that changing constraints produced by physical growth were important considerations when studying human movement. Bayley and Davis (1935) and Norval (1947) reported that children who were taller and had longer legs (and were not overweight) tended to walk earlier than children who were shorter and had shorter legs. In 1982, Kugler et al. proposed that "as a child grows bigger an effectivity such as walking or throwing will pass through a sequence of qualititatively distinguishable forms, where each form is stable over a limited range of growth in the bodily dimensions" (Kugler et al., 1982, p. 10). This led to a new understanding of movement coordination and control during development by taking into account changes in the physical dimensions of the body and the scaled properties of the different limb segments.

Further, Kugler and his colleagues drew together physical biology concepts and the views on perception advanced by Gibson (1979), the Cornell ecological psychologist. They suggested that skilled movement is constrained not only by the physical properties of the skeletal-joint-muscle system, but also by the environment in which the activity is manifested. This contemporary view of motor skill has as its central concern the problem of seeking a means of reducing the many degrees of freedom that are extant in an action system (see also Kugler, 1986; Newell, 1986). It should be pointed out that the more traditional notion of motor skill development that places the burden of control on an executive or schema is helped in no small way by recognizing that the physical constraints on the system naturally reduce the degrees of freedom required for control and, thus, places the role of the executive in a more reasonable light.

How do the physical characteristics of disabled individuals act as constraints on the development of movement skill and performance? In the ensuing pages, we begin by discussing the effect of physical constraints on the movement of nonhandicapped children and continue with a description of growth deviations in the handicapped and the relationship between movement performance and growth deviations. We conclude by discussing some implications of these issues for practitioners working with handicapped individuals and describing how physical constraints might be manipulated to improve movement performance of persons who are handicapped.

Physical Constraints on the Movement of Nonhandicapped Children

There are two major research approaches that have been used in examining the relationship between intrinsic physical constraints and movement performance in nonhandicapped children. First, correlational studies have evaluated the degree of relationships between body size, physique, strength, and motor performance in children (Beunen et al., 1985; Rarick & Oyster, 1964; Seils, 1951). Unfortunately, this type of correlational evidence only provides insight into the relationships between dependent variables and does not allow for any conclusions regarding the actual effect of physical constraints on motor performance. However, the second research approach--the direct manipulation of a morphological variable--does allow for inferences regarding cause and effect. This more definitive type of research is limited at present to studies that focus on the stepping reflex in infants (Thelen et al., 1984).

Studies that have examined correlations between morphological and motor performance measures have indicated that these correlations, in general, are quite low (Beunen et al., 1985; Rarick & Oyster, 1964; Seils, 1951). Rarick and Oyster (1964) determined the correlations between four anthropometric variables (chronological age, skeletal age, height, and weight) and eleven measures of strength and motor performance in second-grade boys. They reported that only 1 of the 11 third-order partial correlations between height and strength/motor performance (with the two types of ages and weight held constant) was greater than .30 (.36 for knee extension strength). Similarly, only 1 of the 11 third-order partial correlations between weight and strength/motor performance (with the two types of ages and height held constant) was greater than .30 (.33 for broad jump, with sign reversed).

Seils (1951) correlated anthropometric variables (chronological age, height, and weight) with seven motor performance measures for 6- to 8-year-old boys and girls and reported results comparable to Rarick and Oyster's (1964). Second-order partial correlations were calculated for height (with age and weight held constant) and weight (with age and height held constant) for each age(3)-gender(2)-performance measure(7) combination (a total of 42 correlations). For height, only 2 of the 42 correlations were greater than .30 (the highest was .46), and for weight, none of the 42 were greater than .30. In both of these studies, the zero-order correlations and lower-order partial correlations also revealed low relationships between physical size and motor performance scores.

Beunen et al. (1985) found a higher relationship between morphology and motor performance than the other two studies. They used multiple regression analyses to determine the relationship between somatotype (endomorphy, mesomorphy, and ectomorphy components) and motor performance (seven items measuring strength, speed, and flexibility) for 12- to 19-year-old Belgian boys. Only two of the mean multiple correlations (averaged across the seven age levels) for the three somatotype components (mean R) were less than .30, with the highest mean R being .52 for the arm pull. As expected, mesomorphy was the most important predictor for nearly all motor items at each age level. In contrast, Szabo, Szmodis, Meszaros, and Pinter (1984) reported that correlations between body build and motor performance were very low for 10- and 14-year-old girls.

The correlational evidence suggests that the relationship between body morphology and motor performance in nonhandicapped children is, in general, low and, at best, moderate (see also Malina, 1975). However, these results must be interpreted with caution since they cannot be used to determine the actual effect of physical constraints on performance. The only studies that have examined the direct manipulation of body morphology on movement behaviour have been carried out by Thelen and her associates.

In these studies, Thelen et al. (1984) elicited stepping responses from 4-week-old infants by holding them under their armpits, tilting them slightly forward, and touching their feet to a solid surface. In Study 2, using a within-subject experimental design with 12 infants, the number of steps taken in one minute under normal conditions was compared with the number of steps taken when a total of 163 g of weight was added to the infants' legs . The number of steps significantly decreased with the added weight, from a mean of

14.2 steps/min to 9.6 steps/min. In Study 3, the number of steps taken by a different set of 12 infants was compared with the number of steps taken when the infants were placed in warm water (up to about mid-torso). The reverse effect was observed, with the number of steps significantly increasing with the mass-decreasing effect of the water from a mean of 10.4 steps/min to 20.3 steps/min. These results support the hypothesis that the well-documented "disappearance" of the stepping reflex may be caused by changes in the physical constraints on the infant (i.e., the leg strength/leg mass ratio) rather than by cortical inhibition.

Although the correlations between morphology and motor performance in children generally are low, the work by Thelen et al. (1984) demonstrates how changes in intrinsic physical constraints can modulate certain aspects of movement behaviour. This result is in line with the hypothesis by Kugler and his colleagues suggesting that "a *continuous* change in a single variable (or combination of variables) may bring about a sudden *qualitative* change in the macro structure of the manifold associated with the variable(s)" (Kugler et al., 1982, p. 64). Thus, a small change in a physical parameter of the body may push the parameter value beyond a critical point, causing a dramatic change in particular movement patterns. Examples of how changes in environmental or task variables may elicit such qualitative changes in the movement behaviour of children have been provided by Halverson (1966).

Growth Deviations in Handicapped Individuals

Many handicapping conditions, such as Down's Syndrome and spina bifida, are accompanied by aberrations in physical growth characteristics. Some of the more common handicapping conditions are described below, organized by basic etiology.

Chromosomal Aberrations

The most common chromosomal disorder in children is Down's Syndrome, with one of the prominent features of this syndrome being short stature. Children with Down's Syndrome fall 2 standard deviations (SDs) below normal for standing height at all ages and become relatively shorter each year until about 15 years (Pryor & Thelander, 1967). Their short stature appears to be attributed more to short leg length rather than to short sitting height (Pryor & Thelander, 1967; Rarick & Seefeldt, 1974). Rarick and Seefeldt (1974) found that the peak height velocity of children with Down's Syndrome occurred at about the same chronological age as nonhandicapped children. They also found that the average increase in height per year for boys from 10 to 19 years of age was only 0.5 cm less than nonhandicapped boys, suggesting that most of the height deficit occurs before 10 years. In Japanese children with Down's Syndrome, Ikeda, Higurashi, Hirayama, Ishikawa, and Hoshina (1977) reported that arm length/stature and leg length/stature ratios were about 2 to 5% less than normal children from 3 to 48 months of age. Finally, the secular trend in growth which is clearly evident in nonhandicapped Japanese infants, was not exhibited in Down's Syndrome infants (Hoshi, Ashizawa, & Ikeda, 1979).

Other chromosomal problems which are characterized by growth disorders include Turner's syndrome (XO), which affects only females, and Klinefelter's syndrome (XXY), which affects only males (Rallison, 1986). Girls with Turner's syndrome tend to be significantly shorter than normal at all ages, while boys with Klinefelter's syndrome tend to be excessively tall and slim, with long limbs and a low upper-body/lower-body ratio.

Congenital Anomalies

Growth deviations in five types of congenital anomalies are discussed in this subsection: (a) abnormalities caused by drug therapy, irradiation, or virus infections of mothers early in gestation, (b) spina bifida (myelomeningocele), (c) cerebral palsy due to hypoxia at birth, (d) neurological deficits or minimal brain dysfunction due to hypoxia of short duration, and (e) mental retardation, not including Down's Syndrome.

Pryor and Thelander (1967) reported that children born to mothers who were given drug therapy or radiation or had virus infections early in their pregnancies had normal increases in height until 5 years of age. At this point, increases in height for both boys and girls were less than normal, until there was a significant difference in height at age 10 (a difference of about 1-2 SDs). Pryor and Thelander also observed that body width measurements, such as chest width and bi-iliac diameter, were in greater deficit than body length measurements.

Children with myelomeningocele from 1 to 16 years of age were shown to have mean upper-body and lower-body lengths that were significantly less than the heights of nonhandicapped children of the same age (Duval-Beaupere, Kaci, Lougovoy, Caponi, & Touzeau, 1987). In general, upper-body lengths were less than 1 SD below the nonhandicapped mean, while lower-body lengths dropped to 3+ SDs below the mean by 13 to 15 years of age. The degree of growth deficit correlated with the level of the spinal cord lesion only up until 7 years, such that the higher the lesion, the greater the growth deficit (Duval-Beaupere et al., 1987). In addition, Rosenblum, Finegold, and Charney (1983) found that 65% of their 99 patients with myelomeningocele had an armspan greater than the length predicted from their total body heights. This difference was more prevalent in children with higher-level damage. Finally, the degree of growth deficits in children with myelomeningocele was similar to that found in children with paraplegia caused by spinal-cord injury (Duval-Beaupere, Lougovoy, Trocellier, & Lacert, 1983).

Children with cerebral palsy due to hypoxia at birth appear to have deficits both in height and width measurements. Pryor and Thelander (1967) observed that height was about even with the mean for nonhandicapped children up to 2 years of age and then gradually decreased to about 2 SDs below the mean around 13 to 15 years. This pattern was similar for width measures in boys, but the width measures for girls were quite normal until about 10 years, when they rapidly matched the deficit shown in boys. For children with neurological deficits or minimal brain dysfunction, no growth deviations were found (Pryor & Thelander, 1967). Also, no differences in height or weight were shown in hyperactive boys, although they had significantly less fat and a significantly lower body mass index (kg/m^2) than their nonhandicapped peers (McGee, Birkbeck, & Silva, 1985).

Children who are mentally retarded, but who are not afflicted with Down's Syndrome, are significantly shorter than nonhandicapped children of the same age (Dobbins, Garron & Rarick, 1981; Kugel & Mohr, 1963; Mosier, Grossman, & Dingman, 1965; Rarick, Dobbins & Broadhead, 1976). Mosier and his co-workers collected anthropomorphic measurements from 2,472 institutionalized mentally retarded persons and reported that, from 2 years of age to adulthood, mean standing heights were about 1 SD below normal means. A similar pattern emerged for weight and width measures, with little differences between males and females. They also found a positive correlation between growth measures and IQ. Moreover, the data presented by Kugel and Mohr (1963) supported the hypothesis that the degree of physical retardation is related to the cause of mental retardation.

Rarick and his associates (Dobbins et al., 1981; Rarick et al., 1976) reported that mildly mentally retarded children were significantly shorter than their normal peers (about 0.2-0.3 SDs less), but not significantly different in weight. This greater amount of weight per unit of height in the children who were mentally retarded was accounted for by significantly higher fat skinfolds (about 1.0-2.0 SDs higher) and significantly greater width measurements (about 0.2-0.8 SDs wider).

Extrinsic Disorders

A child may have normal potential for growth, but growth may be impeded by an "extrinsic" factor, such as a nutritional or systemic disorder. In this category of growth deviations, if the extrinsic factor is removed, "catch-up" growth may occur and a normal pattern of growth may be attained. These extrinsic disorders can exist in isolation or may interact with other handicapping conditions.

Chronic malnutrition is the most prevalent and preventable cause of short stature (Rallison, 1986). Malnutrition may be related to economic hardship, social adversity, or gastrointestinal disease. When nutrition reaches an adequate level, catch-up growth usually occurs, although it is limited in time to normal periods of growth (Stoch & Smythe, 1976). In addition, shortened stature may occur as an outcome of negative psychosocial environments, which also may involve inadequate nutrition (Rallison, 1986). An example of this is "deprivation dwarfism," a syndrome characterized by extreme short stature, a voracious appetite, and a significant delay in sexual maturation (Silver & Finkelstein, 1967). This condition has been observed in children who have experienced emotional and psychological deprivation.

Disorders of almost any of the organ systems of the body may adversely affect physical growth in children (Rallison, 1986). Mehrizi and Drash (1962) reported that out of 890 children with a variety of congenital heart lesions, 27% fell below the 3rd percentile and over 50% were below the 16th percentile in height and weight. However, the correction of heart defects has been shown to be followed by catch-up growth (Suoninen, 1971). Decreased growth also may exist with obstructive lung disease, although it may be difficult to determine whether the decreased growth is produced by too little caloric intake, too much caloric output, or hypoxia (Rallison, 1986). In a longitudinal study of children with asthma, Kaplan, Brush, and Mascie-Taylor (1987) found that asthmatic children weighed less and had lower body mass indexes at 11 years than normal same-aged peers. However, these differences did not exist at 7 years and disappeared by 16 years.

Most children with renal disease exhibit reduced height; more over, short stature may be the initial reason for evaluating renal functioning (Rallison, 1986). Potter and Greifer (1978) summarized data from several studies and found that the heights of children with various types of kidney disease fell below the 3rd percentile from 36 to 67% of the time, with the height deficit being greatest in those children with congenital kidney disease.

Endocrine disorders may cause growth to be less than or greater than normal (Rallison, 1986). Reduced growth may be a product of hypothyroidism, hypopituitarism, isolated growth hormone deficiency, somatomedin deficiency, or excess cortisol production (Cushing's syndrome). On the other hand, excessive growth may be caused by pituitary gigantism (acromegaly), hyperthyroidism, or excess adrenal androgens.

Movement Performance and Growth Deviations in Persons who are Handicapped

Many handicapped children have some type of growth deviation which may put them at a disadvantage in terms of moving effectively and efficiently within their environment. Indeed, a deficit in growth may be the critical feature in some handicapping conditions, such as achondroplasia, Morquio syndrome, Turner's syndrome, or malnutrition. However, there has been very little research that has investigated the relationship between morphological deviations and motor performance. Notable exceptions to this general void are studies by Rarick and his colleagues focusing on the motor performance of mildly mentally retarded children (Dobbins et al., 1981; Rarick et al., 1976) and a study by Malina and Buschang (1985) investigating the effect of shortened stature due to malnutrition on motor performance.

Dobbins et al. (1981) compared 6- to 9-year-old mildly mentally retarded (mean IQ = 67) and nonhandicapped boys in terms of 12 motor performance measures and 7 anthropomorphic measures. They found that the boys who were mentally handicapped performed significantly poorer on all motor performance items (0.3-1.3 SDs below the normal mean) and were significantly shorter (0.3 SD below), fatter (1.0-2.1 SDs above), and wider at the pelvic region (0.7 SD above). They did not differ from their nonhandicapped peers in weight or biacromial width. However, when the effect of the anthropometric variables was statistically partialled out by using a multivariate covariate analysis, the significant differences on 5 out of the 12 performance measures disappeared. The 7 items for which significant differences remained (tire run, scramble, standing broad jump, vertical jump, softball throw, and right and left grip strength), in general, were more complex and required a higher degree of coordination than the other 5 items (35- and 150-yd dash, knee flexion and extension strength, and sit-ups). Thus, when differences in physical constraints were controlled for, the differences in motor performance between mentally retarded and nonhandicapped boys were markedly reduced, particularly in tasks requiring low degrees of coordination.

The project carried out by Rarick et al. (1976) involved six groups of subjects: (a) 6- to 9-year-old mildly retarded boys and girls, (b) 10- to 13-year-old mildly retarded boys and girls, and (c) 6- to 9-year-old nonhandicapped boys and girls. The anthropometric differences between the young retarded children and the nonhandicapped children (matched by chronological age) were similar to those found by Dobbins et al. (1981). The retarded children were significantly shorter (0.2 SDs below the normal mean) and fatter (0.8-2.2 SDs above), but were not significantly different in weight. On the motor performance tasks, the young mentally retarded children were significantly poorer ($p < .01$) than their same-aged peers in 10 out of 12 strength and endurance items, in 10 out of 11 muscular power and gross-body coordination items, and in all 12 fine visual-motor coordination and balance items.

Factor analyses carried out by Rarick and his colleagues indicated that the constraints imposed by body size on motor performance was similar for all groups of boys, but not for the three groups of girls. The 48 individual anthropometric and motor performance items reduced to five to seven basic factors, with one of the factors for all groups being termed "fat or dead weight." Another factor, termed "strength-power-body size," was found to be included in the factor set for all groups, but the "body size" component of this factor was missing for the two groups of mentally retarded girls. Thus, the important influence of body size on simple strength tasks in mildly mentally retarded boys that was reported by Dobbins et al. (1981) was confirmed, while the effect of body size on motor performance in mildly mentally retarded girls appeared to be low. The reason for this gender difference was unclear.

Finally, the relationship between body size and motor performance of undernourished children in Oaxaca, Mexico was determined by Malina and Buschang (1985). When compared against children of the same age from Philadelphia, these 6- to 15-year-old Zapotec children were shorter and lighter and had poorer scores in grip strength, the 35-yard dash, the standing broad jump, and the softball throw-for-distance. When differences in height and weight were controlled for by comparing the performances of children in the two groups with the same heights and weights, differences in the broad jump, and the dash (boys) were minimized at younger ages and in grip strength at all ages. However, the Zapotec children performed below the expectations based on body size at older ages in the dash (after 9 years for boys and all ages for girls) and the broad jump (after 12 years). When height and weight were equal, the Zapotec children threw the softball farther than the Philadelphia children at all ages. Thus, diminished body size caused by malnutrition negatively influenced strength, running, jumping, and throwing, even though the second-order partial correlations between height and motor performance (with age and weight held constant) and between weight and motor performance (with age and height held constant) were generally low (ranging from .13 to .39).

From this limited sample of mentally handicapped and undernourished children, the importance of intrinsic physical constraints on movement performance in handicapped children tentatively has been established. Further, the relative influence of physical constraints on the performance of movement activities in the handicapped children appeared to be quite similar to that found in nonhandicapped children, at least for the mildly mentally retarded boys and the Zapotec boys and girls.

Implications for Practitioners

In this chapter, we have sought to demonstrate that physical constraints interact directly with motor skill development. In fact, it might be argued that such constraints are singularly the most important component when studying the development of coordination, control, and performance. Associated directly with physical constraints is the notion of geometric similarity, the assumption that all linear dimensions of the body are proportional in children of all sizes. These proportions change dramatically from conception through the first several years of life but, during the elementary-school years, become less variable across age (Robins, Brody, Hogan, Jackson, & Greene, 1928). The concepts of physical constraints and geometric similarity are important not only in the study of growth and development in normal individuals, but also is an important consideration for practitioners working with disabled individuals.

Asmussen and Heeboll-Nielsen (1955) sought to describe the geometric relationships between one specific linear dimension (total body height) and such parameters as length of legs, total surface area, respiratory area of the lungs, cross-section areas of blood vessels and muscles, and even motor performance scores. The general hypothesis was that linear measures, areas, volumes, and performance scores could be expressed as some power function of the total body height. For example, strength should increase by height to the second power since strength is proportional to the cross-sectional area of the relevant muscle(s). The results for a group of preadolescent boys indicated that the hypothesized power functions accurately predicted a wide variety of anthropomorphic, energy expenditure, and strength measures. However, there are several confounds in the type of research, including the experience and maturation of the nervous system.

Similarly, McMahon and Bonner (1983) used allometry to examine the effect of the scaling-up of body size on speed and characteristic activities of a wide variety of animals. Their findings illustrate that the size of an animal influences not only its location in the environment, but also the characteristics of its mating and food-gathering behaviours. The effect of size and the associated problems of gravity, and the effects of scale are important considerations that determine modes of locomotion, speed of locomotion, and the relationship between body mass and metabolism in all animals. Further, there is convincing evidence that physical constraints, particularly size, are important predictors of both life style and life expectancy.

The work by Asmussen and Heeboll-Nielsen (1955) and McMahon and Bonner (1983) suggest that height should be accounted for when planning movement programs for all children, whether normal or disabled. While there exists discrepancies in the predictability of movement performance on the basis of body size, it is nevertheless important for the practitioner to record the percentile rating (or other relative value) for each individual's height, particularly for those individuals who score near critical values (e.g., specified values for program entry) on standardized motor assessment tests. When evaluating the motor status of an individual, physical and biological characteristics of the individual, along with chronological age should be considered when determining the program needs of all children.

An individual who is considered to be "exceptional" on the basis of scoring 1.5 SDs above or below the mean on a motor assessment test, such as the Bruininks-Oseretsky Test of Motor Proficiency (Bruininks, 1978), may actually be "average," when all factors are taken into consideration. The practitioner should be reminded that motor test scores alone are insufficient for determining the programmatic needs of either nonhandicapped and handicapped persons. Subtle variations in body morphology beyond some critical point may result in the emergence of some abnormal motor behaviours. A motor behaviour that appears outside an accepted range of normality may in fact be the most adaptive behaviour for that particular individual given the particular constraints of the performer and the environment.

The environment itself, in the terminology of Gibson (1979), affords a variety of movement opportunities which the individual directly comprehends. Recent research indicate that adults are able to accurately perceive their own capacity for action and limits of action in relation to present environment constraints (Mark & Vogele, 1987; Warren, 1984; Warren & Whang, 1987). Thus, the practitioner must carefully observe specific motor behaviours in light of variations across individuals in physical parameters, chronological age, experience in the particular activity, and the exact environmental context.

Manipulation of Physical Constraints to Improve Movement Performance in Handicapped Persons

In some situations, intrinsic physical constraints may be modified or changed to improve movement performance in persons with particular handicapping conditions. For example, orthotics and prosthetics--which have come to mean "an addition to" and "a replacement of," respectively--have been used since ancient times to improve mobility and performance (Meyer, 1974). Orthotics and prosthetics may be designed to match the normal structural constraints of the body or to modify structural constraints to produce more functional behaviour. This latter design principle is exemplified by ankle-foot orthoses prescribed for persons with paresis, spasticity, and/or muscle imbalance. The normal range of inversion-eversion may be restricted to produce greater mediolateral stability; a plantar-flexion stop may be used to allow the toe to clear the ground during the swing phase; a dorsiflexion stop may be included to simulate normal gastrocnemius and soleus function (Lehmann, 1979).

A properly-designed ankle-foot orthosis has been demonstrated to significantly improve the locomotor performance of patients with hemiparesis. Corcoran, Jebsen, Brengelmann, and Simons (1970) observed that hemiparetic patients without orthoses had a markedly higher oxygen consumption than normal persons locomoting at the same speeds. However, with a standard double-upright orthosis, they found that their range of ambulation speeds doubled, their "comfortable" speed occurred at a higher velocity, and their oxygen consumption was slightly reduced. With a similar group of patients, Lehmann, Condon, Price, and deLateur (1987) also showed that the use of an ankle-foot orthosis significantly increased walking speed and that the speed was dependent on the amount of plantarflexion allowed.

Other manipulations of intrinsic physical constraints to improve the movement performance of handicapped persons include adding weights to the limbs to reduce tremor in patients with a variety of pathologies (Chase, Cullen, Sullivan, & Ommaya, 1965; Morgan, 1975; Morgan, Hewer, & Cooper, 1975) and restraining one limb to reduce athetoid movements in persons with cerebral palsy (Nwaobi, 1987). Morgan (1975), for example, reported that when an optimal weight was attached to an ataxic limb, 20 out of 31 patients showed a significant reduction of incoordination. Further, weights placed on the lower limbs and waist produced some improvement in the gait of 11 out of 14 patients and even allowed one severely disabled patient to walk independently, which previously he was unable to do. An explanation based simply on the increase of inertia in the system (which would dampen tremor) appears to be inadequate since there were optimum placements and optimum amounts of weights for improving coordination that varied considerably for different patients.

In a single-case study, Nwaobi (1987) found that the voluntary control of the dominant arm in an 8-year-old boy with athetoid cerebral palsy improved when the contralateral arm was restrained close to the trunk. In a task involving 10 repetitions of touching a switch at the midline of the body from a starting position at the side of the body (requiring shoulder adduction and abduction), electromyographic activity in the deltoids markedly decreased in both limbs and performance time was 27% faster when the restraint was applied, compared to the no-restraint condition. Although some of the strategies described in these studies are still in an experimental stage, they provide examples of how the movement functioning of child with various handicapping conditions might be improved through the manipulation of their intrinsic physical constraints.

Summary

It has only been in the recent past that researchers and theoreticians have begun to recognize the importance of physical constraints on movement skill development and movement performance in children. This chapter provided not only a historical view of the status of physical constraints in the study of normal motor development, but extended some of the contemporary ideas related to this issue to the movement skill and performance potential and limits of persons with selected handicapping conditions. A better understanding of how physical constraints can affect movement behaviour, particularly in persons who are handicapped, can lead to more accurate assessment of motor functioning, more effective movement education programming, and insight into how physical constraints might be manipulated to improve movement functioning.

Author Notes

1. Send request for reprints to Allen W. Burton, School of Physical Education and Recreation, University of Minnesota, Minneapolis, Minnesota, USA, 55455.

References

Asmussen, E. & Heeboll-Nielsen, K. (1955). A dimensional analysis of physical performance and growth in boys. *Journal of Applied Physiology, 7,* 593-603.

Bayley, N., & Davis, F. C. (1935). Growth changes in bodily size and proportions during the first three years: A developmental study of sixty-one children by repeated measurements. *Biometrika, 27,* 26-87.

Beunen, G., Claessens, A., Ostyn, M., Renson, R., Simons, J., & Van Gerven, D. (1985). Motor performance as related to somatotype in adolescent boys. In R. A. Binkhorst, H. C. G. Kemper, & W. H. M. Saris (Eds.), *Children and exercise XI* (pp. 279-284). Champaign, IL: Human Kinetics.

Bruininks, R. H. (1978). *Bruininks-Oseretsky Test of Motor Proficiency.* Circle Pines, MN: American Guidance Service.

Bruner, J. S., & Bruner, B. M. (1968). On voluntary action in the hierarchical structure. *International Journal of Psychology, 3,* 239-255.

Chase, R. A., Cullen, J. K., Sullivan, S. A., & Ommaya, A. K. (1965). Modification of intention tremor in man. *Nature, 206,* 485-487.

Connolly, K. (1970). Skill development: Problems and plans. In K. Connolly (Ed.), *Mechanisms of motor skill development* (pp. 3-16). London: Academic Press.

Connolly, K. (1973). Factors influencing the learning of manual skills by young children. In R. A. Hinde & J. Stevenson-Hinde (Eds.), *Constraints on learning* (pp. 337-363). New York, NY: Academic Press.

Corcoran, P. J., Jebsen, R. H., Brengelmann, G. L., & Simons, B. C. (1970). Effects of plastic and metal leg braces on speed and energy cost of hemiparetic ambulation. *Archives of Physical Medicine and Rehabilitation, 51,* 69-77.

Dobbins, D. A., Garron, R., & Rarick, G. L. (1981). The motor performance of educable mentally retarded and intellectually normal boys after covariate control for differences in body size. *Research Quarterly for Exercise and Sport, 52,* 1-8.

Duval-Beaupere, G., Kaci, M., Lougovoy, J., Caponi, M. F., & Touzeau, C. (1987). Growth of trunk and legs of children with myelomeningocele. *Developmental Medicine and Child Neurology, 29,* 225-231.

Duval-Beaupere, G., Lougovoy, J., Trocellier, L., & Lacert, P. (1983). Trunk and leg growth in children with paraplegia caused by spinal cord injury. *Paraplegia, 21,* 339-350.

Gibson, J. J. (1979). *The ecological approach to visual perception.* Boston, MA: Houghton-Mifflin.

Halverson, L. E. (1966). Development of motor patterns in young children. *Quest, 6,* 44-53.

Hoshi, H., Ashizawa, K., & Ikeda, Y. (1979). Secular trend in growth in infants with Down's syndrome. *Human Biology, 51,* 289-297.

Ikeda, Y., Higurashi, M., Hirayama, M., Ishikawa, N., & Hoshina, H. (1977). A longitudinal study on the growth of stature, lower limb and upper limb length in Japanese children with Down's syndrome. *Journal of Mental Deficiency Research, 21,* 139-151.

Kaplan, B. A., Brush, G., & Mascie-Taylor, C. G. N. (1987). The relationship of childhood asthma and wheezy bronchitis with height, weight and body mass index. *Human Biology, 59,* 921-931.

Kugel, R. B., & Mohr, J. (1963-64). Mental retardation and physical growth. *American Journal of Mental Deficiency, 68,* 41-48.

Kugler, P. N. (1986). A morphological perspective on the origin and evolution of movement patterns. In M. G. Wade & H. T. A. Whiting (Eds.), *Motor development in children: Aspects of coordination and control* (pp. 459-520). Dordrecht: Martinus Nijhoff.

Kugler, P. N., Kelso, J. A. S., & Turvey, M. T. (1980). On the concept of coordinative structures as dissipative structures: I. Theoretical line. In G. E. Stelmach & J. Requin (Eds.), *Tutorials in motor behavior* (pp. 3-47). Amsterdam: North-Holland.

Kugler, P. N., Kelso, J. A. S., & Turvey, M. T. (1982) On the control and co-ordination of naturally developing systems. In J. A. S. Kelso & J. E. Clark (Eds.), *The development of movement control and co-ordination* (pp. 5-78). New York, NY: John Wiley & Sons.

Lehmann, J. F. (1979). Biomechanics of ankle-foot orthoses: Prescription and design. *Archives of Physical Medicine and Rehabilitation, 60,* 200-207.

Lehmann, J. F., Condon, S. M., Price, R., & deLateur, B. J. (1987). Gait abnormalities in hemiplegia: Their correction by ankle-foot orthoses. *Archives of Physical Medicine and Rehabilitation, 68,* 763-771.

Malina, R.M. (1975). Anthropometric correlates of strength and motor performance. *Exercise and Sport Sciences Reviews, 3,* 249-274.

Malina, R. M., & Buschang, P. H. (1985). Growth, strength and motor performance of Zapotec children, Oaxaca, Mexico. *Human Biology, 57,* 163-181.

Mark, L. S., & Vogele, D. (1987). A biodynamic basis for perceived categories of action: A study of sitting and stair climbing. *Journal of Motor Behavior, 19,* 367-384.

McGee, R., Birkbeck, J., & Silva, P. A. (1985). Physical development of hyperactive boys. *Developmental Medicine and Child Neurology, 27,* 364-368.

McMahon, T. A., & Bonner, J. T. (1983). *On size and life.* New York, NY: Scientific American Library.

Mehrizi, A., & Drash, A. (1962). Growth disturbance in congenital heart disease. *Journal of Pediatrics, 61,* 418-429.

Meyer, P. R. (1974). Lower limb orthotics. *Clinical Orthopaedics and Related Research, 102,* 58-71.

Morgan, M. H. (1975). Ataxia and weights. *Physiotherapy, 61,* 332-334.

Morgan, M. H., Hewer, R. L., & Cooper, R. (1975). Application of an objective method of assessing intention tremor - a further study on the use of weights to reduce intention tremor. *Journal of Neurology, Neurosurgery, and Psychiatry, 38,* 259-264.

Mosier, H. D., Jr., Grossman, H. J., & Dingman, H. F. (1965). Physical growth in mental defectives: A study in an institutionalized population. *Pediatrics, 36,* 465-519.

Newell, K. M. (1986). Constraints on the development of coordination. In M. G. Wade & H. T. A. Whiting (Eds.), *Motor development in children: Aspects of coordination and control* (pp. 341-360). Dordrecht: Martinus Nijhoff.

Norval, M. A. (1947). Relationship of weight and length of infants at birth to the age at which they begin to walk alone. *Journal of Pediatrics, 30,* 676-678.

Nwaobi, O. M. (1987). Nondominant arm restraint and dominant arm function in a child with athetoid cerebral palsy: Electromyographic and functional evaluation. *Archives of Physical Medicine and Rehabilitation, 68,* 837-839.

Potter, D. E., & Greifer, I. (1978). Statural growth of children with renal disease. *Kidney International, 14,* 334-339.

Pryor, H. B., & Thelander, H. E. (1967). Growth deviations in handicapped children: An anthropometric study. *Clinical Pediatrics, 6,* 501-512.

Rallison, M. L. (1986). *Growth disorders in infants, children, and adolescents.* New York, NY: John Wiley & Sons.

Rarick, G. L., Dobbins, D. A., & Broadhead, G. D. (1976). *The motor domain and its correlates in educationally handicapped children.* Englewood Cliffs, NJ: Prentice-Hall.

Rarick, G. L., & Oyster, N. (1964). Physical maturity, muscular strength, and motor performance of young school-age boys. *Research Quarterly, 35,* 523-531.

Rarick, G. L., & Seefeldt, V. (1974). Observations from longitudinal data on growth in stature and sitting height of children with Down's syndrome. *Journal of Mental Deficiency Research, 18,* 63-78.

Robins, W. J., Brody, S., Hogan, A. G., Jackson, C. M., & Greene, C. W. (1928). *Growth.* New Haven, CT: Yale University Press.

Rosenblum, M. F., Finegold, D. N., & Charney, E. B. (1983). Assessment of stature of children with myelomeningocele, and usefulness of arm-span measurement. *Developmental Medicine and Child Neurology, 25,* 338-342.

Seils, L. G. (1951). The relationship between measures of physical growth and gross motor performance of primary-grade children. *Research Quarterly, 22,* 244-260.

Silver, H. K., & Finkelstein, M. (1967). Deprivation dwarfism. *Journal of Pediatrics, 70,* 317-324.

Stoch, M. B., & Smythe, P. M. (1976). A 15-year developmental study of effects of severe undernutrition during infancy on subsequent physical growth and intellectual functioning. *Archives of Disease in Childhood, 51,* 327-336.

Suoninen, P. (1971). Physical growth of children with congenital heart disease: Pre- and post-operative study of 355 cases. *Acta Paediatrica Scandinavica, Supplement 225,* 1-50.

Szabo, T., Szmodis, I., Meszaros, J., & Pinter, A. (1984). Somatotype, growth, and motor performance in 10-year-old girls taking part in elevated level physical education at school. In J. Ilmarinen & I. Valimaki (Eds.), *Children and sport: Paediatric work physiology* (pp. 37-41). Berlin: Springer-Verlag.

Thelen, E., Fisher, D. M., & Ridley-Johnson, R. (1984). The relationship between physical growth and a newborn reflex. *Infant Behavior and Development, 7,* 479-493.

Wade, M. G. (1976). Developmental motor learning. *Exercise and Sport Sciences Reviews, 4,* 375-394.

Warren, W. H., Jr. (1984). Perceiving affordances: Visual guidance of stair climbing. *Journal of Experimental Psychology: Human Perception and Performance, 10,* 683-703.

Warren, W. H., Jr., & Whang, S. (1987). Visual guidance through apertures: Body-scaled information for affordances. *Journal of Experimental Psychology: Human Perception and Performance, 13,* 371-383.

Wickstrom, R. L. (1970). *Fundamental motor patterns.* Philadelphia, PA: Lea & Febiger.

Problems in Movement Control
G. Reid (editor)

A PROBLEM SOLVING APPROACH TO MOVEMENT SKILL ACQUISITION: IMPLICATIONS FOR SPECIAL POPULATIONS

M. Bouffard
Department of Physical Education and Sport Studies
University of Alberta

and

A. E. Wall
Department of Physical Education
McGill University

To cope efficiently in numerous movement situations people must have appropriate movement competencies. Handicapped persons are usually less competent than their nonhandicapped peers in movement situations (Bruininks, 1974; Rarick, 1973; Watkinson & Wall, 1982). Consequently, handicapped persons have more frequent problems of adaptation in movement situations than their nonhandicapped peers. It is often more difficult for them to successfully cope with environmental problems.

The acquisition of movement skills has been viewed as depending upon problem solving processes by many theorists of movement skill acquisition (e.g., see Bernstein, 1967; Bruner, 1973; Fitts & Posner, 1967; Gentile, 1972; Newell, 1978; Newell & Barclay, 1982; Requin, Semjen & Bonnet, 1984; Wall, 1986; Wall, McClements, Bouffard, Findlay, & Taylor, 1985). In other words, movement situations often contain problems that must be solved. The interplay of the performer and the environment creates a problem to be solved by a movement task (Keogh & Sugden, 1985). The availability and use of appropriate resources will determine, to a large extent, the degree of adaptation of the person to the environment.

Research on movement skill development has focused mainly on two different levels of analysis: (a) the movement level and, (b) the action level. Newell (1978) makes the following distinctions between movement and action:

> Movements generally refer to the motion of the body and limbs produced as a consequence of the spatial and temporal pattern of muscular contractions. Body movement can also occur, however, independently of the performer's efforts through the creation of an imbalance of forces acting externally on the body. Regardless of the cause of movement, the spatial and temporal pattern can be described rather precisely through kinematics. In contrast, space and time are not usually relevant criteria for actions. Rather, actions are identified by the goal to which are directed (e.g., open the door, lift the weight, etc.) or by specifying certain criteria to which the performer complies in what he does (e.g., walking, hopping, etc.). As a consequence, a variety of potential movements may be *generated* to complete any one act (Bernstein, 1967), and by the same token, a variety of movements may be *identified* as a particular act. (p. 42)

The number of possible solutions to movement problems is limited by a number of factors. Intelligence or the capacity to solve problems is always a product of the interaction between genetic and environmental factors (Zigler & Cascione, 1984). Our genetic inheritance determines a range of potential outcomes (Lerner, 1986), and the observed phenotype depends upon the particular environmental experiences of each person (Bouchard & Malina, 1983; Hirsch, 1970; Lerner, 1986). Hirsch (1970) called this the norm-of-reaction concept: "The same genotype can give rise to a wide array of phenotype depending upon the environment in which it develops" (p. 73). In other words, heredity sets the upper and lower limits for the development of our phenotypes; but environmental experiences play a central role in determining our characteristics within this range (Lerner, 1986).

Further, as noted by Arend (1980), the boundaries of adaptability are limited by morphological, biomechanical, and environmental factors. Arend (1980) and Wall et al. (1985) noted that an important aspect of movement skill development is the acquisition of knowledge about these factors which may be used to control the neuromotor system in relation to the desired goal.

In this paper, we will focus on the problem solving processes involved before, during and after the execution of action in movement situations. As noted by Requin et al. (1984), when the regulation of movement activities are viewed from a problem solving perspective, "it becomes possible to consider movement activities in a broader perspective of active and adaptive exchanges between an organism and its environment. Such exchanges result not only in a transformation of the environment, but also (and in some cases mainly) in the transformation of the organism, since it acquires, in the course of its activity, a better and more reliable knowledge of the surrounding world as well as of its own possibilities" (pp. 490-491). In turn, this knowledge provides the means for new adaptations in the environment.

This review will be limited to the execution of action by handicapped persons; a particular emphasis will be given to mildly mentally handicapped individuals in movement situations. Studies related to the execution of action by mentally retarded persons in movement situations are relatively lacking. To our knowledge, no studies deal with ecologically valid movement tasks; tasks that are most likely to appear relevant to mentally handicapped people.

In the following section, the key steps involved during the problem solving process are outlined. Factors responsible for the inferior performance of developmentally delayed people on problem solving tasks will be discussed thereafter. Implications of this view for future research will then be presented.

Characteristics of the Problem Solving Process

The problem solving process can be partitioned into a number of inter-related steps occurring before, during, or after the execution of action. These steps include the identification of the problem, the definition of representation of the problem, the construction of an appropriate plan that would guide plan execution and finally, the evaluation of one's progress toward the goal (Bransford, 1984; Pea, 1982).

Problem Identification

Problem identification or problem finding is often the first step toward problem solution. Problems must be identified; otherwise, solutions are unlikely to be proposed (Bransford, 1984).

Problem Representation

To generate an appropriate problem representation, the performer must know what the initial state actually is. That is, the problem solver should have information about the pre-response state of the musculature (Schmidt, 1975) and, as well, encode relevant perceptual and/or contextual information. Without it, the performer most likely cannot generate appropriate inferences about what actions are possible. Further, the problem solver must understand the goal state or "what by means of his activity, the situation must become" (Bernstein, 1967, p. 148), note the difference between the initial state and the goal state, and know and understand the constraints on planning (Pea, 1982).

An accurate representation of the problem is essential to the planning process; without it, an appropriate solution cannot be found. For example, if a person playing table-tennis does not understand where he or she should return the ball (goal state), does not note his or her position in relation to the ball (initial state), does not consider the difference between the initial conditions and the desired goal, does not know that the ball must be returned, with the racket, according to the rules of table-tennis (constraints on planning), then the possibility of finding a solution to the movement problem seems impossible.

Plan Construction

This step is essential to eliminate the differences between what the movement situation actually is and what it must become (Bernstein, 1967). When an appropriate representation of the problem has been created, the planner can ask whether a method for solving the problem is known (Polya, 1945). This may economize plan construction. If no plan appears to be available, then the person will have to explore alternative approaches to solve the problem.

Pea (1982) argues that the notion of a strict hierarchical, top-down, process view of planning has met with disfavour during recent years. His view of plan construction is represented by the following points: (a) The formulation of an effective plan requires plan simulation in which alternative plans can be evaluated by the planner. (b) Simulating a plan is a complex process which requires knowledge about effects of a plan (foresight) once it is executed. (c) During plan simulation or plan execution one may be required to redefine the initial goal state according to the feedback received. (d) Plan construction is an iterative process that includes a sequential cycling of initial proposal, simulation, evaluations and revisions until a suitable plan emerges that will reach the intended goal state. (e) Plan construction is an iterative multi-decision process that requires decisions ranging from the abstract to the concrete level.

Plan Execution

Plan execution may range from easy to difficult. Moving a chess piece from position A to B is usually an easy task. However, in many movement situations the time constraints (e.g., returning a spike in volleyball) or the complexity of the movement sequence (e.g., gymnastic sequence) is so great that plan execution is frequently a difficult matter. Moreover, although a plan can be correctly executed, the performer may fail to solve the movement problem because he or she has selected the wrong plan (Schmidt, 1982, 1988). Finally, plan execution may be difficult or impossible in certain cases of movement disorders (e.g., cerebral palsy, apraxia).

Evaluation of Progress

Progress evaluation can occur during all of the above stages, as well as after the plan has been executed. Learners must look back and evaluate the effect of their own activities. As Wessells (1982) noted, the problem solver must:

> Evaluate one's progress toward the goal. This requires making decisions about whether the problem has been solved, whether progress toward the goal has occurred, and whether the current strategy [plan] should be executed further of should be abandoned. These decisions are no doubt tied closely to the type of strategy [plan] that has been chosen. (pp. 323-324)

Although all five steps are involved in problem solving, they are not necessarily executed in the strict linear order described above. The planning of a solution may lead to a better definition of the problem. A plan that is difficult or impossible to execute might be abandoned in favour of a more appropriate one; hence, the early steps of the problem solving process might be repeated a number of times (Wessells, 1982).

In summary, the problem solving process can be partitioned into a number of interrelated steps: problem identification, problem representation, plan construction and execution, and evaluation of progress. Failure at any of these steps may lead to inappropriate problem solution. We argue that for efficient movement adaptation to occur, the learner, often guided by an expert (e.g., parents, teacher, coach), must go through these different steps to learn appropriate movement skills.

Automatization can facilitate the emergence of more advanced competencies; it has some adaptive value. As noted by Brown (1987), "a great deal of the development that occurs with increasing expertise (age) is the result of processes that were originally controlled, effortful, and laborious becoming automated" (p. 81). As new capacity becomes available, more complex problems can be undertaken, more complex task analysis is possible, and former movement sequences can be organized into higher order units. Further, Campione, Brown, and Ferrara (1982) concluded that "there is sufficient work to invite the inference that in these areas of 'automatic' cognitive functioning, retarded persons differ from average learners, if at all, by such small amounts that the variations are trivial" (p. 402). When variations in the knowledge base of the person are taken into account, it appears that mentally handicapped and nonhandicapped perform comparably on tasks that try to assess the automatic, or passive, operations of the system.

Differences between handicapped and nonhandicapped are usually observed on effortful non-routine tasks that demand strategic control (problem solving tasks). These tasks are usually done slowly under deliberate conscious control

(Norman & Shallice, 1980, 1986). Adequate problem solutions depend on the availability and accessibility to appropriate knowledge, the use of appropriate control processes, and an adequate level of motivation. A discussion of these factors follows.

Inappropriate Problem Solutions by Developmentally Delayed

Inappropriate problem solution by developmentally delayed persons have been attributed to three major sources: (a) deficient knowledge base or lack of access to it, (b) lack of use or inappropriate use of control processes, and (c) motivational factors. Evidence for each of these positions will be presented.

The Knowledge Base

Numerous empirical studies have supported the conclusion that what a person knows determines, to a large extent, the problems that a person can solve (e.g., Chi, 1978; Chi & Koeske, 1983; Kirk, 1981; Siegler, 1983). As noted by Glaser (1988):

> The problem-solving difficulty of novices can, to a large extent, be attributed to the inadequacies of their knowledge bases, and not to limitations in their processing capabilities, such as the inability to use problem-solving heuristic. Novices show effective heuristic; however, the limitations of their thinking derive from their inability to infer further knowledge from the literal cues in the problem statement. By contrast, for experts these inferences are necessarily generated in the context of the knowledge structure they have already acquired. (pp. 24-25)

A useful heuristic distinction has been made between declarative knowledge and procedural knowledge. Declarative knowledge refers to factual information stored in memory, such as knowing about balls, knowing about bicycles, knowing about Newtonian mechanics (Bouffard, 1986; Chi, 1987; Wall, 1986). An important type of declarative knowledge has been labelled metacognitive knowledge. This "cluster is roughly concerned with a person's knowledge about his own cognitive resources and the compatibility between himself as a learner and the learning situation" (Brown, & Campione, 1981, p. 521).

Procedural knowledge is knowledge about how to do things. For example, knowing how to throw a ball, how to do addition, or to ride a bike, would be examples of procedural knowledge. Procedural knowledge includes skills, rules, algorithms, heuristic, procedures, and plans. Some procedural knowledge is "concerned primarily with self-regulatory mechanisms during an ongoing attempt to learn or solve problem" (Brown & Campione, 1981, p. 521). These cognitive activities have been referred to as "executive functions" or "metacognitive skills" (Brown & Campione, 1981; Wall et al., 1985).

Another cluster of procedural knowledge includes strategies. A strategy is a set of decisions that determines what sequences of action are needed to perform to ensure certain forms of outcome (Bruner, Goodnow, & Austin, 1956; Chi, 1978). Some strategies like planning, checking, monitoring, testing, revising, and evaluating are metacognitive skills. Some other strategies, like rehearsing and selective abstraction of the environment features, are not part of the metacognitive cluster.

The availability of knowledge, its organization as well as the quality of the representation of the problem are essential to problem solution (Siegler, 1983). Glaser (1984) contends that:

> The relationship between the structure of the knowledge base and problem solving process is mediated through the quality of the representation of the problem. We define a problem representation as a cognitive structure corresponding to a problem that is constructed by a solver on the basis of domain-related knowledge and its organization. At the initial stage of problem analysis the problem solver attempts to "understand" the problem by constructing an initial problem representation. The quality completeness and coherence of this internal representation determine the efficiency and accuracy of further thinking. And these characteristics of the problem representation are determined by the knowledge available to the problem solver and the way the knowledge is organized. (p. 98).

Knowledge accessibility

The knowledge base available in long-term memory constitutes the resources that the problem solver *might* be able to use in solving a problem. However, to solve movement problems, the relevant knowledge must be both available and accessible. A major problem for developmentally delayed children is that "available knowledge, either declarative or procedural, does not guarantee flexible access to and use of those resources" (Campione, 1987, p. 134). Accessibility to knowledge and skills is frequently essential to problem representation, plan construction and execution, and progress evaluation. "The important role that prior experience plays in comprehension and problem solving ultimately depends on the problem solver's ability to spontaneously access that knowledge at the appropriate time and apply it in a productive way to the new situation" (Stein, 1986, p. 432). Inaccessibility may seriously constrain or impair inferential processes (Holland, Holyoak, Nisbett, & Thagard, 1986).

According to Brown and her colleagues (Brown, 1982; Campione et al., 1982), a key characteristic of intelligent behaviour is the "ability to use flexibility and appropriately the information and skills available to the system" (Campione et al., 1982, p. 456). Based on the work of Pylyshyn (1978), they distinguish between two types of access: multiple and reflective. Multiple access refers to the ability to use information or knowledge flexibility under variable conditions. Reflective access refers to the "ability to 'mention as well as use' the components of the system" (Campione et al., 1982, p. 456).

The relative lack of multiple access to the products of learning by the mentally handicapped "is reported so often that 'welding' has been described as a characteristic feature of the learning of retarded children" (Brown & Campione, 1981, p. 522). The problem of multiple access appears to be central to strategy maintenance. In numerous memory studies it has been found that the performance of the mentally retarded will improve if appropriate strategies are taught (for review see Borkowski & Büchel, 1983; Campione, 1987). However, if they are not explicitly required to use the strategy taught, they frequently do not use it. Moreover, their spontaneous use of the instructed strategy (or some minor modification of it) to a new situation is frequently absent. This lack of transfer is more likely to occur if "explicit instruction in self-regulatory mechanisms is not provided. When training does include instruction in both the use and control of the desired skill(s), training attempts are successful" (Brown & Campione, 1981, p. 523).

The ability to consciously describe and discuss one's cognitive activities (reflective access) has been mainly studied through self-report techniques. Although some difficulties are associated with the use of these methods (Brown, 1987; Ericsson & Simon, 1984), a general conclusion is that immature learners are poorly informed about the working of their own information processing system (Campione et al., 1982; Wellman, 1985). Due to their frequent lack of awareness, developmentally delayed persons cannot identify that a problem exist. Consequently, they will not try to solve problems.

Metacognitive Knowledge and Skills

The term metacognition is certainly a fuzzy concept that has been controversial over the years (Brown, 1987; Brown & Campione, 1981; Flavell, 1987). However, theorists like Becker (1975) and Bobrow and Norman (1975), "have come to agree that an important requirement of any functioning system is that it include the *capacity for self-awareness, or accurate knowledge and understanding of its own weakness and properties* [emphasis added]" (Campione et al, 1982, p. 433).

Conscious metacognitive knowledge is believed to be central to an understanding of human flexibility.

> If the child is aware of what is needed to perform effectively then that child can take steps to meet demands of a learning situation more adequately. If, however, the child is not aware of his or her own limitations as a learner or of the complexity of the task at hand, then he or she can hardly be expected to take preventive actions in order to anticipate or recover from problems. (Campione et al., 1982, p. 433)

Brown (1977, 1978) suggested that efficient metacognitive control requires that learners: (a) analyze the problem at hand and characterize it in relation to the knowledge they have available, (b) reflect upon what one knows or does not know and how that may affect a solution, (c) recognize and predict their capacity limitations, (d) select and schedule suitable problem solving strategies, (e) monitor and control the operation of the strategies that are used, and (f) evaluate the success or failure of the entire problem solving operation in relation to the demands of the task.

Research done during the last decade has shown that such self-regulatory behaviour increases with age and experience (Campione, 1987; Flavell & Wellman, 1977; Kopp, 1982). A slower development rate of metacognitive skills has been found with mentally handicapped person (Borkowski & Büchel, 1983; Campione et al., 1982).

To our knowledge, no similar research has been completed in the cognitive-motor domain. Norman and Shallice's (1986) theory of action suggests, however, that the voluntary control an individual has over his or her own cognitive processes is certainly central to problem solving. This is not to say that metacognitive skills are the only factors involved during the problem solving process. The knowledge base, the availability of strategies, the accessibility of domain-specific knowledge, and motivation are also key factors.

Strategies

The relative lack of using spontaneous strategies to appropriately solve memory problems has been frequently demonstrated within the mentally retarded population (for a review see Campione, 1987; Reid, 1986). The relevance of strategies in cognitive-motor skill learning has also received support from experimental studies with nonhandicapped people (Gallagher & Thomas, 1984; Shea, 1977).

The relative lack of spontaneous use of strategies by the mentally retarded has been observed in short-term motor memory tasks (Reid, 1980a; Sugden, 1978). The inference of a rehearsal deficit in the memory processes of retarded persons does not suggest a structural limitation but a failure to employ control processes. This hypothesis has been supported by Reid (1980b) who found that a general strategy program helped in a short-term motor memory task.

In summary, numerous studies have shown that mentally retarded persons do not spontaneously use appropriate strategies to solve memory problems. When appropriate strategies are taught to these people, and they are required to use them, their performance is frequently better. Further, studies done on the use of strategies by mentally handicapped in movement situations are generally lacking.

Belmont and Butterfield (1977), however, argue that to determine the degree of success of any memory strategy training program it must be evaluated against three basic criteria of effectiveness: (a) performance must improve as the result of training, both in terms of accuracy and in terms of activities (strategies) used to effect this accuracy; (b) the effect of the training program must be durable; it is obviously desirable to show that what has been trained can be detected after a reasonable time period has elapsed; (c) training must result in generalization to a class of similar situations where the trained activity would be appropriate, for without evidence of breadth of transfer, the practical utility of any training program is doubtful.

Some evidence for maintenance exists in the literature. Recent studies have shown that extended training can result in durability of a trained behaviour over a period of months and even years (for a review see Campione, 1987). The tendency to maintain a trained behaviour appears to be related to developmental level as very young or retarded individuals are more likely to abandon the strategy than are more knowledgeable people.

The criterion of success that presents the most problem is generalization, or transfer to appropriate situations. Although there is some controversy over what constitutes a suitable transfer task, there is general agreement that flexible generalization to new situations has been lacking. Evidence for generalization was obtained by Brown, Campione, and Barclay (1979) in a study with educable mentally retarded children. One year following the original training with two memory strategies (anticipation and rehearsal) involving a self-checking component, the younger children showed no effect of the training, whereas the older group both maintained the trained strategies and generalized it effectively to a novel situation involving recall of gist prose passages.

To our knowledge, the only research program concerned with the generalizability of strategies in the cognitive-motor domain appears to be the preliminary work completed by Singer and his associates with non-handicapped persons (Brown, Singer, Cauraugh & Luciarello, 1985; Singer & Cauraugh, 1984, 1985; Singer, Cauraugh, Luciarello, & Brown, 1985; Singer & Suwanthada, 1986).

The limited evidence available now in the cognitive-motor domain suggests that appropriate strategies are, to some extent, generalizable across tasks. We are not aware of any similar studies completed with developmentally delayed people.

In general, strategy maintenance and, more specifically, generalization with the mentally retarded population has been obtained only when instructions are relatively complete (Brown, 1987; Campione, 1987). After reviewing the existing literature, Campione (1987) concluded that "teaching (older) retarded children self-checking routines in conjunction with memory strategies leads to impressive immediate training effects, extremely durable outcomes, and evidence for generalized applications of those training experiences" (p. 135).

In our view these successful programs have three complementary dimensions. First, an appropriate strategy is taught. Second, people are trained to use relevant metacognitive skills like checking, planning, monitoring, testing, revising, and evaluating. Third, they give the immature learner more information about the working of their own mind. This can lead to the development of a more comprehensive theory about the functioning of their own information processing system. The restructuring of such personal theories of the mind is possibly central to strategy generalization.

Lifestyle and Self-Regulation

It is well documented that the lifestyle of mentally retarded people is frequently different from that of their non-retarded peers (for a review see Watkinson & Wall, 1982). They are frequently listless and inactive: most of their leisure activities are passive and solitary in nature (Cheseldine & Jeffree, 1981; Watkinson & Wall, 1982). Unfortunately this lifestyle is likely to lead to an impoverished coping repertoire.

First, due to the relative lack of active and adaptive exchanges with the environment, the performer may not acquire knowledge relevant to the solutions of movement problems. Second, a solitary lifestyle may impair the development of problem solving skills. Vygotsky (1978) argued a great deal of learning occurs in social settings in which a child interact with experts in a problem solving situation. It is through interpersonal contacts that the child learn to solve problems. To Vygotsky (1978), "learning awakens a variety of developmental processes that are able to operate only when the child is interacting with people in his environment and in cooperation with his peers. Once these processes are internalized, they become part of the child's independent developmental achievement" (p. 90). Parents, teachers, peers, groups, and others may function as "mediators in the learning process, acting as promoters of self-regulation by nurturing the emergence of personal planning as they gradually cede their own direction" (Brown, Bransford, Ferrara, & Campione, 1983, p. 123).

Briefly, according to Vygotsky (1978), self-regulation emerges through the interaction of people with other expert people in their environment. Consequently, the relative social isolation of developmentally delayed people may impair the process of internalization that foster self-regulation.

Motivation and Practice

Practice, either physical or mental, is essential to the solution of movement problems. Although practice alone does not make perfect, it is one of the most important movement-skill learning variables (Sage, 1984; Schmidt, 1988). Many hours of practice are usually necessary, but not sufficient, for skilled performance. Lack of practice by the mentally retarded could be related to such motivational factors as learned helplessness, lack of movement confidence and minimal personal relevance of the task.

In a recent model of the development of movement competence and confidence, Griffin and Keogh (1981, 1982) stressed the importance of success experiences in movement situations. It is these experiences that lead to movement confidence. In their view, movement confidence is a product of a complex "cognitive evaluation of self in relation to task demands" (Griffin & Keogh, 1982, p. 214). Moreover, movement confidence influences the decision of "whether to become involved or not ... how the individual will do, ... [and] whether to continue involvement now and in the future" (Griffin & Keogh, 1982, p. 214). Confident persons are more likely to seek and choose participation than non-confident persons for which it is "less likely that participation performance and behaviour will be satisfying" (Griffin & Keogh, 1982, p. 214).

Although we are not aware of any empirical study having tested Griffin and Keogh's theory with mentally retarded persons, it seems highly plausible that these persons usually lack movement confidence. In general, the proficiency of mildly and moderately mentally retarded people in prerequisite movement skills is considerably below that of their non-retarded peers (Watkinson & Wall, 1982). This lack of prerequisite skills should, according to Griffin and Keogh, directly affect movement confidence. Evidence supporting this viewpoint comes from the studies based on attribution theory. Gibson (1980), using a pursuit rotor task found that mildly mentally handicapped adolescents attributed their success to luck and their failure to ability much more frequently than their non-retarded peers. This perception of lack of ability is likely part of the complex cognitive evaluation leading to movement confidence and, hence participation choice, performance, and persistence in movement situation. "With an impoverished coping repertoire, he [the mentally retarded] is prone to experience failure (punishment) and thus, is likely to develop little trust in his own resources. In turn, he looks to the external environment for support" (Siegel, 1979, p. 31).

Lacking trust in their own capabilities, mentally retarded people may consequently develop the belief that their own efforts are ineffective. Consequently, they may refuse to become involved in new experiences that might alter their own personal theory. Without testing their beliefs, they would remain in a stable state of helplessness (Chapman & Skinner, 1985).

In an attempt to alter the belief that effort is useless, some researchers have developed attribution retraining procedures (see Vallerand & Reid, this book). These programs teach people to attribute failure to insufficient effort, thereby increasing the probability of task persistence when failure occurs (Andrew & Debus, 1978; Gibson, 1980; Schunk, 1981). Although attribution retraining studies have had considerable success, the assumption that effort alone will improve performance and modify personal theories is certainly questionable. Bandura (1977) has suggested that if the individual does not possess the necessary resources for coping with the task, then continued exhortation to try harder may even serve to increase helplessness. Certainly, this type of attribution retraining should be used with care.

Briefly, motivation and the personal theories that the mentally retarded have about themselves are essential to an understanding of the problem solving behaviour of the mentally handicapped person. Personal theories about self and lack of motivation may lead to a failure to retrieve or access relevant knowledge, use appropriate strategies, or use metacognitive skills available and, hence, impair all the steps necessary to solve a problem (Dweck, 1986; Kurtz & Borkowski, 1984).

Future Directions

An important humanistic goal would be to develop better movement skill acquisition programs for developmentally delayed persons. A desirable goal of these programs would be to obtain spontaneous generalization of the trained skill; that is, the learner should apply what they have learned to novel but related problems (Campione, 1987). If appropriate generalization is obtained, then better coping skills have been acquired.

Most likely, generalization will not occur spontaneously; it will have to be prepared. Generalization programs will have numerous components. Brown and Campione (1986) proposed eight guidelines for promoting flexible use of trained skills (for details see their paper). Some of these guidelines are: (a) do a detailed task analysis of both the training and the transfer domain, (b) know the knowledge and skills acquired by your learner, (c) train people to use self-checking routines, (d) train in multiple contexts to finesse the welding problem, (e) provide feedback concerning the effectiveness of the trained skill, (f) provide direct instruction in generalization, and (g) gradually guide the novice to greater levels of participation. It should be underscored that the less mature the learner is, the more complete the training program will have to be.

The effectiveness of these programmes should be evaluated against the criterion of effectiveness outlined by Belmont and Butterfield (1977). First, improvement in performance must be demonstrated. If this step is successful, then maintenance should be studied for, without maintenance, generalization is unlikely to occur. Maintenance from a few weeks to months should be studied. It is to be expected that the more advanced the developmental level of the person, the more likely the person will spontaneously maintain the trained behaviour if this behaviour is congruent with the subject's personal "theory of mind" (Wellman, 1983, p. 36). On the other hand, less developmentally advanced will more likely require specific instruction into self-regulatory skills (Campione, 1987). The most challenging and most important criterion is certainly generalization or transfer of the trained behaviour to other situations. If no generalization is obtained, the obtained effects, although theoretically interesting, will remain of dubious practical significance (Campione, 1987).

The task selected for instruction and transfer will have to be carefully analyzed. Early in skill acquisition, the performer is frequently overloaded (Schmidt, 1988). Teaching the use of strategies at the same time may be useless. Further, in tasks that are relatively brief in duration (e.g., hitting a ball) the possibility of using the deliberate conscious control system during movement execution is almost impossible. As noted by Norman (1986), control by the deliberate conscious control system is relatively slow and serial, and, therefore, is not very effective for some kind of skills required in movement situations. In this case, deliberate conscious control will be involved before and after the plan execution stage.

Classical group studies methodologies are likely to be inappropriate to evaluate the effectiveness of training studies. Available evidences collected with non-handicapped subjects indicate that they frequently use diverse strategies to solve a problem (Newell, 1973; Siegler, 1987). They also use different strategies for different tasks. Further, subjects seem to use a variety of strategies within tasks (Siegler, 1987).

The above finding has methodological implications. First, averaging data over subjects is likely to be inappropriate. It is only when the subjects in a group consistently use a single strategy over an entire experiment that averaging results over subjects is appropriate (Lewin, 1933; Siegler, 1987). Although the above point was made earlier (Lewin, 1933; Newell, 1973), this practice continues to be extremely common (Siegler, 1987). It is worth reemphasizing the inadequacies of this data analysis strategy. Second, averaging over trials for the same subject could be misleading. A knowledge of the strategies actually used by the subject during each trial is essential. Evidences for this point was provided by Siegler (1987) who showed that a data analysis procedure taking into account the strategy used by the subject and averaging data generated by different strategies can lead to different inferences.

If knowledge of the strategies used by the subject is essential to appropriately analyze the results of problem solving studies, how do we know which strategies were used by the subject? "In many situations, simply asking people immediately after each response how they generated their answers may be the best way to separate data produced by different strategies" (Siegler, 1987, pp. 260-261). Although verbal reports have often been criticized (e.g., see Nisbett & Wilson, 1977), the validity of inferences based upon them can be adequate when the subject is not forced to make inferences. Ericsson and Simon (1984) advocated the use of retrospective report. They argued that immediately after the task is completed, while much information is still in short-term memory, subjects often can accurately retrieve considerable episodic information. This is particularly true when episodes are neither too brief nor too long in duration.

Inappropriately used, verbal reports can convey seriously misleading information about what people are doing (Nisbett & Wilson, 1977; Siegler, 1987). This could be particularly true with special populations when the subject cannot give a coherent account of what he or she did during the immediately preceding response.

Although some methods are better than others for answering a research question, none of them is perfect. This is why converging evidences should also be collected using different methodologies. As noted by Cook and Campbell (1979):

> Naive social quantifiers continue to overlook the presumptive, qualitatively judgmental nature of *all* science. ... scientist must continually judge whether a given rival hypothesis will explain the data. Qualitative contextual information (as well as quantitative evidence on tangential variables) has long been recognized as relevant to such judgments. (p. 93)

Researchers should recognize that all our methodological tools are imperfect. It is through converging evidences that plausible inferences could be made.

Summary and Conclusion

To cope efficiently in movement situations people must frequently solve movement problems. For the purpose of this presentation, the problem solving process has been partitioned into five interrelated steps: problem identification; problem representation, plan construction, plan execution, and evaluation of progress. Failure at any of these steps can seriously impair the problem solving process.

The quality of the observed solution is a function of the availability and accessibility of knowledge stored in long-term memory as well as the encoding of relevant information available in the surrounding environment (Holland et al., 1986; Siegler, 1983). Problem representation, plan construction and execution, as well as evaluation of progress are guided by this information. As noted by Glaser (1984), the quality, completeness and coherence of the problem representation is "determined by the knowledge available to the problem solver and the way the knowledge is organized" (p. 98). When an accurate problem representation has been obtained, then the problem solver may search among action plans already available; if none of them appears to be appropriate, inferential processes should be used to develop a more appropriate one. Further, during the plan construction phase available knowledge may be used to infer (anticipate) what is likely to happen if this plan is executed; this may lead to a restructuring of the action plan before plan execution. When the constructed plan seems appropriate, it should then be differentiated into the details necessary for movement (plan) execution. During or after plan execution, evaluation of progress should be conducted. At this stage, the problem solver may discover that the plan is unworkable. This may be due to unanticipated consequences of action or to factors beyond the planners purview (Pea, 1982). The discovery of plan-intrinsic flaws may lead to a better problem representation, plan construction and execution, as well as a new evaluation of progress. This iterative process can be continued forever until an optimal solution to the movement problem is found.

Metacognitive skills like planning, checking, monitoring, testing, revising, and evaluating are involved before, during or after the execution of action. The solution of movement problems is heavily dependent upon the quality of these metacognitive skills. These skills could be acquired through inferential processes (Holland et al., 1986), under adult guidance, or in collaboration with more developmentally advanced peers (Vygotsky, 1978).

The relative lack of practice and social isolation of developmentally delayed persons can only impair the acquisition restructuring and tuning of knowledge (Norman, 1982) used for inferential purposes during the problem solving process.

Studies based on attribution theory (Dweck, 1986; Gibson, 1980) and movement confidence and competence (Griffin & Keogh, 1981, 1982) underscore the driving role of personal beliefs, its influence upon participation, and its effect upon the acquisition, restructuring, and tuning of existing knowledge (Norman, 1982).

A useful avenue of research, from both a theoretical and practical standpoint, is the use of training studies. Training studies should be evaluated against three basic criteria: (a) performance must improve, (b) maintenance of the trained behaviour, and (c) generalization of the behaviour to appropriate situations. Training studies will most likely require a careful analysis of each subject covert behaviour. Further, the use of multiple methods is advocated.

Author Notes

1. We would like to thank Dr. Peter R.E. Crocker for his comments on an earlier draft of this manuscript.

2. Reprint requests should be addressed to Marcel Bouffard, Department of Physical Education and Sport Studies, The University of Alberta, Edmonton, Alberta, Canada, T6G 2H9.

References

Andrew, G. R., & Debus, R. L. (1978). Persistence and the causal perception of failure: Modifying cognitive attributions. *Journal of Educational Psychology, 70,* 154-166.

Arend, S. (1980). Developing the substrates of skillful movement. *Motor skills: Theory into practice, 4,* 3-10.

Bandura, A. (1977). Self-efficacy: Toward a unifying theory of behavioral change. *Psychological Review, 84,* 191-215.

Becker, J. D. (1975). Reflections on the formal description of behaviour. In D. G. Bobrow & A. Collins (Eds.), *Representation and understanding: Studies in cognitive science* (pp. 83-102). New York, NY: Academic Press.

Belmont, J. M., & Butterfield, E. C. (1977). The instructional approach to developmental cognitive research. In R. V. Kail & J. W. Hagen (Eds.), *Perspectives on the development of memory and cognition* (pp. 437-481). Hillsdale, NJ: Lawrence Erlbaum.

Bernstein, N. (1967). *The co-ordination and regulation of movement.* London: Permagon Press.

Bloom, B. S. (Ed.). (1985). *Developing talent in young people.* New York, NY: Ballantine.

Bobrow, D. G., & Norman, D. A. (1975). Some principles of memory schemata. In D. G. Bobrow & A. Collins (Eds.), *Representation and understanding: Studies in cognitive science* (pp. 131-149). New York, NY: Academic Press.

Borkowski, J. G., & Büchel, F. P. (1983). Learning and memory strategies in the mentally retarded. In M. Pressley & J. R. Levin (Eds.), *Cognitive strategy research* (pp. 103-128). New York, NY: Springer-Verlag.

Bouchard, C., & Malina, R. M. (1983). Genetics for the sport scientist: Selected methodological considerations. *Exercise and Sport Sciences Reviews, 11,* 275-305.

Bouffard, M. (1986). *Knowledge, anticipation, and the solution of movement problems by mentally retarded adolescents.* Unpublished doctoral dissertation, The University of Alberta, Edmonton.

Bransford, J. D. (1984). *The ideal problem solver.* New York, NY: Freeman.

Brown, A. L. (1977). Development, schooling, and the acquisition of knowledge. In R. C. Anderson, R. J. Spiro, & W. E. Montague (Eds.), *Schooling and the acquisition of knowledge* (pp. 241-253). Hillsdale, NJ: Lawrence Erlbaum.

Brown, A. L. (1978). Knowing when, where, and how to remember: A problem of metacognition. In R. Glaser (Ed.), *Advances in instructional psychology* (pp. 77-165). Hillsdale, NJ: Lawrence Erlbaum.

Brown, A. L. (1982). Learning and development: The problems of compatibility, access and induction. *Human Development, 25,* 89-115.

Brown, A. L. (1987). Metacognition, executive control, self-regulation, and other more mysterious mechanisms. In F. E. Weinert & R. H. Kluwe (Eds.), *Metacognition, motivation, and understanding* (pp. 65-116). Hillsdale, NJ: Lawrence Erlbaum.

Brown, A. L., Bransford, J. D., Ferrara, R. A., & Campione, J. C. (1983). Learning, remembering, and understanding. In P. H. Mussen (Ed.), *Handbook of child psychology: Vol. 3. Cognitive development* (pp. 77-166). New York, NY: John Wiley & Sons.

Brown, A. L., & Campione, J. C. (1981). Inducing flexible thinking: A problem of access. In M. Friedman, J. P. Das, & N. O'Connor (Eds.), *Intelligence and learning* (pp. 515-529). New York, NY: Plenum Press.

Brown, A. L., & Campione, J. C. (1986). Training for transfer: Guidelines for promoting flexible use of trained skills. In M. G. Wade (Ed.), *Motor skill acquisition of the mentally handicapped: Issues in research and training* (pp. 257-271). Amsterdam: North-Holland.

Brown, A. L., Campione, J. C., & Barclay, C. R. (1979). Training self-checking routines for estimating test readiness: Generalization from list learning to prose recall. *Child Development, 50,* 501-512.

Brown, H. J., Singer, R. N., Cauraugh, J. H., & Luciarello, G. (1985). Cognitive style and learner strategy interaction in the performance of primary and related maze tasks. *Research Quarterly for Exercise and Sport, 56,* 10-14.

Bruininks, R. H. (1974). Physical and motor development of retarded persons. In N. R. Ellis (Ed.), *International review of research in mental retardation Vol. 7,* (pp. 209-261). New York, NY: Academic Press.

Bruner, J. S. (1973). Organization of early skilled action. *Child Development, 44,* 1-11.

Bruner, J. S., Goodnow, J. J., & Austin, G. A. (1956). *A study of thinking.* New York, NY: John Wiley & Sons.

Campione, J. C. (1987). Metacognitive components of instructional research with problem learners. In F. E. Weinert & R. H. Kluwe (Eds.), *Metacognition, motivation, and understanding* (pp. 117-140). Hillsdale, NJ: Lawrence Erlbaum.

Campione, J. C., Brown, A. L., & Ferrara, R. A. (1982). Mental retardation and intelligence. In R. J. Sternberg (Ed.), *Handbook of human intelligence* (pp. 392-490). Cambridge, MA: Cambridge University Press.

Chapman, M., & Skinner, E. A. (1985). Action in development - development in action. In M. Frese & J. Sabini (Eds.), *Goal directed behaviour: The concept of action in psychology* (pp. 200-213). Hillsdale, NJ: Lawrence Erlbaum.

Cheseldine, S. E., & Jeffree, D. M. (1981). Mentally handicapped adolescents: Their use of leisure. *Journal of Mental Deficiency Research, 25,* 48-59.

Chi, M. T. H. (1978). Knowledge structures and memory development. In R. S. Siegler (Ed.), *Children's thinking: What develops?* (pp. 73-96). Hillsdale, NJ: Lawrence Erlbaum.

Chi, M. T. H. (1987). Representing knowledge and metaknowledge: Implications for interpreting metamemory research. In F. E. Weinert & R. H. Kluwe (Eds.), *Metacognition, motivation, and understanding* (pp. 239-266). Hillsdale, NJ: Lawrence Erlbaum.

Chi, M. T. H., & Koeske, R. D. (1983). Network representation of a child's dinosaur knowledge. *Developmental Psychology, 19,* 29-39.

Cook, T. D., & Campbell, D. T. (1979). *Quasi-experimentation: Design & analysis issues for field settings.* Chicago, IL: Rand McNally.

Dweck, C. S. (1986). Motivational processes affecting learning. *American Psychologist, 41,* 1040-1048.

Ericsson, K. A., & Simon, H. A. (1984). *Protocol analysis: Verbal reports as data.* Cambridge, MA: MIT Press.

Fitts, P. M., & Posner, M. I. (1967). *Human performance.* Belmont, CA: Brooks/Cole.

Flavell, J. H. (1987). Speculations about the nature and development of metacognition. In F. E. Weinert & R. H. Kluwe (Eds.), *Metacognition, motivation, and understanding* (pp. 21-29). Hillsdale, NJ: Lawrence Erlbaum.

Flavell, J. H., & Wellman, H. M. (1977). The development of basic memory processes. In R. V. Kail & J. W. Hagen (Eds.), *Perspectives on the development of memory and cognition* (pp. 3-33). Hillsdale, NJ: Lawrence Erlbaum.

Gallagher, J. D., & Thomas, J. D. (1984). Rehearsal strategy effects on developmental differences for recall of a movement series. *Research Quarterly for Exercise and Sport, 55,* 123-128.

Gentile, A. M. (1972). A working model of skill acquisition with application to teaching. *Quest, 17,* 3-23.

Gibson, B. J. (1980). *An attributional analysis of performance outcomes and the alleviation of learned helplessness on motor performance tasks: A comparative study of educable mentally retarded and non-retarded boys.* Unpublished doctoral dissertation, University of Alberta, Edmonton.

Glaser, R. (1984). Education and thinking: The role of knowledge. *American Psychologist, 39,* 93-104.

Glaser, R. (1988). Cognitive science and education. *International Social Science Journal, 115,* 21-44.

Griffin, N. S., & Keogh, J. F. (1981). Movement confidence and effective movement behaviour in adapted physical education. *Motor skills: Theory into practice, 5,* 23-35.

Griffin, N. S., & Keogh, J. F. (1982). A model for movement confidence. In J. A. S. Kelso & J. E. Clark (Eds.), *The development of movement control and co-ordination* (pp. 213-236). New York, NY: John Wiley & Sons.

Hirsch, J. (1970). Behaviour-genetic analysis and its biosocial consequences. *Seminar in Psychiatry, 2,* 89-105.

Holland, J. H., Holyoak, K. J., Nisbett, R. E., & Thagard, P. R. (1986). *Induction: Processes of inference, learning, and discovery.* Cambridge, MA: MIT Press.

Keogh, J., & Sugden, D. (1985). *Movement skill development.* New York, NY: Macmillan.

Kirk, U. (1981). The development and use of rules in the acquisition of perceptual motor skill. *Child Development, 52,* 299-305.

Kopp, C. B. (1982). Antecedents of self-regulation: A developmental perspective. *Developmental Psychology, 18,* 199-214.

Kurtz, B. E., & Borkowski, J. G. (1984). Children's metacognition: Exploring relations among knowledge, process, and motivational variables. *Journal of Experimental Child Psychology, 37,* 335-354.

Lerner, R. M. (1986). *Concepts and theories of human development* (2nd ed.). New York, NY: Random House.

Lewin, K. (1933). Vectors, cognitive processes and Mr. Tolman's criticism. *Journal of General Psychology, 8,* 318-345.

Newell, A. (1973). You can't play 20-questions with nature and win: Projective comments on the papers of the Symposium. In W. G. Chase (Ed.), *Visual information processing* (pp. 463-526). New York, NY: Academic Press.

Newell, K. M. (1978). Some issues on action plans. In G. E. Stelmach (Ed.), *Information processing in motor control and learning* (pp. 41-54). New York, NY: Academic Press.

Newell, K. M., & Barclay, C. R. (1982). Developing knowledge about action. In J. A. S. Kelso & J. E. Clark (Eds.), *The development of movement control and co-ordination* (pp. 175-212). New York, NY: John Wiley & Sons.

Nisbett, R. E., & Wilson, T. D. (1977). Telling more than we can know: Verbal reports on mental processes. *Psychological Review, 84,* 231-259.

Norman, D. A. (1982). *Learning and memory.* San Francisco, CA: Freeman.

Norman, D. A. (1986). Reflections on cognition and parallel distributed processing. In J. L. McClelland, D. E. Rumelhart, & the PDP Research Group. *Parallel distributed processing: Explorations in the microstructure of cognition. Vol. 2. Psychological and biological models* (pp. 531-546). Cambridge, MA: MIT Press.

Norman, D. A., & Shallice, T. (1980). *Attention to action: Willed and automatic control of behaviour.* (Tech. Rep.). San Diego, CA: University of California, Center for Human Information Processing.

Norman, D. A., & Shallice, T. (1986). Attention to action: Willed and automatic control of behaviour. In R. J. Davidson, G. E. Schwartz, & D. Shapiro (Eds.), *Consciousness and self-regulation: Advances in research and theory, Vol. 4,* (pp. 1-18). New York, NY: Plenum Press.

Pea, R. D. (1982). What is planning development the development of? In D. Forbes & M. T. Greenberg (Eds.), *New directions for child development: Children's planning strategies* (No. 18, pp. 5-27). San Francisco, CA: Jossey-Bass.

Polya, G. (1945). *How to solve it.* New York, NY: Doubleday.

Pylyshyn, Z. W. (1978). When is attribution of beliefs justified? *The Behavioral and Brain Sciences, 1,* 593.

Rarick, G. L. (1973). Motor performance of mentally retarded children. In G. L. Rarick (Ed.), *Physical activity: Human growth and development*. New York, NY: Academic Press.

Reid, G. (1980a). Overt and covert rehearsal in short-term motor memory of mentally retarded and nonretarded persons. *American Journal of Mental Deficiency, 85*, 69-77.

Reid, G. (1980b). The effect of memory strategy instruction in the short-term motor memory of the mentally retarded. *Journal of Motor Behaviour, 12*, 221-227.

Reid, G. (1986). The trainability of motor processing strategies with developmentally delayed performers. In H. T. A. Whiting & M. G. Wade (Eds.), *Themes in motor development* (pp. 93-107). Dordrecht: Martinus Nijhoff.

Requin, J., Semjen, A., & Bonnet, M. (1984). Bernstein's purposeful brain. In. H. T. A. Whiting (Ed.), *Human motor actions: Bernstein reassessed* (pp. 467-504). New York, NY: North-Holland.

Sage, G. H. (1984). *Motor learning and control: A neuropsychological approach*. Dubuque, IA: Wm. C. Brown.

Schmidt, R. A. (1975). A schema theory of discrete motor skill learning. *Psychological Review, 82*, 225-260.

Schmidt, R. A. (1982). The schema concept. In J. A. S. Kelso (Ed.), *Human motor behaviour: An introduction* (pp. 219-235). Hillsdale, NJ: Lawrence Erlbaum.

Schmidt, R. A. (1988). *Motor control and learning: A behavioral emphasis* (2nd ed.). Champaign, IL: Human Kinetics.

Schunk, D. H. (1981). Modeling and attributional effects on children's achievement: A self-efficacy analysis. *Journal of Educational Psychology, 73*, 93-105.

Shea, J. B. (1977). Effects of labeling on motor short-term memory. *Journal of Experimental Psychology: Human Learning and Memory, 3*, 92-99.

Siegel, P. S. (1979). Incentive motivation and the mentally retarded person. In N. R. Ellis (Ed.), *Handbook of mental deficiency, psychological theory and research* (2nd ed., pp. 1-61). Hillsdale, NJ: Lawrence Erlbaum.

Siegler, R. S. (1983). How knowledge influences learning. *American Scientist, 71,* 631-638.

Siegler, R. S. (1987). The perils of averaging data over strategies: An example from children's addition. *Journal of Experimental Psychology: General, 116,* 250-264.

Singer, R. N., & Cauraugh, J. H. (1984). The generalization of psychomotor learning strategies to related psychomotor tasks. *Human Learning, 3,* 215-225.

Singer, R. N., & Cauraugh, J. H. (1985). The generalizability effect of learning strategies for categories of psychomotor skills. *Quest, 37,* 103-119.

Singer, R. N., Cauraugh, J. H., Luciarello, G., & Brown, H. J. (1985). Achievement in related psychomotor tasks as influenced by learning strategies. *Perceptual and Motor Skills, 60,* 843-846.

Singer, R. N., & Suwanthada, S. (1986). The generalizability effectiveness of a learning strategy on achievement in related closed motor skills. *Research Quarterly for Exercise and Sport, 57,* 205-214.

Stein, B. S. (1986). Constraints on spontaneous transfer in problem-solving tasks. *Memory and cognition, 14,* 432-441.

Sugden, D. A. (1978). Visual motor short term memory in educationally subnormal boys. *British Journal of Educational Psychology, 48,* 330-339.

Vygotsky, L. S. (1978). *Mind in society: The development of higher psychological processes.* Cambridge, MA: Harvard University Press.

Wall, A. E. (1986). A knowledge-based approach to motor skill acquisition. In M. G. Wade & H. T. A. Whiting (Eds.), *Motor development in children: Aspects of coordination and control* (pp. 33-49). Dordrecht: Martinus Nijhoff.

Wall, A. E., McClements, J. D., Bouffard, M., Findlay, M. A., & Taylor, M. J. (1985). A knowledge-based approach to motor development: Implications for the physically awkward. *Adapted Physical Activity Quarterly, 2,* 21-42.

Watkinson, E. J., & Wall, A. E. (1982). *The PREP play program: Play skill instruction for mentally handicapped children.* Ottawa: Canadian Association for Health Physical Education and Recreation.

Wellman, H. M. (1983). Metamemory revisited. In. M. T. H. Chi (Ed.), *Trends in memory development* (pp. 31-51). New York, NY: Karger.

Wellman, H. M. (1985). The origins of metacognition. In D. L. Forrest -Pressley, G. E. MacKinnon, & T. G. Waller (Eds.), *Metacognition, cognition, and human performance: Vol 1. Theoretical perspectives.* Orlando, FL: Academic Press.

Wessells, M. G. (1982). *Cognitive psychology.* New York, NY: Harper & Row.

Zigler, E., & Cascione, R. (1984). Mental retardation: An overview. In E. S. Gollin (Ed.), *Malformations of development: Biological and psychological sources and consequences* (pp. 69-94). New York, NY: Academic Press.

Problems in Movement Control
G. Reid (editor)

EMPLOYMENT OF INDIVIDUALS WITH DEVELOPMENTAL DISABILITIES

Phillip D. Tomporowski
Alys M. Hayden
Department of Psychology
University of Alabama

The goals of human engineering are to both "fit the task to the man," thereby maximizing efficiency levels and minimizing error, and to "fit the man to the task" by selecting and training operators for optimal efficiency and identifying subtolerent efficiency levels (Craig, 1984). Considerable efforts have been made by researchers during the past 40 years to understand factors related to efficient job performance and successful employment of workers who fall within the normal ranges of physical and mental capabilities. More recently, there has been an increased interest in understanding factors related to successful employment of workers with physical handicaps (see Erekson & Rotatori, 1986) and with developmental disabilities (Rowitz, 1986; Rusch, 1986). Some of the reasons underlying the interest in employment of developmentally disabled individuals are voiced in terms of humanitarianism (Wolfensberger, 1967), social priorities (Bellamy et al., 1984), or economics (Mithaug, 1979; Weisgerber, Dahl & Appleby, 1981).

A recent symposium on employment for individuals with mental handicaps considered the prognosis for success of programs designed to prepare people with developmental disabilities for the work place (Rowitz, 1986). Several important issues were raised and recommendations were voiced. Of immediate concern was the fact that an estimated 250,000 to 300,000 special education students ages 18 to 25 graduate each year from the public school system and an additional 6,000 individuals with developmental disabilities leave public institutions for community placement (Stark & Kiernan, 1986). The prognosis for successful employment of the majority of these individuals over the next decade is poor. Several factors impede employment of individuals with developmental disabilities. First, individuals with developmental disabilities face growing competition for available jobs. The skill level of adults entering the labour force in the United States has been declining gradually over the past decade and it is predicted to worsen in the next decade (Stark & Kiernan, 1986). Secondly, many middle-income workers now perform lower paying, service-based jobs traditionally targeted for persons with developmental disabilities because of a decline in available jobs in the manufacturing sector (Ferguson & Ferguson, 1986). For the general population, not only will competition for jobs increase but there will be fewer jobs available. This problem is compounded for workers with developmental disabilities. Studies that have evaluated job performance and reasons for job separation in disabled populations have noted that the greatest number of separations were due to lack of motivation, slow work, low quality work, and the need for too much supervision (Hill, Wehman, Hill & Goodall, 1986).

Despite pessimistic economic and employability forecasts, a solution was proposed to the problems faced in preparing individuals with developmental disabilities. The recommendation was to acquire, through research, a better understanding of the factors that contribute to the successful employment of adults with developmental disabilities. The focus of this chapter will be: (a) to review several theoretical approaches to the evaluation of job performance and employment issues and (b) to survey data obtained from theory-driven research conducted to assess work performance and employment of individuals with developmental disabilities. Theory and research will be evaluated with a view toward understanding the worker-job interface; i.e., the "fit" between *job demands* and *worker characteristics*.

Theories of Human Performance and Their Relation to Employment Issues

The study of human movement and the skillful execution of acts has intrigued researchers for many years. Numerous theories have been proposed over the past three decades to explain the basic properties of movement. These theories differ in their level of abstraction; some are essentially descriptive and tend to be inductive in nature while others involve hypothetical processes and are deductive. In addition,some emphasize applied issues while others relate more to basic issues of human performance. Both applied and basic theories of human performance have had an impact on, or have the potential to influence, research conducted with individuals with developmental disabilities.

One approach that has influenced research on employment issues is derived from the broad area of learning theory and applied technology. The *behaviour-analysis approach* is characterized by objective analyses of environmental determinants of behaviour. The focus is placed upon behaviours that can be developed through contingencies of reinforcement (Kazdin, 1975; Rusch & Schutz, 1979). Job performance is viewed as a series of behaviourial responses that can be taught to a worker. Through the objective analysis of task demands and the development of reliable training programs, a worker can acquire the skills necessary to meet job demands (Wehman & McLaughlin, 1980). The behaviourial-analysis approach is oriented toward engineering the performance of the individual. Training programs are developed specifically to teach individuals the skills needed to perform work at a criterion level. Skill development reflects the acquisition of basic motor responses which are then chained together in a hierarchical fashion to form complex responses. Crucial to the acquisition of responses is the systematic application of the principles of behaviour modification.

An alternative theoretical approach to evaluating employment and job analyses issues has been taken by researchers who categorize tasks in terms of the basic abilities required of workers to perform various jobs. Rather than stressing highly detailed individual task analysis techniques, the focus of the *taxonomic approach* is to identify general task dimensions which are applicable to various jobs. Fleishman and his colleagues (1972, 1975, 1978, 1982) have provided perhaps the most comprehensive attempts to describe and interrelate characteristics of tasks and worker ability level. Fleishman's system brings together concepts from experimental psychology, human factors technology, and task analysis. Central to his work has been the development of a task taxonomy which, in Fleishman's view, provides an integrative framework and a common language that is applicable to both applied and basic research activities. The taxonomy categorizes tasks and basic abilities on the basis of experimental and factor analytic methods. Assessment is carried out in the psychometric tradition, i.e., subjects perform numerous tests that are believed to be related to a particular task. The patterns of responses made by subjects on these test batteries are evaluated and basic abilities are identified on the basis of statistical analyses. A considerable amount of data has been gathered by Fleishman which suggests that the taxonomic approach provides a viable method for selecting workers for specific jobs.

A third approach to evaluating employment issues is derived from *cognitive theories* of motor behaviour. This approach is oriented toward the measurement of basic mental operations which govern skilled movement (Schmidt, 1982). Mental operations are viewed to differ from general aptitudes such as spatial ability or sensory-motor ability, as measured by researchers following the taxonomic approach. General aptitudes are based upon aggregate measures whereas mental operations are viewed as elementary processes that underlie performance across a wide range of tasks. Mental operations themselves are not observable acts; rather, they are either actions performed by the mind or the mental instructions for actions (Carr, 1984). The worker is viewed as an operator functioning as an information processor and whose behaviour is hypothesized to be the end product of a series of computer-like stages of mental activity. The operator responds to environmental conditions through a stimulus identification component, evaluates environmental conditions through a response-selection component, and selects an act on the basis of a response programming component. Cognitive theories of motor behaviour attempt to explain observed changes in behaviour. For example, the movement of novice workers is characterized by stiff, jerky, inefficient acts; with practice, however, the novice's performance becomes a well-coordinated chain of sensory, perceptual, cognitive, and motor mechanisms. Further, as skill levels increase, the amount of attention required of the worker to complete the task lessens and the acts become more automatic in nature. Observing systematic changes in patterns of motor movement and timing ability has led to the development of several stage-type theories of information processing.

In summary, employment-related research has been guided by three theory-driven approaches. The behaviour-analysis approach focuses on applied issues and addresses topics directly related to the employment of workers with developmental disabilities. The taxonomic approach uses psychometric techniques to identify factors which interrelate worker abilities and task demands. The taxonomic system is seen as a way of addressing both applied and basic research issues. It can be used for selecting and placing workers on the basis of how well their abilities "fit" job demands. It also can be used to interpret and predict human performance, in general. The cognitive theory approach focuses on basic research issues and addresses topics related to understanding the processes which underlie motor movement, learning, and skilled performance.

Research Activities Related to Employment Issues

Competitive employment for workers with developmental disabilities has been identified as a goal that can be achieved through training and by changing the attitudes and expectancies of employers (Rusch, 1986). Several studies have identified factors related to successful employment of workers with developmental disabilities (Brickey, Browning & Campbell, 1982; Brickey, Campbell & Browning, 1985; Greenspan & Shoultz, 1981; Greenspan, Shoultz & Weir, 1981; Hill & Wehman, 1979; Kiernan & Ciborowski, 1986; Kochany & Keller, 1981). Two themes dominate these studies. The successful worker is an individual who: (a) possesses the skills necessary to perform the job and (b) is able to cope with the social dynamics inherent in the workplace. For the employer, job productivity and cohesiveness among workers and supervisory staff is essential (Mithaug, 1979). The developmentally disabled worker must be able to acquire job-related skills and to generalize and maintain those skills as work conditions change. Several surveys have revealed that termination of employees who were mentally handicapped was related to slow work performance and an inability to modify behaviours to meet changes in work routines (Hill et al., 1986; Sali & Amir, 1971). Surveys have revealed that employment success is also related to a workers abilities to adjust to the social demands placed upon them by co-workers and supervisors (Cheney & Foss, 1984; Foss & Peterson, 1981; Hill & Wehman, 1979; Hollender, 1974; Salzberg, Likins, McConaughy & Lignugaris/Kraft, 1986).

The approaches which have been taken by various researchers to study issues of task performance and interpersonal relations reflect different theoretical orientations. These approaches and representative research they have generated are reviewed in the following sections.

The Applied Behaviourial Analysis Approach

The view taken by some researchers is that traditional, standardized vocational evaluation techniques are not valid predictors of work potential (Menchetti, Rusch & Owens, 1983). Job performance is neither necessarily related to intelligence nor general traits but, rather, to sets of behaviours which can be taught (Wehman & McLaughlin, 1980). With systematic training techniques and adequate environmental control, many developmentally disabled persons can be taught to perform work at levels which will make them competitive for jobs. It may take longer for some individuals to learn specific skills, but it is assumed there are few manual-type tasks that cannot be trained (Gold, 1972, 1975; Revell, Kriloff & Sarkees, 1980). A second assumption is that the social skills necessary for successful employment can be acquired by developmentally disabled workers through the use of behaviour modification techniques. Wehman and McLaughlin (1980) provide numerous examples for promoting work proficiency in developmentally disabled persons by using a behaviourial approach.

Developmentally disabled individuals can acquire motor behaviour if task demands are assessed and the responses required to perform the task are divided into discrete units which can be chained together in a sequence (Kazdin, 1975). The topography of job-related behaviours has been altered in developmentally disabled persons by using such techniques as verbal instruction paired with modelling correct movement (Bellamy, Peterson & Close, 1975) and stimulus enhancement and cue redundancy (Gold, 1972, 1974). People with poor motor coordination because of cerebral palsy or who display sensory-motor deficits such as spasticity or athetosis may require a prosthesis or a specially arranged instructional environment; however, Wehman and McLaughlin (1980) and others following the behaviourial-analysis approach posit that such physical handicaps can be overcome through systematic training and that most individuals, regardless of the etiology of their disability, can acquire complex work skills.

Once movement patterns are mastered, the next training goal is to modify the individual's behaviour to match job demands. Behaviours performed at rates which are too slow have been increased by the use of verbal prompting (Bellamy et al., 1975), peer modelling (Brown & Pearce, 1970; Kliebhan, 1967) and by manipulation of external reinforcement contingencies such as praise, money, and tokens (Evans & Spradlin, 1966; Huddle, 1967; Hunt & Zimmerman, 1969; McNally, Norusis, Gentz & McConathy, 1983; Schroeder,

1972) and internal self-monitoring contingencies (Ackerman & Shapiro, 1984; Shafer, 1987a).

Successful employment requires that the worker adapt to variations in task demands, work settings, supervisors, and time requirements. Some individuals with developmental disabilities, particularly those who are mentally retarded, have difficulty generalizing their skills to new situations (Stokes & Baer, 1977). Several researchers have proposed that work skills can be generalized and maintained by teaching the developmentally disabled worker core skills that are related to a variety of job situations. Wehman and McLaughlin (1980) suggest that movement sequences such as reading, grasping, and picking up objects serve as the basic elements of general subdomains of motor performance applicable to domestic skills, food service skills, home industry skills, horticulture skills, janitorial skills, and office and clerical skills. Gifford, Rusch, Martin and White (1984) and Wacker and Berg (1986) have outlined methods that can be used to teach mentally retarded and motorically involved individuals to adapt to environmental and task demands and to work independently. Several studies addressing the issue of skill generalization and maintenance have demonstrated the durability of work performance of the developmentally disabled worker (Connis, 1979; Connis & Rusch, 1980; Cuvo, Leaf & Borakove, 1978; Rusch, 1979; Sowers, Rusch, Connis & Cummings, 1980).

Terminating developmentally disabled workers from employment is related to their temperament, emotionality, and failure to follow established social norms (Greenspan & Shoultz, 1981). Antisocial and disruptive behaviours appear to be a greater problem for mildly retarded individuals than for severely or profoundly retarded persons. Hill et al. (1986) suggest that mildly handicapped individuals are more aware of the financial disincentives for handicapped persons in the work place. Given that the level of understanding of one's role in the work force is a characteristic of people with developmental disabilities in general, it is clear that job-training programs must teach social skills as well as job skills. Wehman and McLaughlin (1980) describe several techniques that may be employed to decrease antisocial or disruptive behaviours which can interfere with job productivity.

Recently, applied researchers have tended to emphasize a comprehensive and longitudinal approach to training developmentally disabled individuals termed the *Supported Work Model* (Krauss & MacEachron, 1982; Shafer, 1987b; Whitehead, 1987). This approach integrates job placement, job-site training, and long-term performance assessment. The most efficient way to teach workers the job skills and social skills necessary for successful employment is to instruct them under actual work conditions. The Supported Work Model may be a more ecologically valid approach for preparing developmentally disabled individuals for employment than the traditional sheltered-workshop training. Rather than learning job skills under simulated conditions, the client learns in actual work environments what Rusch (1979) refers to as social-vocational survival skills; i.e., *all* the behaviours necessary to maintain competitive employment.

Historically, the applied-behaviourial approach has played a dominant role in the education and training of developmentally handicapped individuals. Instructional techniques based upon operant learning theory have been used to teach behaviours and skills in a wide variety of situations. Indeed, those teachers and researchers who ascribe to the applied-behaviourial approach have the optimistic view that the quality of life of virtually all individuals can be improved through contingency management. Certainly, these methods have found a place in preparing developmentally handicapped persons for employment.

The Taxonomic Approach

Psychometrics, or methods of measuring stable characteristics of individuals by means of standardized test protocols, has influenced many areas of psychology. The use of tests to measure employees' ability levels and personality traits has been an integral part of industrial and organizational psychology since the early 1900s (Hilgard, 1987). Psychometric methods also have been employed by researchers interested in developing job taxonomies for individuals with developmental disabilities. The assessment of handicapped persons' psychomotor, behaviourial, and cognitive abilities is seen as a critical part of vocational planning and rehabilitation (Revell et al., 1980).

Most researchers have taken approaches similar to Fleishman's, in which test batteries are given to measure workers' basic ability factors and task factors. Fleishman (1975) identified 11 distinctive perceptual-motor abilities and nine physical proficiency abilities that were related to specific types of work; however, these data were based, for the most part, on the performance of military personnel. Research conducted with individuals with developmental disabilities reflects the importance of job-related abilities and social/interpersonal abilities. Pruitt (1977), for example, identified several characteristics related to successful employment of people with developmental handicaps. These characteristics include:

Specific and general motor skills
Physical capacity and work tolerance
Educability and trainability
Work adjustment
Social skill and work habits
Personality and temperament
Values and attitudes
Motivation and needs

These factors are believed to be stable individual characteristics which are amenable to measurement and may serve to predict work success. Likewise, Schreiner (1978) analyzed factors related to work performance of mentally retarded adults. He suggested that a general ability factor, composed of cognitive, visual-motor, and sorting ability, is predictive of employment success. Numerous tests have been developed to assess the basic abilities of individuals with developmental disabilities (see Botterbusch, 1974; Revell et al., 1980).

The taxonomic approach to predicting job success in developmentally disabled populations is not without criticism (Bechtoldt, 1962; Menchetti et al., 1983). Many inventories constructed to predict job success have been judged psychometrically deficient (Diamond, 1978a, 1978b; McLaughlin, 1985). Reviews of psychometric-type vocational research have identified several weaknesses in the use of traditional test protocols to predict retarded individuals' vocational success (Gold, 1975; Wolfensberger, 1967). Some of the problems cited include poor design and control, lack of cross validation, and low correlations between predictor and criterion variables. Indeed, Jackson (1968) found groups of studies reporting nonsignificant, positive, negative, and curvilinear relations between IQ scores of retarded individuals and successful employment. Clearly, progress in the taxonomic approach to predicting job success will depend upon psychometrically sound protocols that can be used with individuals with various developmental handicaps.

There is agreement that, in isolation, psychometric measures of personality and intelligence factors, deemed important during the "testing movement" of the 1950s and 1960s, are poor predictors of employment potential. However, modern taxonomic approaches have the potential to identify the behaviourial assets and deficits of developmentally handicapped individuals and to direct training and educational programs. Measures of motor abilities, in particular the Oseretsky Test of Motor Proficiency, the Bender Visual-Motor Gestaldt test, and the Purdue Pegboard test, appear to be related consistently to employment success. Further, psychometric tests can be used as part of ongoing training programs to mark progress (Wehman & McLaughlin, 1980).

Another method of assessment used by test-oriented researchers to predict developmentally disabled individuals' employment potential is the laboratory work sample method. This technique requires the worker to complete a number of brief job-simulation tasks. The advantage of the work sample method is that it provides the evaluator with an objective assessment of the worker's skill level, behaviour, and motivation in situations similar to those encountered in actual work conditions. Work samples have been shown to be particularly useful in evaluating the psychomotor skills of potential workers. Several work samples test batteries are available commercially; a number of these tests are described in Table 1. They have been designed for various types of developmental disabilities and focus on a variety of vocational areas.

Table 1: Work Samples

Work Samples	Measures	Population	Norms
AAMD-Becker Reading-Free Vocational Interest Inventory (RFVII)	11-areas-males 8 areas-females	Educable mentally retarded at high school level	1050 workers
Hester System	28 factors in 7 areas	Physically and mentally handicapped rehabilitation clients	Not available
McCarron-Dial Work Evaluation System	17 work samples in 5 areas	Mentally ill and mentally retarded	200 developmentally disabled adults
Philadelphia Jewish Employment and Vocational Service Work Sample System (JEVS)	28 work samples in 10 areas	Disadvantaged persons	1100 clients in 32 U.S. facilities
Pre-Vocational Readiness Battery (VALPAR 17)	5 areas	Mentally retarded	Not interpretable
Singer Vocational Evaluation System	20 work samples	Physically disabled and mildly retarded	Not interpretable
TOWER System (Testing, Orientation, and Work Evaluation in Rehabilitation	93 work samples in 14 areas	Physically and emotionally disabled	Not available
Valpar Component Work Sample Series (VALPAR)	16 work samples	Industrially injured workers	Not available

(continued...)

Work Samples	Measures	Population	Norms
Vocational Information and Evaluation Work Samples (VIEWS)	16 work samples in 4 areas	Mildly, moderately and severely retarded	104 developmentally disabled (aged 16-61)
Vocational Interest and Sophistication Assessment (VISA)	7 areas-males 4 areas-female	Mentally retarded adolescents and young adults	Not available
Wide Range Employment Sample Test (WREST)	10 work samples in 2 areas	Sheltered workshop clients	General population, sheltered workshop employees, and competitively employed workers

The disadvantage of the work sample method is that the protocols often lack measures of validity and reliability; further, some researchers view the work sample technique as misrepresenting actual work conditions since they fail to address motivational and social demand issues.

The taxonomic approach to evaluating the "fit" of the worker to the job has an established place in the study of employment issues. Despite the challenges made by some researchers, the psychometric assessment of abilities and skills is used extensively in personnel selection and job training. The taxonomic approach is seeing a revival with the development of the Supported Work Model. Psychometric methods provide relatively quick and inexpensive indices of individual attributes and tests can serve as personnel selection devices.

The cognitive-theory approach

Researchers who evaluate human motor performance from a cognitive or information processing approach focus on the "mental machinery" which underlies observed behaviour. Movements are the end product of a series of mental processes which are believed to function in a computer-like fashion. Environmental events are perceived, decisions are made, and responses are initiated by mental processes which exist within the individual. Some of these processes are believed to be structural or "hard wired"; they are invariant, fixed attributes of a the information processing system. Governing the activities of "hard wired" mental mechanisms are controlling or "executive" processes which direct movement on the basis of learned rules and strategies. Observed differences in the performance of individuals have been explained in terms of structural deficits, control deficits, and their interaction.

Most cognitive theories of motor behaviour propose that the information processing components which underlie complex motor behaviour are organized in a hierarchical fashion. Higher level executive-type cognitive control processes initiate simpler, lower-level motor programs or subroutines (Adams, 1971; Keele, 1968; Schmidt, 1975; Singer, 1980). Motor programs are those aspects of movement which are highly automated and, once initiated by higher-level processes, are executed with minimal conscious effort. Executive-type control processes, on the other hand, serve a generative function in which sets of rules are evaluated and used by the individual to organize and plan movements. Higher-level processes are controlling processes which demand attentional resources of the individual and depend upon feedback from the environment to modify ongoing behaviour (Posner & Snyder, 1975; Schneider & Fisk, 1983).

The research conducted on structural and control processes has direct relevance to employment issues for developmentally handicapped individuals. As discussed earlier, job termination for developmentally handicapped individuals is related to slow productivity and the need for too much supervision. Inefficient productivity may be related to the speed with which a worker performs a job and, thus, may reflect structural process deficits. Poor job performance, i.e., the failure of a worker to follow instructions or adapt to changes in job demands, may reflect control process deficits.

Mentally retarded individuals perform more slowly on simple, nonproblem solving tests that measure reaction time than do nonretarded individuals (Maisto & Baumeister, 1984; Vernon, 1986; Zelaznik & Aufderheide, 1986). The reaction-time paradigm has been used extensively to evaluate the role specific stages of information processing have on performance. Individuals who are mentally retarded are slower than nonretarded individuals in perceptual scanning (Lally & Nettelbeck, 1980; Nettelbeck, 1985; Nettelbeck & McLean, 1984; Phillips & Nettelbeck, 1985), information encoding and memory processes (Maisto & Jerome, 1977), and speed of information processing (Saccuzzo, Kerr, Marcus & Brown, 1979). Mentally retarded individuals also appear to be less efficient in their abilities to initiate movements that nonretarded individuals (Kirby, Nettelbeck & Western, 1982; Wade, Newell & Wallace, 1978).

These data have prompted some researchers to suggest that performance differences between retarded and nonretarded individuals are related primarily to the speed of executing basic information processes. Fast processing of information implies efficient use of memory capacity; slow processing promotes less efficient learning, weak formation of associations, more variable performance, and poor generalization of skills (Vernon, 1986). Nettelbeck, Cheshire and Lally (1979) observed a significant correlation between scanning speed and performance on an industrial sewing task of subjects with IQ scores between 60 and 95. Slower scanning speeds were related to the number of errors made by workers, particularly as the speed of the tasks increased.

Skilled performance depends upon the efficient integration of a variety of basic operations; it is also goal directed. Criterion-level job performance requires that a worker choose and plan a sequence of responses that accomplishes the task. In many jobs the worker must employ control processes to perform the task efficiently. Control processes enable the individual to select, modify, and integrate stored information in a way that can be used to solve problems. Examples of controlled strategic actions include rehearsal of information in memory use of mnemonic elaboration, chunking, imagery, and associative clustering. These strategies have been shown to facilitate the learning and retention of both verbal skills (Borkowski & Cavanaugh, 1981; Borkowski, Reid & Kurtz, 1984; Butterfield & Belmont, 1975; Campione & Brown, 1984) and motor skills (Ho & Shea, 1978; Reid, 1980; Shea, 1977).

Individual differences in verbal and motor performance are related to the extent to which persons spontaneously employ control processes and strategies. A characteristic of mentally retarded persons is their failure to employ strategies and to generalize behaviour learned in one setting to a different setting (Borkowski & Cavanaugh, 1981; Brown, 1974; Campione & Brown, 1984). Considerable research has assessed whether strategic behaviour can be taught. Brown and Campione (1986) provide a guideline for promoting generalization of motor learning that is based upon their research with mildly retarded persons. Of particular interest is the similarities between their generalization techniques and those proposed by applied-behaviour theorists. They state, "A list of eight guidelines that has influenced our own work was published in 1978, and it is remarkably similar to those emerging from the applied behaviour analysis school, even though the two groups of researchers did not cross reference each other, and were not aware of the similarity" (p. 260).

Several cognitive theories posit that control processes are effortful mental acts which expend attentional capacity (Kahneman, 1973; Schneider & Shiffrin, 1977; Shiffrin & Schneider,1977). They suggest that the attentional resources available to an individual are limited and that the amount of attentional capacity varies among individuals. Thus, a worker who is required to act simultaneously upon two or more tasks to perform a job efficiently must be able to divide limited attentional resources among the tasks. When attentional capacity fails to meet task demands, performance efficiency deteriorates. The poor performance of mentally retarded individuals on tasks that demand the use of strategies and effortful processing is proposed to be due, at least in part, to limited attentional capacity (Carr, 1984).

Attentional capacity also influence an individual's ability to detect changes in environmental conditions which are not directly related to the task at hand. While a worker must be able to concentrate on the job, he/she must also be able to shift job behaviours contingent upon external signals or cues. Behaviourial flexibility depends upon the ability of the individual to continuously monitor environmental cues. Mentally retarded individuals are less adept than nonretarded in monitoring signals that occur infrequently (Baumeister, Wilcox & Greeson, 1969; Tomporowski & Allison, 1988). These findings suggest that these workers may be more inflexible in the face of changing task requirements than nonretarded workers.

Marteniuk (1979) provides an instructional framework for rehabilitative training based upon cognitive motor learning theory. Using Fitts' (1964) three-stage theory of motor learning, Marteniuk describes motor skill acquisition and specifies how educators may arrange their training programs to promote learning. During the first stage of training, referred to as the cognitive phase, the educator should instruct the learner to approach a new task as a problem to be solved. The learner must "understand" what is required to perform the task. The individual's cognitive appraisal of task demands can be enhanced by the use of verbal instruction, visual cues, and proprioceptive feedback. Also, the attention of the learner should be directed toward critical movement cues and movement patterns. During the second, or associative phase, the learner shifts from attempting to evaluate what acts are appropriate for the performance of the task to refining the chosen motor movements involved in performing the task. Movement components become more efficient and they gradually come under control of higher-level executive processes. The trainer should ensure that the learner practices the motor skill. The learner should be given considerable visual and proprioceptive feedback during this stage and taught to interpret environmental cues that predict certain behaviourial changes; i.e.,to be able to adapt to variation in work situation. In the third, or autonomous stage, movement patterns come under increasing control of executive processes; skilled acts are conducted smoothly with little attention devoted to the specific acts performed to complete the task. The learner must be instructed not to attend to individual steps involved in performing the task. Indeed, the direction of attention of the learner to the details of the task may interfere with efficient performance.

Cognitive theories of behaviour have important implications to the employment of people with developmental disabilities. These theories identify specific processes that are hypothesized to underlie behaviour; skilled work performance demands the integration of sensory, cognitive, and motor processes. When one or more of these processes are disrupted by injury, disease, or congenital factors, skilled performance is influenced detrimentally. Research driven by cognitive theories of behaviour provides a way of identifying those processes that most affect the performance in an individual with a developmental disability. Once deficits are identified, cognitive theory also provides a direction for ameliorating the disordered process. Marteniuk's (1979) attempt to relate cognitive theory to rehabilitation is an example of how basic theory can be used to address applied issues and problems. Likewise, the instructional and generalization techniques described by Brown and Campione (1986), provide educators with approaches for preparing the developmentally handicapped person for employment.

Successful employment of developmentally handicapped individuals also requires their abilities to meet the social demands present in the workplace. Cognitive theorists have addressed the issues of mentally retarded individuals' social competence but, as pointed out by Sternberg and Spear (1985) the study of how mentally handicapped individuals "fit" into their social environment has neither received much attention nor been investigated in a systematic fashion. Early work by Zigler and Balla (1972) evaluated factors that influenced the motivation and persistence of mentally retarded children. On the basis of a series of studies (see Zigler & Balla, 1982), they proposed that the ability of mentally retarded individuals to adjust to society will be hampered by their history of social deprivation, which may lead to either increased desire for social contact or wariness about interacting with others, and by their history of experiences of failure, which will lower their level of aspiration. Mentally retarded individuals are more likely to depend upon external sources of direction than to rely on their own abilities. Sternberg and Spear (1985) posit that an individual strives to maintain an optimal fit in society. Under normal conditions, people attempt to shape their environment to correspond to their unique abilities and needs. People with developmental disabilities who are placed in a position where job demands exceed their abilities have little opportunity to control their work environment or to alter work demand; they do, however, have the option to quit or to be terminated from their job. Unfortunately, little cognitive-based research has been conducted that evaluates how developmentally handicapped individuals function in the context of employment.

Information processing theories have had an impact on business and industry in the United States and Europe. McCormick (1979) has developed a comprehensive job analysis inventory that combines the taxonomic approach with the cognitive-theory approach. The Position Analysis Questionnaire (McCormick, Jeanneret & Mecham, 1969) evaluates jobs with respect to task demands, environmental demands, and worker abilities in a fashion not unlike Fleishman's. McCormick's inventory, however, also evaluates work demands in light of cognitive processes. He proposes that virtually all jobs have four operational functions in common: information receiving, information storage, information processing and decision making, and action functions. While these four functions are found in ally types of tasks, the role of each function varies. Some jobs involve continuous repetition of movement and may demand minimal information processing and decision-making demands, but require considerable movement and action functions. Other jobs may require highly sophisticated sensory systems to perform a job efficiently, but require only minimal motor involvement.

An inventory similar to McCormick's has been developed in Germany by Rohmert and Landau (1983). Their Ergonomic Job Analysis classifies jobs on the basis of three factors: the physical characteristics of the job, the environmental demands in the workplace, and information processing demands inherent in the task. They view optimal work performance as the interaction of task factors and subject factors; efficient performance is dictated by the dynamic interaction of individual abilities, cognitive processes, and task performance.

Both the Position Analysis Questionnaire and the Ergonomic Job Analysis protocols have been evaluated extensively to determine their reliability and validity with nonhandicapped workers. The protocols have been used for worker selection, placement, job classification, rehabilitation, and job design. The protocols have not been used, however, to evaluate the work potential of developmentally handicapped individuals.
Historically, the cognitive approach to evaluating motor behaviour is quite new. Only in the past decade has an interest in studying motor skill deficiencies of the mentally handicapped arisen (Wade, 1986). Nevertheless, the theories of cognition in the field of psychology that have emerged recently can be expected to exert growing influence on industrial and employment issues.

Future Directions

The direction of future human engineering research is driven by a clear mandate. The goal is to both fit the task to the worker and the worker to the task. The three approaches to selecting and preparing developmentally handicapped individuals for employment evaluated in this review have followed this mandate. In each of the approaches the actions of the applied researchers have been based upon a well-founded theoretical orientation. There are, however, several areas that beg the attention of both basic and applied researchers.

Studies addressing employment issues have been conducted, for the most part, with mentally retarded individuals. Further, many of the studies following the applied-behaviourial approach have been limited, by design, to individuals who are severely retarded. The findings obtained from these studies have been generalized to other types of developmental disabilities; however, direct evaluations of the characteristics of individuals with such disabilities as cerebral palsy, learning disabilities, and emotional disturbances are lacking. Likewise, the study of individual differences in cognitive functioning has been limited primarily to those who are mentally handicapped. Most of these studies have focused on verbal learning and the results are often generalized to motor learning. The assumption that verbal and motor learning are governed by the same set of laws is open to question, however (Adams, 1983). It is clear that additional research which evaluates the characteristics of individuals who exhibit various types of developmental handicaps is needed. Also, research methodologies need to address directly motor movement issues which are related to employment.

Progress made to date for employing people with developmental handicaps has placed society at a critical juncture. Given that handicapped individuals can be taught the job-related and social skills necessary for employment, their acceptance into the work force will hinge ultimately upon the willingness of employers to hire handicapped workers. While there is a continued need for theory-driven laboratory research, there is also a pragmatic concern that must be addressed. Without the existence of employment opportunities to drive research, the study of employment issues will exist only as an academic exercise. The limitations of employment often results from the availability of support systems and employment opportunities rather than the functional skills of the handicapped worker.
The developmentally handicapped person's role in the workplace may lie in the effectiveness of longitudinal, multidimensional training programs such as the Supported Work Model. This model seeks to overcome barriers that impede successful employment. Job success can be improved in several ways. Some of these methods include educating and preparing the employer and coworkers to integrate the handicapped individual into the work force, designing work environments which enhance productivity, modifying work conditions to match the characteristics of the employee, and making use of prosthetic aids, devices, and new technology to enhance work performance. Each of a these proposals invites evaluation and research. Given the continued emphasis in the United States and other Western governments towards providing employment opportunities for handicapped individuals (Gaylord-Ross, 1987), data will be needed to make meaningful decisions about employment issues as they relate to developmentally disabled workers.

Summary

The quality of life for individuals with developmental handicaps depends upon the same factors that are important for all people. One factor that contributes greatly to the quality of life is gratification obtained from being successfully employed. This fact has been recognized by those who provide services to developmentally handicapped persons and it has led to an emphasis being placed on preparing them for gainful employment.

The methods currently used to enhance the employability of developmentally handicapped individuals reflects three approaches to the study of employment issues; these are the behaviour-analysis approach, the taxonomic approach, and the cognitive-theory approach. Each approach is based upon a set of assumptions which has directed research that has produced important information related to employment issues. However, for those interested in assisting the developmentally handicapped individual obtain employment, an integrated approach to the study of employment issues is lacking.

It is clear that the developmentally handicapped individual will have to meet a variety of physical, cognitive, and social demands in order to become successfully employed. It is suggested that research be conducted which evaluates the ability of developmentally disabled individuals to meet these interrelated demands.

Author Notes

1. Send requests for reprints to Phillip Tomporowski, Department of Psychology, University of Alabama, P.O. Box 2968, Tuscaloosa, Alabama, USA, 35487.

References

Ackerman, A. M., & Shapiro, E. S. (1984). Self-monitoring and work productivity with mentally retarded adults. *Journal of Applied Behavior Analysis, 17,* 403-407.

Adams, J. A. (1971). A closed-loop theory of motor learning. *Journal of Motor Behavior, 3,* 111-150.

Adams, J. A. (1983). On the integration of the verbal and motor domains. In R. A. Magill (Ed.), *Memory and control of action* (pp. 3-13). New York, NY: North-Holland.

Baumeister, A. A., Wilcox, S., & Greeson, J. (1969). Reaction times of retardates and normals as a function of relative stimulus frequency. *American Journal of Mental Deficiency, 73,* 935-941.

Bechtoldt, H. P. (1962). Factor analysis and the investigation of hypotheses. *Perceptual Motor Skills, 14,* 319-342.

Bellamy, G. T., Peterson, L., & Close, D. (1975). Habilitation of the severely and profoundly retarded: Illustrations of competence. *Education and Training of the Mentally Retarded, 10,* 174-186.

Bellamy, G. T., Rhodes, L. E., Wilcox, B., Albin, J. M., Mank, D. M., Boles, S. M., Horner, R. H., Collins, M., & Turner, J. (1984). Quality and equality in employment services for adults with severe disabilities. *Journal of the Association for the Severely Handicapped, 9,* 270-277.

Borkowski, J. G., & Cavanaugh, J. C. (1981). Metacognition and intelligence. In M. P. Friedman, J. P. Das & N. O. O'Connor (Eds.), *Intelligence and learning* (pp. 253-258). New York, NY: Plenum Press.

Borkowski, J. G., Reid, M. K., & Kurtz, B. E. (1984). Metacognition and retardation: Paradigmatic, theoretical, and applied perspectives. In P. H. Brooks, R. Sperber, & C. McCauley, (Eds.), *Learning and cognition in the mentally retarded* (pp. 55-75). Hillsdale, NJ: Lawrence Erlbaum.

Botterbusch, K. F. (1974). Test use in vocational evaluation. *Vocational Evaluation and Work Adjustment Bulletin, 7,* 6-9.

Brickey, M. P., Browning, L. J., & Campbell, K. M. (1982). Vocational histories of sheltered workshop employees placed in projects with industry and competitive jobs. *Mental Retardation, 20,* 52-57.

Brickey, M.P., Campbell, K. M., & Browning, L. J. (1985). A five-year follow up of sheltered workshop employees placed in competitive jobs. *Mental Retardation, 23,* 67-73.

Brown, A. L. (1974). The role of strategic behavior in retardate memory. In N. R. Ellis (Ed.), *International review of research in mental retardation* (Vol. 7, pp. 55-111). New York, NY: Academic Press.

Brown, A. L., & Campione, J. C. (1986). Training for transfer: Guidelines for promoting flexible use of trained skills. In M. G. Wade (Ed.), *Motor skill acquisition of mentally handicapped: Issues in research and training* (pp. 257-271). New York, NY: North-Holland.

Brown, A. L., & Pearce, E. (1970). Increasing production rate of trainable retarded students in a public school simulated workshop. *Education and Training of the Mentally Retarded, 5,* 15-22.

Butterfield, E. C., & Belmont, J. M. (1975). Assessing and improving the executive cognitive functions of mentally retarded people. In I. Bialer & M. Steinlicht (Eds.), *Psychological issues in mentally retarded people* (pp. 277-318). Chicago, IL: Aldine.

Campione, J. C., & Brown, A. L. (1984). Learning ability and transfer propensity as sources of individual differences in intelligence. In P. H. Brooks, R. Sperber & C. McCauley (Eds.), *Learning and cognition in the mentally retarded* (pp. 265-293). Hillsdale, NJ: Lawrence Erlbaum.

Carr, T. H. (1984). Attention, skill, and intelligence: Some speculations on extreme individual differences in human performance. In P. H. Brooks, R. Sperber & C. McCauley (Eds.), *Learning and cognition in the mentally retarded* (pp. 189-215). Hillsdale, NJ: Lawrence Erlbaum.

Cheney, D., & Foss, G. (1984). An examination of social behaviors of mentally retarded workers. *Education and Training of the Mentally Retarded, 19,* 216-221.

Connis, R. T. (1979). The effects of sequential cues, self-recording, and praise on the job task sequencing of retarded adults. *Journal of Applied Behavior Analysis, 12,* 355-361.

Connis, R. T., & Rusch, F. R. (1980). Programming maintenance through sequential withdrawal of social contingencies. *Behavior Research of Severe Developmental Disabilities, 1,* 249-260.

Craig, A. (1984). Human engineering: The control of vigilance. In J. S. Warm (Ed.), *Sustained attention in human performance* (pp. 247-291). New York, NY: John Wiley & Sons.

Cuvo, A. J., Leaf, R. B., & Borakove, L. S. (1978). Teaching janitorial skills to the mentally retarded: Acquisition, generalization, and maintenance. *Journal of Applied Behavior Analysis, 11,* 345-355.

Diamond, E. E. (1978a). Vocational interest and sophistication assessment (Review by J. J. Parmicky, H. Kahn, & A. D. Burdett). In O. K. Buros (Ed.), *The eighth mental measurement yearbook* (Vol. II, pp. 1631-1632). Highland Park, NJ: Gryphon Press.

Diamond, E. E. (1978b). AAMD-Becker Reading-free vocational interest inventory (Review by R. L. Becker). In O. K. Buros (Ed.), *The eighth mental measurement yearbook* (Vol. II, pp. 1535-1536). Highland Park, NJ: Gryphon Press.

Erekson, T. L., & Rotatori, A. F. (1986). *Accessibility to employment training for the physically handicapped.* Springfield, IL: Charles C. Thomas.

Evans, G. W., & Spradlin, J. E. (1966). Incentives and instructions as controlling variables of productivity. *American Journal of Mental Deficiency, 71,* 129-132.

Ferguson, D. L., & Ferguson, P. M. (1986) The new victors: A progressive policy analysis of work reform for people with very severe handicaps. *Mental Retardation, 24,* 331-338.

Fitts, P. M. (1964). Perceptual-motor skills learning. In A. W. Melton (Ed.), *Categories of human learning* (pp. 244-285). New York, NY: Academic Press.

Fleishman, E. A. (1972). On the relation between abilities, learning, and human performance. *American Psychologist, 27,* 1017-1032.

Fleishman, E. A. (1975). Toward a taxonomy of human performance. *American Psychologist, 30,* 1127-1149.

Fleishman, E. A. (1978). Relating individual differences to the dimensions of human tasks. *Ergonomics, 21,* 1007-1019.

Fleishman, E. A. (1982). Systems for describing human tasks. *American Psychologist, 37,* 821-834.

Foss, G., & Peterson, S. L. (1981). Social-interpersonal skills relevant to job tenure for mentally retarded adults. *Mental Retardation, 19,* 103-106.

Gaylord-Ross, R. (1987). Vocational integration for persons with mental handicaps: A cross-cultural perspective. *Research in Developmental Disabilities, 84*, 531-548.

Gifford, J., Rusch, F., Martin, J., & White, D. (1984). Autonomy and adaptability: A proposed technology for maintaining work behavior. In N. R. Ellis & N. W. Bray (Eds.), *International review of research on mental retardation* (Vol.12, pp. 285-318). New York, NY: Academic Press.

Gold, M. W. (1972). Stimulus factors in skill training of the retarded on a complex assembly task; Acquisition, transfer, and retention. *American Journal of Mental Deficiency, 76,* 517-526.

Gold, M. W. (1974). Redundant cue removal in skill training for the mildly and moderately retarded. *Education and Training of the Mentally Retarded, 9,* 5-8.

Gold, M. W. (1975). Vocational training. In J. Wortis (Ed.), *Mental retardation and developmental disabilities* (Vol. 7, pp. 254-264). New York, NY: Brunner/Mazel.

Greenspan, S., & Shoultz, B. (1981). Why mentally retarded adults lose their jobs: Social competence as a factor in work adjustment. *Applied Research in Mental Retardation, 2,* 23-28.

Greenspan, S., Shoultz, B., & Weir, M. M. (1981). Social judgement and vocational adjustment of mentally retarded adults. *Applied Research in Mental Retardation, 2,* 335-346.

Hilgard, E. R. (1987). *Psychology in America: A historical survey.* New York, NY: Harcourt Brace Jovanovich.

Hill, M., & Wehman, P. (1979). Employer and non-handicapped coworker perceptions of moderately and severely retarded workers. *Journal of Contemporary Business, 8,* 107-112.

Hill, J. W., Wehman, P., Hill, M., & Goodall, P. (1986). Differential reasons for job separation of previously employed persons with mental retardation. *Mental Retardation, 24,* 347-351.

Ho, L., & Shea, J. B. (1978). Levels of processing and the coding of position cues in motor short-term memory. *Journal of Motor Behavior, 10,* 113-121.

Hollender, J. W. (1974). Prediction of work adjustment for adolescent male educable retardates. *Journal of Counseling Psychology, 21,* 164-165.

Huddle, D. D. (1967). Work performance of trainable adults as influenced by competition, cooperation, and monetary reward. *American Journal of Mental Deficiency, 72,* 198-211.

Hunt, J. G., & Zimmerman, J. (1969). Stimulating productivity in a simulated sheltered workshop setting. *American Journal of Mental Deficiency, 74,* 43-49.

Jackson, R. N. (1968). Employment adjustment of educable mentally handicapped ex-pupils in Scotland. *American Journal of Mental Deficiency, 72,* 924-930.

Kahneman, D. (1973). *Attention and effort.* Englewood Cliffs, NJ: Prentice Hall.

Kazdin, A. E. (1975). *Behavior modification in applied settings.* Homewood, IL: Dorsey Press.

Keele, S. W. (1968). Movement control in skilled motor performance. *Psychological Bulletin, 70,* 387-403.

Kiernan, W. E., & Ciborowski, J. (1986). Survey of employment for adults with developmental disabilities. *Remedial and Special Education, 7,* 25-30.

Kirby, N. H., Nettelbeck, T., & Western, P. (1982). Locating information processing deficits of mildly mentally retarded young adults. *American Journal of Mental Deficiency, 87,* 338-343.

Kliebhan, J. (1967). Effects of goal setting and modelling on job performances of retarded adolescents. *American Journal of Mental Deficiency, 72,* 220-226.

Kochany, L., & Keller, J. (1981). An analysis and evaluation of the failures of severely disabled individuals in competitive employment. In P. Wehman (Ed.), *Competitive employment: New horizons for severely disabled individuals* (pp. 181-198). Baltimore, MD: Paul H. Brookes.

Krauss, M., & MacEachron, A. (1982). Competitive employment training for mentally retarded adults: The supported work model. *American Journal of Mental Deficiency, 86,* 650-653.

Lally, M., & Nettelbeck, T. (1980). Intelligence, inspection time, and response strategy. *American Journal of Mental Deficiency, 84,* 553-560.

Maisto, A. A., & Baumeister, A. A. (1984). Dissection of component processes in rapid information processing tasks: Comparison of retarded and nonretarded people. In P. H. Brooks, R. Sperber, & C. McCauley (Eds.), *Learning and cognition in the mentally retarded* (pp. 165-188). Hillsdale, NJ: Lawrence Erlbaum.

Maisto A. A., & Jerome, M. A. (1977). Encoding and high-speed memory scanning of retarded and nonretarded adolescents. *American Journal of Mental Deficiency, 82,* 282-286.

Marteniuk, R. G. (1979). Motor skill performance and learning: Considerations for rehabilitation. *Physiotherapy Canada, 31,* 187-202.

McCormick, E. J. (1979). *Job analysis: Methods and applications.* New York, NY: AMACOM.

McCormick, E. J., Jeanneret, P. R., & Mecham, R. C. (1969). *The development and background of the Position Analysis Questionnaire.* Lafayette, IN: Purdue University.

McLaughlin, P. J. (1985). Career counseling for the mentally retarded adolescent. *Personnel, 62,* 61-66.

McNally, R. J., Norusis, P. L., Gentz, S. A. & McConathy, L. C. (1983). The use of self-delivered reinforcement and group contingency management to increase productivity of severely retarded workers. *Psychological Reports, 52*, 499-503.

Menchetti, B. M., Rusch, F. R., & Owens, D. (1983). Vocational training. In J. L. Matson & S. E. Breuning (Eds.), *Assessing the mentally retarded* (pp. 247-284). New York, NY: Brune & Stratton.

Mithaug, D. E. (1979). Negative employer attitudes toward hiring the handicapped: Fact or fiction. *Journal of Contemporary Business, 8*, 19-26.

Nettelbeck, T. (1985). Inspection time and mild mental retardation. In N. R. Ellis & N. W. Bray (Eds.), *International review of research in mental retardation* (Vol. 13, pp. 109-141). New York, NY: Academic Press.

Nettelbeck, T., Cheshire, F., & Lally, M. (1979). Intelligence, work performance, and inspection time. *Ergonomics, 22*, 291-297.

Nettelbeck, T., & McLean, J. (1984). Mental retardation and inspection time: A two-stage model for sensory registration and central processing. *American Journal of Mental Deficiency, 89*, 83-90.

Phillips, C. J., & Nettelbeck, T. (1985). Mild mental retardation and memory scanning. In N. R. Ellis & N. W. Bray (Eds.), *International review of research in mental retardation* (Vol. 13, pp. 144-179). New York, NY: Academic Press.

Posner, M. I., & Snyder, C. R. (1975). Attention and cognitive control. In R. L. Solso (Ed.), *Information processing and cognition* (pp.55-85). Hillsdale, NJ: Lawrence Erlbaum.

Pruitt, W. A. (1977). *Vocational (work) evaluation.* Menomonie, WI: Walt Pruitt.

Reid, G. (1980). The effects of memory strategy instruction in the short term memory of the mentally retarded. *Journal of Motor Behavior, 12*, 221-227.

Revell, W. G., Kriloff, L. J., & Sarkees, M. O. (1980). Vocational evaluation. In P. Wehman, & P. J. McLaughlin (Eds.), *Vocational curriculum for developmentally disabled person* (pp.75-94). Baltimore, MD: University Press.

Rohmert, W., & Landau, K. (1983). *A new technique for job analysis.* London: Taylor & Francis.

Rowitz, L. (Ed.). (1986). Symposium on employment for people with mental retardation. *Mental Retardation, 24,* 329-356.

Rusch, F. R. (1979). A functional analysis of the relationship between attending to task and producing in an applied restaurant setting. *The Journal of Special Education, 13,* 399-411.

Rusch, F. R. (Ed.). (1986). *Competitive employment issues and strategies.* Baltimore, MD: Paul H. Brookes.

Rusch, F. R., & Schutz, R. P. (1979). Non-sheltered competitive employment of the mentally retarded adult: Research to reality? *Journal of Contemporary Business, 8,* 85-98.

Saccuzzo, D. P., Kerr, M., Marcus, A., & Brown, R. (1979). Input capability and speed of processing in mental retardation. *Journal of Abnormal Psychology, 4,* 341-345.

Sali, J., & Amir, M. (1971). Personal factors influencing the retarded person's success at work: A report from Israel. *American Journal of Mental Deficiency, 76,* 42-47.

Salzberg, C. L., Likins, M., McConaughy, E. K., & Lignugaris/Kraft, B. (1986). Social competence and employment of retarded persons. In N. R. Ellis & N. W. Bray (Eds.), *International review of research in mental retardation* (Vol. 14, pp. 225-257). New York, NY: Academic Press.

Schmidt, R. A. (1975). A schema theory of discrete motor skill learning. *Psychological Review, 82,* 225-260.

Schmidt, R. A. (1982). *Motor control and learning.* Champaign, IL: Human Kinetics.

Schneider, W., & Fisk, A. D. (1983). Attention theory and mechanisms for skilled performance. In R. A. Magill (Ed.), *Memory and control of action* (pp. 119-143). New York, NY: North Holland.

Schneider, W., & Shiffrin, R. M. (1977). Controlled and automatic human information processing: I. Detection, search, and attention. *Psychological Review, 84,* 1-66.

Schreiner, J. (1978). Prediction of retarded adults' work performance through components of general ability. *American Journal of Mental Deficiency, 83,* 77-79.

Schroeder, S. (1972). Parametric effects of reinforcement frequency, amount of reinforcement, and required response force on sheltered workshop behavior. *Journal of Applied Behavior Analysis, 5,* 431-441.

Shafer, M. S. (1987a). Supported competitive employment: The use of self management programming in the follow-along process. *Journal of Rehabilitation, 53,* 31-36.

Shafer, M. S. (1987b). Competitive employment for workers with mental retardation. In M. Hersen, R. M. Eisler & P. M. Miller (Eds.), *Progress in behavior modification* (pp.86-107). New York, NY: Academic Press.

Shea, J. B. (1977). Effects of labeling on motor short-term memory. *Journal of Experimental Psychology: Human Learning and Memory, 3,* 92-99.

Shiffrin, R. M., & Schneider, W. (1977). Controlled and automatic human information processing: II. Perceptual learning, automatic attending, and a general theory. *Psychological Review, 84,* 127-190.

Singer, R. N. (1980). Motor behavior and the role of cognitive processes and learner strategies. In G. E. Stelmach & J. Requin (Eds.), *Tutorials in motor behavior* (pp. 591-603). New York, NY: North Holland.

Sowers, J., Rusch, F. R., Connis R. T. & Cummings, L. E. (1980). Teaching mentally retarded adults to time manage in a vocational setting. *Journal of Applied Behavior Analysis, 13,* 119-128.

Stark, J. A., & Kiernan, A. J. (1986). Symposium overview: Employment for people with mental retardation. *Mental Retardation, 24,* 329-338.

Sternberg, R. J., & Spear, L. C. (1985). A triarchic theory of mental retardation. In N. R. Ellis & N. W. Bray (Eds.), *International review of research in mental retardation* (Vol. 13, pp. 301-326). New York, NY: Academic Press.

Stokes, T. F., & Baer, D. M. (1977). An implicit technology of generalization. *Journal of Applied Behavior Analysis, 10,* 349-367.

Tomporowski P. D. & Allison, P. (1988). Sustained attention of adults with mental retardation. *American Journal of Mental Retardation, 92,* 525-530.

Vernon, P. A. (1986). Speed of information-processing, intelligence, and mental retardation. In M. G. Wade (Ed.), *Motor skill acquisition of the mentally handicapped: Issues in research and training* (pp. 113-129). New York, NY: North-Holland.

Wacker, D. P., & Berg, W. K. (1986). Generalizing and maintaining work behavior. In F. R. Rusch (Ed.), *Competitive employment issues and strategies* (pp. 129-140). Baltimore, MD: Paul Brookes.

Wade, M. G. (1986). Introduction. In M. G. Wade (Ed.), *Motor skill acquisition of the mentally handicapped: Issues in research and training* (pp. 3-4). New York, NY: North-Holland.

Wade, M. G., Newell, K. M., & Wallace, S. A. (1978). Decision time and movement time as a function of response complexity in the motor performance of retarded persons. *American Journal of Mental Deficiency, 83,* 135-144.

Wehman, P., & McLaughlin, P.J. (1980). *Vocational curriculum for developmentally disabled persons.* Baltimore, MD: University Press.

Weisgerber, R. A., Dahl, P. R., & Appleby, J. A. (1981). *Training the handicapped for productive employment.* London: Aspen.

Whitehead, C. W. (1987). Supported Employment: Challenge and opportunity for sheltered workshop. *Journal of Rehabilitation, 53,* 23-28.

Wolfensberger, W. (1967). Vocational preparation and occupation. In A. A. Baumeister (Ed.), *Mental retardation: Appraisal, education and rehabilitation* (pp. 232-273). Chicago, IL: Aldine.

Zelaznik, H. N., & Aufderheide S. K. (1986). Attentional and reaction time analysis of performance: Implications for research with mentally handicapped individuals. In M. G. Wade (Ed.), *Motor skill acquisition of the mentally handicapped: Issues in research and training* (pp. 131-153). New York, NY: North-Holland.

Zigler, E., & Balla, D. (1972). Developmental course of responsiveness to social reinforcement in normal children and institutionalized retarded children. *Developmental Psychology, 6,* 66-73.

Zigler, E., & Balla, D. (1982). Motivational and personality factors in the performance of the retarded. In E. Zigler & D. Balla (Eds.), *Mental retardation: The developmental difference controversy (pp.* 9-26). Hillsdale, NJ: Lawrence Erlbaum.

Problems in Movement Control
G. Reid (editor)

MOTIVATION AND SPECIAL POPULATIONS: THEORY, RESEARCH, AND IMPLICATIONS REGARDING MOTOR BEHAVIOUR

Robert J. Vallerand
Laboratoire de Psychologie Sociale
Université du Québec à Montréal

and

Greg Reid
Department of Physical Education
McGill University

Physical activities represent some of the most popular types of activities with children (Ryan, Vallerand, & Deci, 1984). According to one report (Roberts, 1984), well over 20 million North American children participate regularly in diverse types of physical activities. While most children experience pleasure and inherent satisfaction in learning and performing new forms of movement (Vallerand, Deci, & Ryan, 1987), this may not be so for an estimated 12 to 15 percent of all children who experience various types of handicaps (Bowd, McDougall, & Yewchuk, 1982). The motor performance of most of these youngsters is usually below age expectations (Bruininks & Bruininks, 1977; Rarick, Dobbins, & Broadhead, 1976); a number of reasons having been posited to explain such performance deficits (see Reid, 1987). It is likely that the rewards these children derive from participation are minimal, with frustration and feelings of incompetence dominating (Alley & Deshler, 1979). These in turn may lead to a desire to cease participation in physical activity.

Over the past two decades, much work has been conducted in order to help special populations benefit from involvement in physical activity. Basically, treatment approaches have fallen into three broad categories: biological, cognitive, and behaviourial (see Smith, 1986; Torgesen, 1986), with behaviourial analysis being the most popular approach. While the above research has led to advances in our understanding of some of the factors likely to influence the learning of physical movement by persons with a disability, these approaches, and most notably the behaviourial approach, have been recently criticized. For instance, Cohen (1986) suggests that programs based on behaviour modification principles are ill equipped to facilitate the self-regulated learning and performance of educational tasks (see also Paris & Oka, 1986). Because the emphasis of the behaviourial approach is on extrinsic reinforcement, children learn to behave in order to receive rewards but not as self-determined individuals interested in engaging in human movement. In addition, much research (see Deci & Ryan, 1980, 1985, 1987 for reviews) has demonstrated that the use of extrinsic incentives can undermine, rather than facilitate, performance on and interest in activities which are intrinsically motivating. While it might be successful in the short run, in the long run, the behaviour modification approach may turn exceptional children away from the very activities we wish to promote.

It is our belief, that in order to be fully successful, approaches to physical activity for special populations must take into consideration the emotional and motivational components of human experience. As suggested by Deci and Chandler (1986, p. 589), "the most important thing the (exceptional) field could do is adopt a motivational perspective that recognizes the developing human being, that is organismic in nature, that considers the fit between child and environment, and that promotes a more holistic, active-organism approach to the education of children". So far, the motivational approach has been sorely neglected.

The issue of motivation toward motor activities with special populations deserves closer attention for several reasons. First, the study of motivation would help us understand the experiential and social factors that regulate behaviours of these individuals. Although it is generally accepted that exceptional children display low levels of motivation (e.g., Harter, Silon, & Pike, 1981; Haywood & Switzky, 1986), it must be recognized that very little scientific evidence exists on this topic with respect to motor tasks. Second, a better grasp of motivation may help understand the failure cycle to which exceptional children fall prey (Alley & Deschler, 1979) and which results in reduced participation and dropping out of physical activities. Specifically, we believe that failure undermines exceptional learners' perceptions of competence which in turn decrease their motivation toward physical activities. Low motivation toward activities, in turn, ensures that a low output will be obtained during the next interaction with the task, thereby leading to failure again, and so on. Third, and finally, paying attention to motivational considerations may suggest ways to restructure educational environments so as to enhance fun, enjoyment, and other desirable consequences associated with the learning of physical activities (see Vallerand, 1981; Vallerand et al., 1987).

The purpose of this chapter is to propose the adoption of a theory of motivation for the study of human movement with special populations and to show how the theory may be amenable to a better understanding of the factors which regulate the motor behaviour of such individuals. It is believed that using a motivational approach to the study of special populations may lead to significant scientific and practical advances for the field. The chapter is divided into four sections. In the first section, we present the different types of motivation which underlie Deci and Ryan's (1985, 1987) self-determination theory. In the second section, we review research on the determinants and consequences of motivation and show how these may be relevant to conditions experienced by handicapped learners. In the third section we present practical implications based on the motivational approach. Finally, the chapter ends on a discussion on future directions for research and a few concluding thoughts.

Motivation and Special Populations: A Proposed Theoretical Framework

Motivation refers to the forces that initiate, direct, and sustain behaviour (Petri, 1981) and has been studied from several perspectives. For example, some perspectives have focused on instinctual drives (e.g., Freud, 1923/1962), whereas others have focused on environmental contingencies (Skinner, 1953). While radically different, these two positions nevertheless share a fundamental assumption: people are passive organisms who react to internal or external stimuli. In this section we outline a more recent theoretical perspective that considers the individual as an active organism striving for effective interactions with the environment in a context of autonomy (Deci,1975; Deci & Ryan, 1985, 1987). This perspective distinguishes between intrinsic, extrinsic, and amotivation. These different types of motivation are described below.

Intrinsic, Extrinsic, and Amotivation

Intrinsically motivated behaviours are engaged in for their own sake--for the pleasure and satisfaction derived from their performance (Deci, 1971). They are voluntarily performed in the absence of material rewards or constraints (Deci & Ryan, 1985, 1987). The child who engages in ice skating for the inherent pleasure derived from doing so is intrinsically motivated toward that activity. Intrinsic motivation is thought to stem from the needs to feel competent and self-determined (Deci, 1975; Deci & Ryan, 1985). Activities that lead the individual to experience feelings of competence and/or self-determination are intrinsically rewarding and are likely to be performed again.

On the other hand, extrinsically motivated behaviours are performed to receive or avoid something once the activity is terminated, and are not performed for their inherent experiential aspects (Deci, 1975; Kruglanski, 1978). It was originally thought that extrinsic motivation referred exclusively to nonself-determined behaviour -- to behaviour that could only be prompted by external contingencies. More recently, however, Deci, Ryan and their colleagues (Connell & Ryan, 1986; Deci & Ryan,1985; Ryan, Connell, & Deci,

1985; Ryan, Connell, & Grolnick, in press) have proposed that there are different types of extrinsic motivation, some of which may be self-determined. Deci and Ryan distinguish four types of extrinsic motivation, namely external regulation, introjection, identification, and integration.

External regulation occurs when behaviour is externally regulated (usually through rewards or constraints). For example, children may participate in activities because they feel urged to do so by the teacher. In this case, an activity that can or should be fun is performed in order to avoid negative consequences (e.g., criticisms from the teacher). The motivation is extrinsic because the reason for participation lies outside the activity itself. Furthermore, the behaviour is not chosen or self-determined. External regulation may also be fuelled by a desire for rewards. For example, a child might agree to play with the other children in order to receive a prize promised by the teacher. In this case the motivation is still extrinsic and nonself-determined, but the instigating factor is the desired reward (e.g., the promised toy) rather than a constraint. Regardless of whether the goal of behaviour is to obtain rewards or to avoid sanctions, the individual experiences an obligation to behave in a specific way, and feels controlled by the reward or by the constraint (Deci & Ryan, 1985).

With *introjected regulation*, individuals begin to internalize the reasons for their actions. Thus, the source of control is inside the individual. However, this form of internalization while internal to the person is not truly self-determined since it is limited to the internalization of external contingencies. Rewards or constraints are now imposed by the individual and not by others. The individual is internally controlling (Ryan, 1982). Thus, a child might say, " I play with the others because I feel guilty when I don't". Beliefs and controls are now internalized, although these are not self-determined and are experienced as pressure and tension toward specific aims.

In contrast, *identified regulation* occurs when a behaviour is valued by the individual and is perceived as being chosen by oneself. Behaviour is internally regulated but in a self-determined way. An example would be children who practice a specific movement because they believe that this will eventually improve their ability in sport. The motivation is extrinsic because the activity is not performed for itself but as a means to an end (to improve their motor control). However, the behaviour is nevertheless self-determined: the individual has *decided* that practising the activity is beneficial. The child experiences a sense of direction and purpose, instead of obligation and pressure, in performing the behaviour.

The last type of extrinsic motivation is *integration*. At this level the person does the behaviour willingly and the self-regulation is consistent with the individual's self-concept. At this level, the individual experiences the greatest level of self-determination for extrinsically motivated behaviours. For instance, a child might say, "I'm a child who likes to be smart; therefore I've decided to play in this game which can help improve my 'smartness'". Typically, this highest level of self-determined extrinsic motivation is only attained by adults with highly integrated self-concepts. It is therefore not generally assessed in children.

Apart from intrinsic and extrinsic motivation, Deci and Ryan (1985) claim that a third construct, *"amotivation"*, must be considered to fully understand human behaviour. Individuals are amotivated when they perceive a lack of contingency between their behaviour and outcomes. There is an experience of incompetence and lack of control. Amotivated behaviours are neither intrinsically nor extrinsically motivated: they are nonmotivated. There are no rewards (neither intrinsic nor extrinsic) and participation in the activity will eventually cease. Amotivated behaviours are the least self-determined because there is no sense of purpose, and no expectation of reward or of the possibility of changing the course of events. An amotivated child might say, "I can't come to see why I should play at this game; I'm no good and it won't do a thing for me". At this stage, learned helplessness (Abramson, Seligman, & Teasdale, 1978) can result from amotivation.

In sum, a distinction has been made between six types of motivation with varying degrees of self-determination. Intrinsically motivated behaviours are the most self-determined whereas amotivated behaviours are the least self-determined. Because very little work has been conducted on the motivation of handicapped and unsuccessful children toward motor behaviour, from this perspective, it is difficult to determine the type of motivation which may characterizes them. In addition, it should be made clear that motivation may vary for a given individual depending on the situation and the activity. However, based on the more general literature on academically handicapped and retarded children which reveals that these children hold an external locus of control orientation (Lawrence & Winchell, 1975), low levels of self-esteem (Chapman, 1988) and perceived control (Smith, Adelman, Nelson, Taylor & Phares, 1987), as well as an extrinsic personality orientation (Haywood, 1968a, b), it is likely that exceptional children are generally characterized by nonself-determined forms of motivation and may be at times amotivated. This does not mean that these children cannot display self-determined forms of motivation. Indeed, with the appropriate context and on certain tasks they can be regulated out of identified and integrated regulation, and may even become intrinsically motivated. However, it would appear that intrinsic motivation is not the main mover for these children (Haywood & Switzky, 1986). Let us now turn to the determinants and consequences of these various types of motivation.

Consequences and Determinants of Intrinsic, Extrinsic, and Amotivation

Intrinsic, extrinsic, and amotivation are related to determinants and consequences. That is, they are influenced by various situational and personal variables and in turn lead to various types of cognitive, affective, and behaviourial consequences. Below, we consider some of these determinants and consequences with a special emphasis on those which may be important for education in the context of physical activity.

Consequences of Intrinsic, Extrinsic, and Amotivation

Given that behaviour can be intrinsic, extrinsic, or amotivated, what are the consequences of these kinds of motivation for exceptional learners in human movement? Because the different kinds of motivation are supposedly on a continuum from high to low self-determination (Deci & Ryan, 1985), and because self-determination is associated with enhanced psychological functioning (Deci, 1980), one would expect a corresponding pattern of consequences. That is, one might expect intrinsic motivation to have the most positive consequences, followed by the self-determined forms of extrinsic motivation (integration and identification), nonself-determined types of extrinsic motivation (introjection and external regulation) and finally amotivation. External regulation and especially amotivation are hypothesized to lead to the most negative consequences.

Research conducted in experimental settings tends to support the above hypothesis. Performing activities out of intrinsic motivation (relative to nonself-determined types of extrinsic motivation) leads to several consequences of interest for the learning of human movement. For instance, intrinsic motivation is associated with greater cognitive flexibility, enhanced conceptual learning, greater interest, a more positive emotional tone, and higher self-esteem. In addition, intrinsic motivation also leads to higher creativity, performance and persistence (see Deci & Ryan, 1985, 1987, for reviews).

Results from a personality perspective by Haywood and his colleagues also support the findings from the social psychological perspective presented above. Such research reveals that retarded children with an intrinsic personality orientation (children who generally perform an activity for reasons associated with the task itself) learn better than those with an extrinsic personality orientation (children who generally participate in an activity for incentives not associated with the task, such as rewards, or threats; Haywood & Wachs, 1966). Trait intrinsic motivation has been found to be more important as children's IQ decreases. For instance, average IQ and educable mentally retarded children with an intrinsic personality orientation have been found to have achievement scores about one full school year higher than comparable children with an extrinsic personality orientation; a difference usually associated with at least 20 IQ points (Haywood, 1968b). While these latter results pertain to classroom performance and learning, similar results would be expected with physical activities.

There has been much less research on the self-determined types of extrinsic motivation because the distinction between the various forms of extrinsic motivation has only recently been made. However, emerging evidence indicates that self-determined forms of extrinsic motivation (i.e., identified and integrated regulation) are associated with positive consequences, although less so than intrinsic motivation (Blais, Sabourin, Boucher, & Vallerand, 1988; Connell & Ryan, 1986; Grolnick & Ryan, 1987; Vallerand & Bissonnette, 1988; Vallerand, Blais, Brière, & Pelletier, 1989; Vallerand & O'Connor, 1989).

Finally, amotivation has been found to have strong negative effects on a host of cognitive, affective, and behaviourial variables. For instance, it is associated with reductions in concentration, self-esteem, life satisfaction, performance, and persistence (Boggiano & Barrett, 1985; Vallerand & Bissonnette, 1988; Vallerand et al., 1989; Vallerand & O'Connor, 1989). In sum, the hypothesis that there are increasingly positive consequences as one moves from amotivation to intrinsic motivation has been confirmed in several studies in psychology. However, only one study, to the best of our knowledge, has tested this hypothesis within the context of physical activity. In that study (Brière, Vallerand, Blais, & Pelletier, 1988), amateur athletes from several sports completed a questionnaire assessing the various forms of motivation postulated by self-determination theory, except for integration. Athletes also completed scales tapping various types of consequences such as concentration, locus of control in sport, positive emotions experienced during participation in their sport, interest in their sport, and time spent in pleasant sport activities. Results from correlational analyses supported the hypothesis that there are increasingly positive consequences as one moves from amotivation to intrinsic motivation. Consistently, the most positive correlations were obtained between intrinsic motivation and positive outcomes, whereas the most negative correlations were found between amotivation and outcomes. Correlations involving the other types of motivation were in between these extremes, in line with predictions from the theory (Deci & Ryan, 1985).

Several of the consequences reviewed above are pertinent to physical activity with special populations. These children often show a lack of self-esteem, interest, control, and satisfaction (Chapman, 1988; Deshler & Schumaker, 1986; Kistner, Haskett, White, & Robbins, 1987). In light of the above research, and Haywood and Switzky's (1986) findings that special populations are characterized by an extrinsic personality orientation, it is plausible to assume that these consequences are engendered by nonself-determined forms of motivation and possibly by amotivation toward physical activity. However, perhaps the most severe problem that is generally encountered in physical activity with special populations is that of lack of persistence in physical activity. Indeed, since one of the major goals of physical activity within special education is to help children develop into self-regulating individuals (Paris & Oka, 1986) during the learning of basic human movement and to enjoy the practice of such activities (Lewko, 1978), this goal becomes unreachable if children refuse to engage in the activity at all. Recent studies reveal that motivation plays an important role in the persistence of activities. In two recent studies in education, it was found that students who dropped out of a compulsory course (Vallerand & Bissonnette, 1988) and of high school all together (Daoust, Vallerand, & Blais, 1988) were less intrinsically motivated, less identified and integrated, and more amotivated toward school-related activities than persistent students. These basic findings have been recently replicated in the context of sport where it was found that swimmers who intended to quit swimming had lower levels of intrinsic motivation and identification and higher levels of external regulation and amotivation than swimmers who intended to pursue swimming (Pelletier, Brière, Vallerand, & Blais, 1988).

Clearly, motivation plays an important part in persistence and other types of consequences in physical activity. Given the importance of these consequences for the teaching of adapted physical activity, it becomes important to better understand the determinants of the various types of motivation. A thorough understanding of the triggering motivational factors should facilitate the learning and enjoyment of human movement. We now turn to the study of these determinants.

Determinants of Intrinsic, Extrinsic, and Amotivation

According to the present theoretical approach, the human being is an active organism motivated by the needs to feel competent and self-determining. Individuals desire to be effective (White, 1959) and self-determining (deCharms, 1968; Deci, 1980) in their attempts to explore, grow, and develop. This innate tendency to grow, however, may be facilitated, stalled, or stopped because of the organism's vulnerability to being influenced by the environment. Several theories have been proposed in order to explain these social influences on the person's motivation (see Deci & Ryan, 1985; Vallerand et al., 1987). However, the most complete formulation appears to be cognitive evaluation theory (see Vallerand & Halliwell, 1983).

Since human motivation is based in the needs for self-determination and competence, cognitive evaluation theory (Deci, 1975; Deci & Ryan, 1980, 1985) suggests that any event which affects people's feelings and perceptions of self-determination or of competence can affect the various forms of motivation. Further, every event, whether a reward, a structure, or a communication, has three functional aspects; a controlling aspect, and informational aspect, and an amotivational aspect. Whenever one of these three aspects is perceived as being salient by the person, motivation will be affected by one of two factors: the perceived locus of causality and perceptions of competence. We now discuss the two processes in turn and present relevant research.

Perceived causality. Factors that lead to an internal perceived locus of causality enhance feelings of self-determination, which in turn enhance intrinsic motivation. On the other hand, when individuals perceive situations to be controlling, the perceived locus of causality becomes more external, self-determination is diminished, and intrinsic motivation is decreased. For example, providing children with choice regarding which activities to engage in should produce an internal locus of causality which should enhance intrinsic motivation. On the other hand, controlling children through the use of rewards ("If you play this game, you'll get a nice toy") should lead to an external locus of causality, which should eventually undermine intrinsic motivation.

Research has consistently supported these hypotheses. Experiences which undermine one's sense of self-determination such as providing rewards in the form of money (Deci, 1971), prizes (Harackiewicz, 1979), food (Ross, 1975), and good player awards (Lepper, Greene, & Nisbett, 1973) all tend to decrease intrinsic motivation. These findings have been replicated in the context of physical activity as well. For example, Orlick and Mosher (1978) tested the effects of receiving an award on children's subsequent intrinsic motivation toward an interesting motor task (the stabilometer). First, the children had a free-choice period (during which intrinsic motivation was measured). Then, children played in order to receive a trophy (task-contingent reward condition) or for no reason at all (control condition). Intrinsic motivation was again measured during a free-choice period which followed the imposition of experimental conditions. Results revealed that, in line with the findings mentioned previously, subjects in the reward condition displayed a decrease in intrinsic motivation from the pre- to post-session. Other studies using motor tasks have also obtained similar findings (Halliwell, 1978; Thomas & Tennant, 1978).

The negative effects on intrinsic motivation has not been restricted to material rewards. Other studies, mostly from psychology laboratories, have revealed that deadlines (Amabile, Dejong, & Lepper, 1976), surveillance (Lepper & Greene, 1975), threats (Deci & Cascio, 1972), and competing to win at all costs (Deci, Betley, Kahle, Abrams & Porac, 1981a; Vallerand, Gauvin, & Halliwell, 1986a) also undermine self-determination and intrinsic motivation. It thus appears that external events that tend to pressure people to behave in specific ways and that are experienced as being controlling also tend to undermine intrinsic motivation. Although we believe that these findings also apply to special populations, no study to date has replicated these findings with such populations in the context of physical activity and this represents an important research agenda for the future.

When the controlling aspect of the event is low, and autonomy support is conveyed by the context, the perceived locus of causality can then become more internal. Self-determination and intrinsic motivation can then be augmented. Thus, research suggests that enhancing self-determination through choice opportunities increases intrinsic motivation toward cognitive (e.g., Swann & Pittman, 1977; Zuckerman, Porac, Lathin, Smith, & Deci, 1978) and motor tasks (Brawley & Vallerand, 1986; Thompson & Wankel, 1980).

Promoting self-determination should also enhance self-determined forms of extrinsic motivation: the individual will experience a sense of purpose and direction in the performance of activities that are not inherently interesting (Ryan et al., 1985). Conversely, a decrease in feelings of self-determination should increase nonself-determined extrinsic motivation and eventually amotivation, because the individual may become dependent upon others to provide direction. For example, encouraging exceptional children to feel responsible for practising less interesting activities should lead to an internal locus of causality which should augment self-determined types of extrinsic motivation toward these activities (see Eghrari & Deci, 1986). On the other hand, if students are simply told to engage in the tasks without encouragement for self-responsibility or clear rationale for doing so, there is a risk of inducing an external locus of causality which could enhance nonself-determined forms of extrinsic motivation, dependence on the teachers, and perhaps eventually amotivation.

While research has yet to focus explicitly on the link between self-determination and motivation with special populations, recent studies are nevertheless supportive. For instance, in one study (Smith et al., 1987), special education students either took part in a regular program or in an experimental program which encouraged perceived personal control. Results showed that students in the experimental program reported higher levels of perceived control and more positive attitudes toward school than students in the regular program. Similar results have also been obtained with low-achieving students (deCharms, 1976). Furthermore, a program which encourages active participation in learning from the children's part has been found to increase performance (Pratton & Hales, 1986). It is therefore likely that providing exceptional children with opportunities for self-determination increases their intrinsic motivation and self-determined extrinsic motivation, which in turn should produce beneficial outcomes. Children provided with opportunities for autonomy should have higher levels of intrinsic and self-determined extrinsic motivation towards the practice of physical activities and may engage in such activities more frequently and with more zest, leading them to derive more satisfaction and meaning from their performance. However, this remains to be empirically tested with this specific population.

Perceived competence. Perceptions of competence (Deci, 1975; see also Roberts, 1984) and self-efficacy (Bandura, 1977) also have an impact on intrinsic motivation, especially when the informational aspect of the event is salient. The informational aspect of the event is said to be salient when individuals receive information relevant to their competence at a meaningful task for which they feel personal causation of self-determination. For example, positive competence feedback and success experiences enhance intrinsic motivation (e.g., Blanck, Reis, & Jackson, 1984; Sansone, 1986; Vallerand, 1983; Vallerand & Reid, 1984, 1988). Several studies in the context of physical activity have supported this effect. For instance, Weinberg and Jackson (1979) provided subjects with success or failure feedback following performance on the stabilometer motor task. Results revealed that subjects in the success condition reported higher levels of intrinsic motivation than subjects in the failure condition. Other research supports the cognitive evaluation theory postulate that perceptions and feelings of competence mediate between the effects of positive feedback and success experiences on intrinsic motivation (Harter & Connell, 1984; Vallerand & Reid, 1984, 1988).

Research with special populations is in agreement with such findings. In a study with learning disabled students, Lincoln and Chazan (1979) reported that these students perceived themselves as less competent and intrinsically motivated in the school domain than regular students. In other studies, the impact of different remedial programs on perceptions of competence and intrinsic motivation were assessed (Bandura & Schunk, 1981; Fuchs, Fuchs, & Tindal, 1986). For instance, in the Bandura and Schunk study, students with important difficulties in mathematics were assigned to different self-directed learning conditions of either distal (long term) goals, proximal (short term) goals, no goals or no treatment. In the distal condition, subjects were simply told to complete the entire set of 42 pages of math problems by the end of the seventh and final session. Subjects in the proximal goal condition were encouraged to set themselves the goal of completing at least six pages of math problems each session. Finally, subjects in the other two conditions did not receive any mention of goals. Assessment of subjects included perceived self-efficacy (or perceived confidence) and intrinsic motivation. It was hypothesized that students in the proximal goal condition would perceive themselves as more competent and intrinsically motivated than subjects in the other groups because the program would enable them to experience several instances of success. Repeated success was hypothesized to enhance students' perceptions of competence which in turn would increase their intrinsic motivation. Results supported the authors' hypotheses. It thus appears likely that perceived competence affects handicapped learners' intrinsic motivation in a similar fashion as it affects that of regular students.

An important consideration with the competence feedback, is that it must be given in a context of self-determination, otherwise it will be perceived as controlling and nonself-determined types of extrinsic motivation will be enhanced at the expense of intrinsic motivation (Fisher, 1978; Ryan, 1982). Thus, congratulating students for having freely engaged in physical activities should promote feelings of competence which should increase intrinsic motivation. On the other hand, continually telling students that they are doing good work because their initiatives serve to reduce the teacher's workload could eventually lead to feelings of being controlled, which should reduce intrinsic motivation and facilitate nonself-determined forms of extrinsic motivation. In such instances, students may not engage in such activities anymore unless prodded by the teacher.

Finally, when the amotivating aspect of the event is salient, individuals perceive no control over the environment, feel incompetent, and their intrinsic motivation is reduced (Deci & Ryan, 1985). For instance, research suggests that negative competence feedback undermines one's sense of competence and decreases intrinsic motivation (Vallerand & Reid, 1984, 1988; Weinberg & Jackson, 1979). In one study, Vallerand and Reid (1984) assessed the effects of positive, negative, and no-verbal feedback on intrinsic motivation toward the stabilometer motor task. Following a pretest, subjects were assigned to one of the three feedback conditions. Results revealed that negative verbal feedback (e.g., "You're not doing very well on this task") decreased subjects' intrinsic motivation relative to the pretest scores as well as relative to the other two groups. When experienced on a regularly basis, negative feedback can eventually lead to amotivation and withdrawal (Boggiano & Barrett, 1985; Peterson & Seligman, 1984). It is believed that this may apply to children who have experienced a prolonged history of failure with respect to several school-related activities, including physical activity.

Another variable which affects perceived competence, and thus indirectly motivation is the attribution emitted by the child to explain his or her performance. It has been repeatedly shown that internal attributions for one's success increase feelings of competence, while the same attributions for one's failure decrease competence percepts (see Weiner, 1985). Perceptions and feelings of competence in turn enhance intrinsic motivation, while feelings of incompetence undermine it (Vallerand & Blais, 1986; Vallerand & Reid, 1984, 1988) and should eventually lead to amotivation. Normally-achieving children usually attribute their success to internal factors but their failure to external factors. Such a strategy allows them to preserve their intrinsic interest in the activity, even in the face of failure. However, learning-disability students are more likely to attribute failure to their lack of ability and their success to external factors such as luck or the teacher's help (Jacobsen, Lowery & DuCette, 1986; Pearl, 1982; Pearl, Bryan & Donahue, 1980). It thus follows that the intrinsic and self-determined forms of motivation of these children are likely to be low and to remain low following both success and failure. Research by Schunk (1989) has shown that in instances where students have developed a faulty attributional style, ability attributional feedback from the teacher (e.g., "You're good at this") may help students internally attribute their success, experience feelings of competence, persist longer at the task and eventually perform better on it (see Schunk & Cox, 1986). In light of the above findings, research along those lines with special populations on motor tasks would therefore appear important as it might lead to useful applications.

Individual differences. Cognitive evaluation theory (Deci & Ryan, 1985) posits that the effects of various situational variables on motivation are produced through the meaning that these variables convey to the individual. Most of the studies reviewed so far have explored this concept by manipulating the event or its context, thereby making the controlling, informational, or amotivating aspect more salient. However, individuals also carry with them idiosyncratic ways of perceiving situations and events, and these differences can affect the extent to which the controlling and informational aspects of events are salient for them. Recent research suggests that these individual differences may modify substantially the effects of various situational variables on motivation.

One such variable is locus of control. One's locus of control can be internal or external. The locus of control is internal when one has the beliefs that outcomes that occur are contingent upon one's actions. On the other hand, individuals have an external orientation of control when they believe that they have no effects on events that happen to them (e.g., Rotter, 1966). Much research with mentally handicapped and learning disabled children, reveals that they generally possess an external locus of control (Lawrence & Winchell, 1975; Smith et al., 1987) and that such an external orientation mitigates the positive effects of various social motivators such as positive feedback (Heitman & Justen, 1980).

In a recent study, Earn (1982, Exp. 1) explored the interactive effects of locus of control and rewards on intrinsic motivation toward puzzles. In a first study, internal and external locus of control subjects were randomly assigned to work on a puzzle task under conditions of ambiguous rewards or no rewards. It was predicted that when rewards were presented in an ambiguous way, such that it was not clear whether they were controlling or informational, they should increase intrinsic motivation for internals and decrease intrinsic motivation for externals. Results supported the hypothesis. Earn suggested that internals tend to interpret rewards as informational because of their beliefs in influencing their environment, whereas externals tend to interpret them as controlling, because they are used to have no control over the environment. Consequently, rewards increase the intrinsic motivation of internals but decrease that of externals. Results of a second study by Earn (1982, Exp. 2) supported his interpretation.

Another personality variable which has received some attention is that of the intrinsic personality orientation. Trait intrinsic motivation refers to a general tendency to do things out of intrinsic motivation. For instance, Boggiano and Barrett (1985) ascertained the effects of success and failure feedback on intrinsically and extrinsically oriented students. The authors postulated that positive feedback to extrinsics would be experienced as more controlling and would therefore decrease intrinsic motivation, whereas positive feedback would be experienced as informational for intrinsics and would therefore enhance their intrinsic motivation. Results confirmed their hypothesis. It was found that positive feedback led to higher levels of intrinsic motivation for the intrinsically oriented than for the extrinsically-oriented children. In addition, although the extrinsics displayed a decrease of intrinsic motivation following the failure feedback, the intrinsics did not. Apparently, the intrinsics interpreted failure as a challenge which enhanced their interest toward the activity.

Similar findings have been obtained with mentally handicapped children. For instance, research by Haywood and Switzky has shown consistently that children with an intrinsic personality orientation work harder, persist longer, explore more, and perform better under task incentive conditions (e.g., under low pressure to perform), whereas extrinsic personality orientation children display the above characteristics under extrinsic incentive condition (e.g., conditions wherein rewards are offered for performance; Haywood & Weaver, 1967; Switzky & Haywood, 1974; see also Haywood & Switzky, 1986 for a review).

Overall, the above findings suggest that it may be particularly difficult to facilitate the intrinsic and self-determined forms of motivation of exceptional children. Indeed, since "facilitative" variables such as success feedback may be interpreted in a controlling way, while undermining variables such as rewards and failure feedback may be interpreted even more negatively, it would appear that enhancing self-determined forms of motivation in exceptional children is a particular challenge. We will discuss this further in the section on implications.

The impact of teachers. So far, we have discussed the impact of a host of situational variables on motivation. However, in the context of physical activity, many of these variables are under the influence of the teacher. It would therefore appear that depending on the teacher, these variables may be used in a controlling or in a supportive and informative way. Through their behaviours, teachers can also either control the children's behaviour or support their autonomy. The former condition would be predicted to facilitate a more external perceived locus of causality in their pupils, while the latter would be predicted to facilitate a more internal one. Deci, Ryan and their colleagues (Deci, Schwartz, Sheinman, & Ryan, 1981c) have devised an instrument (The Problems in School Questionnaire) to assess the teachers' style of relating to children and then related it to the children's intrinsic motivation, perceived competence, and self-esteem. Results revealed that students of controlling teachers displayed less intrinsic motivation, perceived competence, and self-esteem than children of autonomy-supportive teachers (see Deci, Nezlek, & Sheinman, 1981b). These findings have been replicated in the realm of sport where it was found that athletes who perceived their coach to be more informational had higher intrinsic motivation and self-esteem than those who perceived their coach to be more controlling (Vallerand & Pelletier, 1985).

In another study, Pelletier and Vallerand (1985) presented swimmers with descriptions of hypothetical swimming coaches who varied in terms of their controlling versus autonomy-supportive style. Swimmers were then asked to indicate what their motivation would be if they had each of these coaches. Results indicated that athletes would be most intrinsically motivated with the autonomy-supportive coach but most externally regulated with the controlling coach. Finally, in the Pelletier et al. (1988) study discussed earlier, students' perceptions of their coaches along the dimensions of control and autonomy support were also assessed. Results revealed a coherent picture of the relationship between the perceived coaching style and students' motivation. Specifically, perceptions of autonomy support from the coach were found to positively relate to intrinsic and self-determined forms of extrinsic motivation while perceptions of a controlling style was positively related to nonself-determined forms of extrinsic motivation and to a lesser extent to amotivation. Finally, the autonomy-supportive style was also negatively associated with amotivation.

As applied to the teaching of human movement, these findings suggest that students' perceptions of their teachers have potent effects on their motivation. It appears that different dimensions of teaching behaviours may relate to students' different types of motivation. An autonomy-supportive interpersonal style may facilitate intrinsic and self-determined types of extrinsic motivation as well as prevent amotivation. On the other hand, a controlling teaching style may encourage dependency and nonself-determined forms of extrinsic motivation and perhaps facilitate amotivation. Thus, an autonomy-supportive style should be encouraged. However, it should be underscored that the above findings have been obtained with very specific types of physical activity (sports) and populations (regular athletes). Research is needed to reproduce these findings within the context of other types of physical activity and with special populations.

In light of the importance of the coach's behaviour on athletes' intrinsic motivation, Vallerand and Pelletier (1985; see also Vallerand et al., 1987) attempted to identify some of the determinants of coaches' interpersonal behaviours and have postulated a model to capture the interplay among several variables that influence the athletes' intrinsic motivation within the context of the coach-player relationship. It is our belief that this model holds as well for the teacher-student relationship within the context of adapted physical education. This model is depicted in Figure 1. As can be seen, the model proposes that students' intrinsic motivation is a function of the teachers' behaviour and/or students' perceptions of such behaviour, mediated by perceived competence and self-esteem. As can also be seen in Figure 1, three determinants of teachers' behaviours have been identified so far. A first source of influence deals with the teachers' generalized interpersonal style (controlling/autonomy support), which is believed to be a part of their personality. Research in classrooms (Deci et al., 1981c; Deci, Spiegel, Ryan, Koestner & Kauffman, 1982; Ryan & Grolnick, 1986) and sports (Pelletier & Vallerand, 1985; Vallerand & Pelletier, 1985) suggests that this variable may also be important in adapted physical activity settings.

A second important source of influence on a teacher's behaviour resides in the situation or context in which the teacher operates. To the extent that teachers feel pressured and controlled by their context, they are predicted to respond by being more controlling toward their students. Recent research (Deci et al., 1982; Harackiewicz & Larson, 1986) reveals that this is more likely to occur if the teacher's job or salary depended on students' performance.

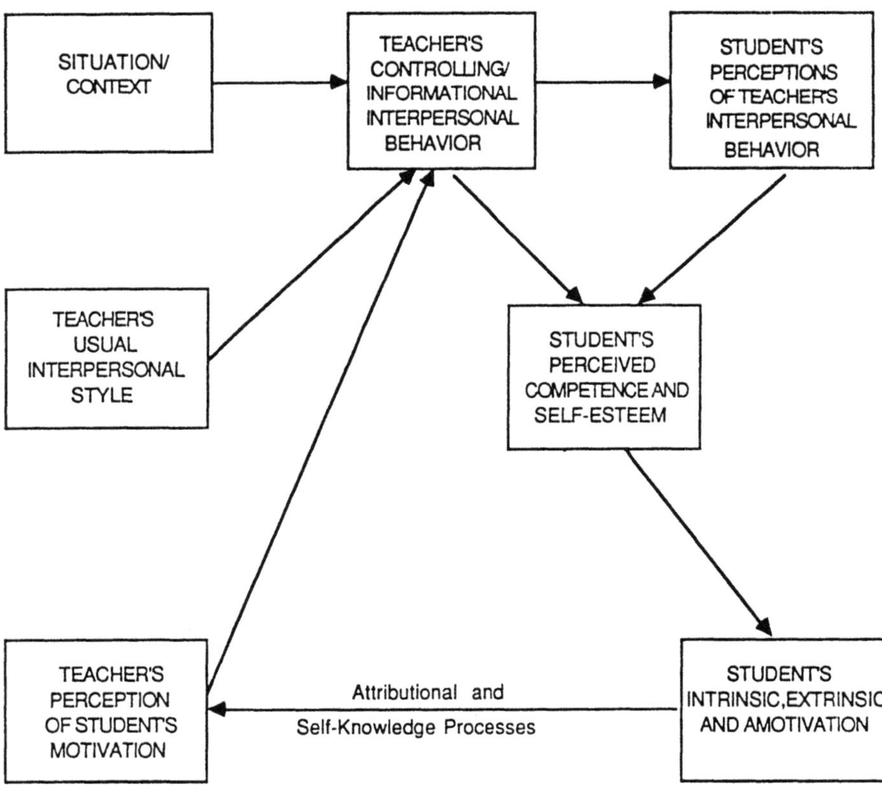

Figure 1: Vallerand and Pelletier's (1985) model of the determinants of the teacher's behaviors and how these may affect the intrinsic, extrinsic, and amotivation of the student.

Finally, a third source of influence on teachers' behaviour concerns their perceptions of their students' motivation. Several studies in the context of physical activity have shown that teachers' expectations regarding students' performance lead them to behave differently toward the students which in turn affects the actual performance of the latter individuals (Horn, 1984; Martinek, 1981; Martinek & Karper, 1984; Rejeski, Daracott, & Hutslar, 1979). This phenomenon has been termed the "self-fulfilling prophecy" (Rosenthal & Jacobson, 1968). A vast amount of research conducted in classroom (Rosenthal & Rubin, 1978) and laboratory settings (Snyder, 1984; Snyder, Tanke, & Berscheid, 1977) has shown that such effects are pervasive and can take place even if the initial perceptions are false. Thus, to the extent that teachers perceive students to be intrinsically motivated and self-determined, they should be more likely to act in an autonomy-supportive way. On the other hand, perceiving students as extrinsically motivated should lead teachers to act in a controlling way in order to ensure that expected behaviours are executed as expected. This may be especially important with special populations. These students are often labelled as "unmotivated" or "tough to teach". [Although this may be true for many of them (see Tzuriel & Haywood, 1985), it is certainly not true for all children.] The teacher may come in with these beliefs in mind and may adjust his or her behaviours to suit the beliefs. In so doing, the beliefs in low levels of student motivation may turn into reality, thereby killing whatever motivation was left in the child.

A recent laboratory study by Pelletier and Vallerand (1989) has attempted to show how this "beliefs create reality" sequence operates in a teaching context by leading teachers to believe that the student they were about to teach how to solve interesting puzzles was either intrinsically or extrinsically motivated (in this case through external regulation). Results showed that teachers who were (falsely) led to believe that the student was extrinsically motivated became controlling toward the student which, in turn, led the latter to become less intrinsically motivated toward the puzzles. On the other hand, teachers who thought that they were interacting with an intrinsically motivated student became more autonomy supportive and instilled intrinsic motivation in their students. Thus, beliefs about the student's motivation had turned into reality.

In sum, it appears that teachers' behaviours toward their students can have profound influences on the latter's motivation. The proposed model of Vallerand and Pelletier (1985) appears to account well for the accumulated data and seems to provide with a reasonable account of the existing situation in adapted physical activity. However, research is needed to test more directly some of the above hypotheses with exceptional children in the context of human movement.

Practical Implications

In light of the research presented in this chapter we are now in a better position to derive a certain number of practical implications for the teaching of physical activity to handicapped and unsuccessful students. These implications can be regrouped under three headings: (a) promoting self-determination, (b) promoting feelings of competence, and (c) teachers' orientations toward children. These are discussed in turn.

Promoting Self-Determination

In 1978, Lewko suggested that, "The goal of having handicapped children demonstrate desire to participate in sport-recreation activities of their own accord ... should be the major socialization goal for handicapped children in sport" (p. 273). In effect, Lewko is suggesting that one of the major goals of adapted physical activity should be to encourage children to become self-determined and intrinsically motivated toward physical activity. We could not agree more. If children are to profit from the physiological and psychological benefits derived from sustained participation in physical activity (Browne & Mahoney, 1984; Taylor, Sallis, & Needle, 1985), they need to develop the necessary motivation to help them go through failure experiences with renewed energy to grow and to develop. Self-determination can provide such energy. Thus, one of our tasks must deal with the promotion of self-determination. In this regard, research suggests that a certain number of variables must be used with extreme caution. This is the case of material rewards. The negative effects of participation-contingent rewards (those offered to lead the student to engage in the activity) on intrinsic motivation are well known. They induce a shift toward an external locus of causality and thus lead to intrinsic motivation decrements (see Deci & Ryan, 1985, 1987, for reviews).

However, the above findings have been generally obtained with children with a high interest in the activity (see Deci & Ryan, 1985). Thus, participation-contingent rewards are not recommended with the latter individuals. However, additional research (e.g., Loveland & Olley, 1979; McLoyd, 1979) reveals that participation-contingent rewards may be helpful in leading children with low initial interest in the activity to engage more frequently in it. It thus follows that for some persons with disabilities, for instance, who are functioning at an amotivational level, participation-contingent rewards may be necessary in the initial stages. However, teachers should make sure that rewards are removed through fading techniques so that the new behaviour eventually becomes self-determined.

Performance-contingent rewards (those offered when a given level of performance is attained) are a little more tricky. They may convey a message of competence to recipients and thus may enhance their intrinsic motivation (Lopez, 1981). However, it should be recalled that it is the recipients' perceptions of the reward which determine its effects on intrinsic motivation. If recipients perceive the controlling aspect of the reward as highly salient, then even the performance-contingent reward will undermine students' intrinsic and self-determined forms of extrinsic motivation. In addition, these rewards may also convey a message of incompetence and consequently decrease the intrinsic motivation of those who are not good enough to obtain the award (Vallerand, Gauvin, & Halliwell, 1986b). Thus, the use of any type of reward is potentially detrimental to motivation and should be kept at a strict minimum.

Other variables, however, may be used effectively to promote self-determination, interest, and fun toward physical activity. Choice is one such variable. Choice may take various forms depending on students' age and proficiency. Allowing young children to decide which warm-up drills to engage in may be a first step on a road to self-determined participation in physical activity. As students become more mature, they also should be encouraged to try to discover how to perform various movements. Several programs which emphasize active participation (Pratton & Hales,1986), control (Smith et al., 1987), and mastery (Fuchs et al., 1986) from the students' part have been found beneficial in students' learning, performance, and enjoyment. By permitting students to be in charge of some elements inherent in their participation, and to enjoy the process of doing so, teachers allow youngsters to derive ownership from their participation (Cohen, 1986), and may instill positive attitudes toward physical activity which may go a long way toward a life-long involvement in physical exercise.

Goal setting is another variable which may be used effectively in facilitating students' intrinsic and self-determined forms of motivation. This is likely to take place when goals are self-determined (Mossholder, 1980). This is not to say that teachers should let students decide entirely by themselves which goals to set. One must make the difference between a laisser faire and an autonomy-supportive approach to goal setting. In the laisser faire approach, the teacher lets the student decide what is the appropriate goal without providing adequate structure and input to assure that the student is in a position to choose appropriate goals for his or her development. On the other hand, an autonomy-supportive approach allows for the experience of freedom within certain prescribed limits determined in part by the teacher's perceptions of the student's needs. Appropriate limits, especially when presented in a supportive way do not decrease intrinsic motivation toward the activity (Koestner, Ryan, Bernieri, & Holt, 1984). However, they may ensure that the student's will make choices in a context of support which will lead to success experiences in the student's quest for autonomous learning.

An important point to consider with respect to goal setting, is that such an autonomy-supportive approach to goal setting (and choice) must be made gradually. The teacher must be able to gauge when students are ready to accept more responsibility in the self-determining process. Providing too much input too quickly may lead individuals to feel incompetent in the process of being autonomous and may induce amotivation and dependence on the teacher. On the other hand, not providing enough self-determination may provoke frustration and reactance. This gradual increase in self-determination, as handicapped individuals become more competent, is important since, it should increase intrinsic and self-determined forms of motivation toward physical activity. When one takes into consideration exceptional children's history of dependency toward significant others (including teachers), as well as their low levels of intrinsic motivation for new mastery attempts (Lincoln & Chazan, 1979), it becomes rather obvious that initially at least, allowing for too much self-determination can lead to disastrous consequences which may reduce the individual's already low level of interest toward the activity. When properly gauged, however, gradual increases in self-determination should lead to heightened levels of motivation toward the activity. It is encouraging to see that this progression from external guidance to self-determined engagement has been incorporated in recent adapted physical activity programs (Watkinson & Wall, 1982).

Perhaps a few words should be said about competition. We have seen in this chapter that participating in order to beat other participants rather than to better oneself has negative effects on one's intrinsic motivation and fun derived from participation (Deci et al., 1981a; Vallerand et al., 1986a). Thus, teachers should be careful in employing this motivational device: although it may lead to participation in activities, such participation may not be self-determined, and eventually participation under less controlling situations may cease. In addition, competitive contexts often serve to emphasize students' incompetence in the eyes of their peers. When presented in this fashion, competition may not appear as very appealing to unsuccessful students who have a history of failing.

However, it does not have to be this way. Competition does not have to be presented in a context wherein there is only one winner and several losers, and where students feel that they must win at all costs. Teachers should be aware that competition can also be presented as a fun event wherein the presence of competitors allows students to experience excitement while testing their skills. Students should feel that it is acceptable to lose and that one can still grow, learn, and have fun in the process. However, children should also have the opportunity to win. Losing continually entails that one is incompetent, which should eventually undermine intrinsic and self-determined forms of motivation. These last comments underscore the importance of structuring competitive environments so that competitors are evenly matched, and thus can derive fun in the mastery process inherent in competition. When competition is presented in such a fashion, it can have positive effects on intrinsic motivation (Reeve, Olson, & Cole, 1985).

On the other hand, one should recognize that other forms of games and physical activity contexts do exist. Cooperation represents one such context. For instance, Daoust and Vallerand (1987) have shown that cooperation increases intrinsic motivation toward cognitive tasks relative to competition. In addition, cooperative programs have been used with much success in education (Ames, 1984; Aronson & Osherow, 1980; Johnson & Johnson, 1985; Slavin, 1986). Johnson and Johnson (1985) have reported that cooperative structures help to enhance learning disabled and physically handicapped students' sense of self-esteem and attitudes toward school. Several well prepared texts on cooperative games are available in the area of physical activity (Orlick, 1978a, 1978b). In light of the many positive consequences associated with cooperative ventures, teachers should familiarize themselves with such games. Cooperation is therefore recommended in physical activity settings not as much as an alternative but as a complement to competition. We feel that all children, handicapped or not, should learn that it is appropriate to both cooperate and compete. What they have to learn is when it is desirable to compete and when it is to cooperate (Aronson & Osherow, 1980). When children feel self-determined and at ease in their interactions with others, be they cooperative or competitive in nature, fun and interest are likely to flourish as are the various consequences associated with these more self-determined forms of motivation.

Another motivational device which may be used is that of modelling. When using modelling, the teacher may ask an intrinsically motivated student to display his/her interest while performing a given activity. This interest toward the task may be "picked up" by fellow students who may then undergo an increase of intrinsic interest. Recent research (Cellar & Barrett, 1987; Cellar & Wade, 1988) supports this basic interpretation. However, it is our belief that in order to be effective, modelling must be used in a noncontrolling context. Thus, teachers are encouraged not to use the proverbial "See Mary over there - see how she tries to do the task. Why don't you do like her?". Such statements are controlling and in all likelihood will lead modelling to be ineffective. When used in an informational way, however, modelling should be particularly effective.

Promoting Feelings of Competence

As we have demonstrated in this chapter, perceptions and feelings of competence represent another process through which motivation may vary. Several variables have been found to influence feelings of competence, and these should be of concern to teachers. In this regard, verbal feedback represents an important variable to consider. Teachers' feedback is very often the measurement index used by students to assess their competence (Horn & Hasbrook, 1987). Teachers may forget this at times. Negative feedback such as "Why did you miss the movement John? Can't you do anything right?" conveys a clear message. It is tantamount to suggesting that the student is incompetent and worthless. On the other hand, a message such as "Nice try, John. You'll get it next time", acknowledges that it is all right to miss the movement. The student's sense of competence is not being questioned. In addition, the teacher might take the student aside and suggest that some work may be needed in order to improve his/her skills. When such a suggestion is made in the context of support (in an informational way) students do not feel that their self-esteem is on the line. They do not perceive themselves as lesser individuals. Rather, they see the opportunity to grow and better oneself within a context of support from the teacher and peers. This type of performance feedback should therefore help sustain students' intrinsic motivation or at least self-determined forms of extrinsic motivation in the face of failure.

Positive feedback is generally not problematic. Most teachers make ample use of positive feedback when commenting on students' performance (Lewko, 1978). We know that such feedback generally produces positive effects on students' perceived competence and intrinsic motivation. What might be problematic, however, is the context within which positive feedback is used. For instance, if students receive positive feedback only when they perform well, they may feel that all that counts for the teacher is that they perform up to standards. Students may feel controlled and their intrinsic motivation may decrease. Teachers should also be aware that overemphasizing ability praise may not always facilitate intrinsic motivation. At times effort praise may be more suited, especially when the child is attempting to master new movements on his own (Koestner, Zuckerman, & Koestner, 1987). Thus, positive feedback while generally leading the individual to feel competent and intrinsically motivated may also be perceived as being controlling and may at times have deleterious effects on students' intrinsic motivation, especially those who suffer from already low levels of perceived competence and control (Boggiano, Main, & Katz, 1988). It should therefore be used with care.

In addition to providing students with positive and informative feedback, teachers can also arrange physical settings so that children experience success experiences. This is especially important with special populations who have a long history of repeated failure. Success may not happen without some task intervention. In this vein, the use of task analysis which identifies prerequisite skills and subdivides a task into progressively more difficult phases is an effective means to enable the person to be successful. Curriculum models in adapted physical education (e.g., Knowles, Vogel, & Wessel, 1975; Watkinson & Wall, 1982) have adopted the task analysis teaching strategy. The positive effects of this approach can be readily understood in terms of cognitive evaluation theory. Achieving several sub-goals (while failing at a relatively few) should provide one with a sense of competence leading to an increase in intrinsic motivation toward the task and the desire to master new tasks and movements.

Leisure counselling may prove very useful in this context of structuring the physical activity environment. Leisure counselling is the process through which the leisure skills, aspirations, opportunities and needs of an individual are explored (Taylor, 1987). Through dialogue with a counsellor, the goals and barriers to leisure fulfilment are dealt with. Observations and even initial practice of a new activity may help the counsellor and individual select activities which match the person's skills and needs. In this manner, children's feelings and perceptions of competence should be increased thereby leading to high levels of intrinsic motivation toward the new activity. In addition, because the task has been carefully selected, chances are that it will be mastered, eventually boosting the child's overall sense of self-esteem. This in turn should help the child to have a different outlook toward new activities, and lead him or her to freely engage in these activities, feeling that they can be mastered.

While providing positive feedback and structuring tasks to be performed may be sufficient for several unsuccessful learners to feel competent and more motivated to tackle new forms of movement, it may happen that for some individuals these two motivational devices are not sufficient. This is likely to happen with children who display severe cases of failure history and who have come to believe that failure is due to their lack of ability while success is due to luck or other external factors such as help from the teacher. These children have developed a faulty attributional style (Abramson et al., 1978; Weiner, 1985) which prevents them from feeling competent following success, and conversely leads them to feel exaggeratedly incompetent following failure, with the ensuing negative motivational consequences. Past research within the context of physical activity (Vallerand & Blais, 1986; Weinberg & Jackson, 1979), has demonstrated that attributions play an important motivational role through their influence on feelings of competence. Thus, by changing children's faulty attributions it would be feasible to change their perceptions of competence and consequently their motivation toward physical activities.

Much research with regular (see Forsterling, 1986; Peterson & Seligman, 1984) and learning disabled students (Borkowski, Weyhing, & Carr, 1988; Litch & Kistner, 1986) reveals that reattribution training may prove useful in changing children's faulty attributions, improving their feelings of competence and motivation, as well as enhancing their performance. This is likely to occur when success is attributed to exerted effort and failure to lack of effort. This is because effort is an internal but unstable cause (Weiner, 1985). The stability of the cause implies that both success and failure are under the person's control and especially with respect to failure, that it can be changed. According to Forsterling (1986), reattribution training involves four phases: (a) telling and modelling for children that when they fail they must try harder, (b) prompting children to verbalize effort, (c) reinforcing children for such attributions, and (d) linking new attributions to new successes in order to promote their validity (Licht, 1983; Ruble & Boggiano, 1980; Thomas & Pahely, 1982).

While the use of effort attributions in reattribution training has led to several positive consequences, one should be aware of its limits. An important point to consider is that attributions should remain realistic (Schunk, 1989). It is conceivable that continually and indiscriminately admonishing one to try harder on a skilled task in which the person is biologically limited may create frustrations (Fincham, 1983; Grimes, 1981). Simply using more energy is not likely to overcome a deficit or result in satisfaction for the person with such a limitation. Also, effort attributions following failure in which the child has offered a supreme effort could lead to the conclusion that one is highly incompetent and to amotivation (Jacobsen et al., 1986). Remediating the deficit directly with appropriate instruction, goal setting, and being sensitive to real but sometimes modest improvement must accompany effort attributions. In addition, as children become more and more proficient at the task, they should gradually be led to attribute their success to their ability (Schunk, 1989). Because ability is an internal and stable cause (Weiner, 1985), it is more likely to instill a more permanent sense of competence than effort attributions when mastery of the task is eventually accomplished. Ability attributions following success should then be expected to enhance children's feelings of competence and consequently their intrinsic and self-determined forms of motivation. It thus appears that reattribution training represents an important component to a remedial physical activity program. Unfortunately, no study to date has specifically assessed the effects of such training on special populations' motivation toward physical activities and this would represent an important research issue to consider.

Teachers' Orientations Toward Children

Thus far, we have discussed the effects of various variables that are present in the realm of physical activity. We would like to underscore the fact that these variables do not exist in a vacuum. Indeed, the very meaning conveyed by rewards, choice, goal setting, feedback and other variables comes to life through the use teachers make of these variables. This is where we can best discern the controlling from the autonomy-supportive teacher. While both types of teachers might use the above variables in their interactions with students, the controlling teachers use them in order to have students perform as they see fit. For this type of teacher, variables which may generally be considered as informational may be perceived as controlling by students. On the other hand, the autonomy-supportive teacher fosters students' self-determination and supports their attempts toward gradual autonomous mastery. Thus, some motivational tools that are typically perceived as controlling may be considered as informational by students when used by teachers with an autonomy-supportive style.

In light of the many findings reported in this chapter, an autonomy-supportive interactional style is clearly recommended. To develop such an interactional style is not easy. It often involves a change of focus from one's own goals to that of the students. In addition, it may also mean additional work on one's communication skills (e.g., Miller, 1982). An ideal way for physical educators to improve the quality of feedback provided is to ask for supervision during interactions with handicapped individuals. This supervision can be performed by fellow instructors and can lead to interesting exchanges. If this proves impossible to do, however, it becomes very important for teachers to make use of their own sense of awareness in determining when they behave in a controlling or autonomy-supportive fashion. Once one has a good idea of what his or her interactional style is, it becomes easier to implement the desired changes. Teachers should be aware of the various social and personal influences which may impinge on their interactional style with their students. By increasing such an awareness, the teacher may become less affected by such forces and consequently less controlling with the students. The adoption of an autonomy-supportive approach to teaching allows for many rewards which go way beyond the immediate context and is strongly encouraged.

Future Directions and Conclusion

Physical activity is a domain in which intrinsic interest, fun, and excitement should predominate. Unfortunately, for a relatively important percentage of people, such positive consequences are not readily attainable. In this chapter, we have argued that motivation plays a crucial role in allowing individuals to enjoy themselves while learning important movement skills. In so doing, we have reviewed a large portion of research mainly conducted in laboratory and educational settings which demonstrates that when students' self-determination and competence are facilitated, intrinsic and self-determined forms of motivation are enhanced, thereby leading to a host of adaptive consequences. Recent research conducted within the context of sports and physical activity with regular students and athletes supports the relevance of such a literature for adapted physical activity settings. However, it is obvious that research specifically conducted with special populations in physical activity settings is sorely needed. In this regard, three directions seem important. A first one deals with the need to develop the necessary methodology to test hypotheses such as the ones discussed in this chapter. More specifically, this amounts to developing a scale to measure the various types of extrinsic motivation postulated by Deci and Ryan (1985). Some sport motivation questionnaires exist already (Dwyer, Grant, & Fischer, 1988; Weiss, Bredemeier & Shewchuk, 1985). However, these are limited to the measurement of intrinsic motivation and do not assess amotivation and the various types of motivation. Recently, Brière et al. (1988) have developed a scale which measures the various types of motivation postulated by Deci and Ryan in the context of sport. This scale has demonstrated very adequate reliability and validity indices. A similar scale could be developed for the realm of physical activity specifically for special populations. The development of such a scale would appear very important as it would allow to replicate some of the research conducted in other domains, as well as to allow the testing of several new hypotheses specific to the adapted physical activity field.

A second research direction that would appear important for the field of adapted physical activity deals with the assessment of the effects of teachers' orientation on the handicapped learner's motivation. We have seen that teachers' and coaches' interactional styles have important effects on students' and athletes' intrinsic motivation. We need to find out about the effects of teachers' orientations and the processes through which these affect special students' motivation toward physical activity. Which interactional styles are more conducive to self-determined learning in children? Which styles stall children's quest for mastery attempts? These and other questions need to be ascertained.

A third and final research direction pertains to the assessment of the effects of various intervention programs on children's motivation toward physical activity. For instance, what are the effects of task analysis on children's intrinsic, extrinsic, and amotivation? What are the effects of reattribution training on unsuccessful learners' feelings of competence and motivation? Such research may serve to reorient interventions such that those facilitating students' intrinsic and self-determined forms of motivation are favoured over those which encourage students' dependency and nonself-determined forms of motivation.

The intrinsic and self-determined forms of motivation are important for ensuring that enjoyment and long-term involvement in physical activity takes place in special populations. Much research is needed in order to structure physical settings so that they become more conducive to such consequences. It is hoped that the present chapter will help to eventually reach this objective.

Author Notes

1. This paper was prepared while the first author was supported by research grants from Le Fonds pour la Formation des Chercheurs et l'Aide à la Recherche (FCAR Quebec), Le Conseil Québécoise de la Recherche Sociale, and the Université du Québec à Montréal.

2. Send requests for reprints to Robert J. Vallerand, Laboratoire de Psychologie Sociale, Université du Québéc à Montréal, C.P. 8888, Station "A", Montréal, Québec, Canada, H3C 3P8.

References

Abramson, L. Y., Seligman, M. E. P., & Teasdale, J. D. (1978). Learned helplessness in humans: Critique and reformulation. *Journal of Abnormal Psychology, 87,* 49-74.

Alley, G. R., & Deshler, D. D. (1979). *Teaching the learning disabled adolescent: Strategies and methods.* Denver, CO: Love Publishing.

Amabile, T. M., DeJong, W., & Lepper, M. R. (1976). Effects of externally imposed deadlines on subsequent intrinsic motivation. *Journal of Personality and Social Psychology, 34,* 92-98.

Ames, C. (1984). Competition, cooperation, and individual goal strategies: A cognitive-motivational analysis. In C. Ames & R. Ames (Eds.), *Research in motivation in education: Vol.1. Student motivation* (pp. 177-207). New York, NY: Academic Press.

Aronson, E., & Osherow, A. (1980). Cooperation, prosocial behavior, and academic performance: Experiments in the desegregated classroom. In L. Bickman (Ed.), *Applied social psychology annual* (Vol. 2, pp. 163-196). Beverly Hills, CA: Sage

Bandura, A. (1977). Self-efficacy: Toward a unifying theory of behaviorial change. *Psychological Review, 84,* 191-215.

Bandura, A., & Schunk, D.H. (1981). Cultivating competence, self-efficacy, and intrinsic interest through proximal self-motivation. *Journal of Personality and Social Psychology, 41,* 586-598.

Blais, M. R., Sabourin, S., Boucher, C., & Vallerand, R. J. (1988). *Toward a motivational model of couple happiness.* Manuscript submitted for publication.

Blanck, P. D., Reis, H. T., & Jackson, L. (1984). The effects of verbal reinforcement on intrinsic motivation for sex-linked tasks. *Sex Roles, 10,* 369-387.

Boggiano, A. K., & Barrett, M. (1985). Performance and motivational deficits of helplessness: The role of motivational orientations. *Journal of Personality and Social Psychology, 49,* 1753-1761.

Boggiano, A. K., Main, D. S., & Katz, P. A. (1988). Children's preference for challenge: The role of perceived competence and control. *Journal of Personality and Social Psychology, 54,* 134-141.

Borkowski, J. G., Weyhing, R. S., & Carr, M. (1988). Effects of attributional retraining on strategy-based reading comprehension in learning-disabled students. *Journal of Educational Psychology, 80,* 46-53.

Bowd, A., McDougall, D., & Yewchuk, C. (1982). *Educational psychology: A canadian perspective.* Toronto, ON: Gage Pub.

Brawley, L. B., & Vallerand, R. J. (1986). *Effects of choice and gender on intrinsic motivation and self-determination.* Unpublished manuscript, University of Waterloo, Waterloo, Ontario.

Brière, N. M., Vallerand, R. J., Blais, M. R., & Pelletier, L. G. (1988). [Construction and validation of the Sport Motivation Scale (SMS)]. Unpublished raw data.

Browne, M. A., & Mahoney, M. J. (1984). Sport psychology. *Annual Review of Psychology, 35,* 605-625.

Bruininks, V. L., & Bruininks, R. H. (1977). Motor proficiency of learning disabled and nondisabled students. *Perceptual and Motor Skills, 44,* 1131-1137.

Cellar, D. F., & Barrett, G. V. (1987). Script processing and intrinsic motivation: The cognitive sets underlying cognitive labels. *Organizational Behavior and Human Decision Processes, 40,* 115-135.

Cellar, D. F., & Wade, K. (1988). Effect of behaviorial modelling on intrinsic motivation and script-related recognition. *Journal of Applied Psychology, 73,* 181-192.

Chapman, J. W. (1988). Cognitive-motivational characteristics and academic achievement of learning disabled children: A longitudinal study. *Journal of Educational Psychology, 80,* 357-365.

Cohen, M. W. (1986). Intrinsic motivation in the special education classroom. *Journal of Learning Disabilities, 19,* 258-261.

Connell, J. P., & Ryan, R. M. (1986). *Autonomy in the classroom: A theory and assessment of children's self-regulatory styles in the academic domain.* Unpublished manuscript, University of Rochester, Rochester, NY.

Daoust, H., & Vallerand, R. J. (1987). Effets de la coopération sur la motivation intrinsèque. [Effects of cooperation on intrinsic motivation]. *Résumés des Communications de la Société Québécoise de Recherche en Psychologie* (abstract, p. 100).

Daoust, H., Vallerand, R. J., & Blais, M. R. (1988). Motivation and education: A look at some important consequences. *Canadian Psychology, 29*(2a), 172.

deCharms, R. (1968). *Personal causation: The internal affective determinants of behavior.* New York, NY: Academic Press.

deCharms, R. (1976). *Enhancing motivation: Change in the classroom.* New York, NY: Irvington Pubs.

Deci, E. L. (1971). Effects of externally mediated rewards on intrinsic motivation. *Journal of Personality and Social Psychology, 18*, 105-115.

Deci, E. L. (1975). *Intrinsic motivation.* New York, NY: Plenum.

Deci, E. L. (1980). *The psychology of self-determination.* Lexington, MA: DC Heath.

Deci, E. L., Betley, G., Kahle, J., Abrams, L., & Porac, J. (1981a). When trying to win: Competition and intrinsic motivation. *Personality and Social Psychology Bulletin, 7*, 79-83.

Deci, E. L., Nezlek, J., & Sheinman, L. (1981b). Characteristics of the rewarder and intrinsic motivation of the rewardee. *Journal of Personality and Social Psychology, 40*, 1-10.

Deci, E. L., Schwartz, A. J., Sheinman, L., & Ryan, R. M. (1981c). An instrument to assess adults' orientation toward control versus autonomy with children: Reflections on intrinsic motivation and perceived competence. *Journal of Educational Psychology, 73*, 642-650.

Deci, E. L., & Cascio, W. F. (1972/May). *Changes in intrinsic motivation as a function of negative feedback and threats.* Paper presented at the meeting of the Eastern Psychological Association, Boston, MA.

Deci, E. L., & Chandler, C. L. (1986). The importance of motivation for the future of the LD field. *Journal of Learning Disabilities, 19*, 587-594.

Deci, E. L., & Ryan, R. M. (1980). The empirical exploration of intrinsic motivational processes. In L. Berkowitz (Ed.), *Advances in experimental social psychology* (Vol. 13, pp. 39-80). New York, NY: Academic Press.

Deci, E. L., & Ryan, R. M. (1985). *Intrinsic motivation and self-determination in human behavior.* New York, NY: Plenum.

Deci, E. L., & Ryan, R. M. (1987). The support of autonomy and the control of behavior. *Journal of Personality and Social Psychology, 53,* 1024-1037.

Deci, E. L., Spiegel, N. H., Ryan, R. M., Koestner, R., & Kauffman, M. (1982). The effects of performance standards on teaching styles: The behavior of controlling teachers. *Journal of Educational Psychology, 74,* 852-859.

Deshler, D. D., & Schumaker, J. B. (1986). Learning strategies: An instructional alternative for low-achieving adolescents. *Exceptional Children, 52,* 583-590.

Dwyer, J., Grant, P., & Fischer, D. (1988). Convergent and divergent validity of the sports intrinsic motivation scale. *Canadian Psychology, 29*(2a), 218.

Earn, B. M. (1982). Intrinsic motivation as a function of extrinsic financial rewards and subjects' locus of control. *Journal of Personality, 50,* 360-373.

Eghrari, H., & Deci, E. L. (1986). *Facilitating internalization: The effects of informational and controlling contexts.* Unpublished manuscript, University of Rochester, Rochester, NY.

Fincham, F. D. (1983). Clinical applications of attribution theory: Problems and prospects. In M. Hewstone (Ed.), *Attribution theory: Social and functional extensions* (pp. 187-203). Oxford: Blackwells.

Fisher, C. F. (1978). The effects of personal control, competence and extrinsic reward systems on intrinsic motivation. *Organizational Behavior and Human Performance, 21,* 273-288.

Försterling, F. (1986). Attributional retraining: A review. *Psychological Bulletin, 98*(3), 495-512.

Freud, S. (1962). *The ego and the id.* New York, NY: Norton (originally published in 1923).

Fuchs, L. S., Fuchs, D., & Tindal, G. (1986). Effects of mastery learning procedures on student achievement. *Journal of Educational Research, 79,* 286-291.

Grimes, L. (1981). Learned helplessness and attribution theory: Redefining children's learning problems. *Learning Disability Quarterly, 4,* 91-100.

Grolnick, W. S., & Ryan, R. M. (1987). Autonomy in children's learning: An experimental and individual difference investigation. *Journal of Personality and Social Psychology, 52,* 890-898.

Halliwell, W. R. (1978). The effect of cognitive development on children's perceptions of intrinsically and extrinsically motivated behavior. In D. Landers & R. Christina (Eds.), *Psychology of motor behavior and sport* (pp. 403-419). Champaign, IL: Human Kinetics.

Harackiewicz, J. M. (1979). The effects of reward contingency and performance feedback on intrinsic motivation. *Journal of Personality and Social Psychology, 37,* 1352-1363.

Harackiewicz, J. M., & Larson, J. R. (1986). Managing motivation: The impact of supervisor feedback on subordinate task interest. *Journal of Personality and Social Psychology, 51,* 547-556.

Harter, S., & Connell, J. P. (1984). A model of children's achievement and related self-perceptions of competence, control, and motivational orientation. In J. G. Nicholls (Ed.), *The development of achievement motivation* (Vol. 3, pp. 219-250). Greenwich, CT: JAI Press.

Harter, S., Silon, E., & Pike, R. (1981). *Perceived competence, intrinsic versus extrinsic orientation, and anxiety in the educable mentally retarded: A comparison of mainstreaming and self-contained classrooms.* Unpublished manuscript, University of Denver, Denver, CO.

Haywood, H. C. (1968a). Motivational orientation of overachieving and underachieving elementary school children. *American Journal of Mental Deficiency, 72,* 662-667.

Haywood, H. C. (1968b). Psychometric motivation and the efficiency of learning and performance in the mentally retarded. In B. W. Richards (Ed.), *Proceedings of the Congress of the International Association for the Scientific Study of Mental Deficiency* (pp. 276-283). Reigate, England: Michael Jackson.

Haywood, H. C. & Switzky, H. N. (1986). Intrinsic motivation and behavior effectiveness in retarded persons. In N. R. Ellis (Ed.), *International review of research in mental retardation* (Vol. 14, pp. 1-46). New York, NY: Academic Press.

Haywood, H. C., & Wachs, T. D. (1966). Size discrimination learning as a function of motivation-hygiene orientation in adolescents. *Journal of Educational Psychology, 57,* 279-286.

Haywood, H. C., & Weaver, S. J. (1967). Differential effects of motivational orientation and incentive conditions on motor performance in institutionalized retardates. *American Journal of Mental Deficiency, 72,* 459-467.

Heitman, R. J., & Justen, J. E. (1980). Locus of control and social reinforcement in the motor performance of educable mentally retarded students. *Education and Training of the Mentally Retarded, 15,* 204-208.

Horn, T. S. (1984). Expectancy effects in the interscholastic setting: Methodological considerations. *Journal of Sport Psychology, 6,* 60-76.

Horn, T. S., & Hasbrook, C. A. (1987). Psychological characteristics and the criteria children use for self-evaluation. *Journal of Sport Psychology, 9,* 208-221.

Jacobsen, B., Lowery, B., & DuCette, J. (1986). Attributions of learning disabled children. *Journal of Educational Psychology, 78*(1), 59-64.

Johnson, D. W., & Johnson, R. (1985). Motivational processes in cooperative, competitive, and individual learning situations. In C. Ames & R. Ames (Eds.), *Research in Motivation in education: Vol. 2. The classroom milieu* (pp. 249-286). New York, NY: Academic Press.

Kistner, J., Haskett, M., White, K., & Robbins, F. (1987). Perceived competence and self-worth of LD and normally achieving students. *Learning Disability Quarterly, 10,* 37-44.

Knowles, C., Vogel, P. Wessel, J. (1975). Project I CAN: Individualized curriculum designed for mentally retarded children and youth. *Education and Training of the Mentally Retarded, 10,* 155-160.

Koestner, R., Ryan, R. M., Bernieri, F., & Holt, K. (1984). Setting limits in children's behavior: The differential effects of controlling versus informational styles on intrinsic motivation and creativity. *Journal of Personality and Social Psychology, 52,* 233-248.

Koestner, R., Zuckerman, M., & Koestner, J. (1987). Praise, involvement, and intrinsic motivation. *Journal of Personality and Social Psychology, 53,* 383-390.

Kruglanski, A. W. (1978). Endogenous attribution and intrinsic motivation. In M. R. Lepper & D. Greene (Eds.), *The hidden costs of reward: New perspectives on the psychology of human motivation* (pp. 85-107). Hillsdale, NJ: Lawrence Erlbaum.

Lawrence, E., & Winchell, J. E. (1975). Loss of control: Implications for special education. *Exceptional Children, 42,* 483-490.

Lepper, M. R., & Greene, D. (1975). Turning play into work: Effects of adult surveillance and extrinsic rewards on children's intrinsic motivation. *Journal of Personality and Social Psychology, 31,* 479-486.

Lepper, M. R., Greene, D., & Nisbett, R. E. (1973). Undermining children's intrinsic interest with extrinsic rewards: A test of the "overjustification" hypothesis. *Journal of Personality and Social Psychology, 28,* 129-137.

Lewko, J. H. (1978). Significant others and sport socialization of the handicapped child. In F. Smoll & R. Smith (Eds.), *Psychological perspectives in youth sports* (pp. 249-277). Washington, DC: Hemisphere Pubs.

Lincoln, A., & Chazan, S. (1979/Fall). Perceived competence and intrinsic motivation in learning disability children. *Journal of Clinical Child Psychology,* 213-216.

Litch, B. G. (1983). Cognitive-motivational factors that contribute to the achievement of learning-disabled children. *Journal of Learning Disability, 16,* 483-490.

Litch, B. G., & Kistner, J. A. (1986). Motivational problems of learning-disabled children: Individual differences and their implications for treatment. In J. Torgesen & B. Wong (Eds.), *Psychological and educational perspectives on learning disabilities* (pp. 225-255). New York, NY: Academic Press.

Lopez, E. M. (1981). Increasing intrinsic motivation with performance-contingent rewards. *Journal of Psychology, 108,* 59-65.

Loveland, K. K., & Olley, J. G. (1979). The effect of external reward on interest and quality of task performance in children of high and low intrinsic motivation. *Child Development, 50,* 1207-1210.

Martinek, T. (1981). Pygmalion in the gym: A model for the communication of teacher expectations in physical education. *Research Quarterly for Exercise and Sports, 52,* 58-67.

Martinek, T., & Karper, W. B. (1984). The effects of noncompetitive and competitive instructional climates on teacher expectancy effects in elementary physical education classes. *Journal of Sport Psychology, 6,* 408-421.

McLoyd, V. C. (1979). The effects of extrinsic rewards of differential value on high and low-intrinsic interest. *Child Development, 50,* 1010-1019.

Miller, T. W. (1982). Assertiveness training for coaches: The issue of healthy communication between coaches and players. *Journal of Sport Psychology, 4,* 107-114.

Mossholder, K. W. (1980). Effects of externally mediated goal setting on intrinsic motivation: A laboratory experiment. *Journal of Applied Psychology, 65,* 202-210.

Orlick, T. D. (1978a). *Winning through cooperation.* Washington, DC: Hawkins & Associates.

Orlick, T. D. (1978b). *The cooperative sports and games book.* New York, NY: Pantheon.

Orlick, T. D., & Mosher, R. (1978). Extrinsic awards and participant motivation in a sport-related task. *International Journal of Sport Psychology, 9,* 27-39.

Paris, S. G., & Oka, E. R. (1986). Self-regulated learning among exceptional children. *Exceptional Children, 53,* 103-108.

Pearl, R. (1982). LD children's attributions for success and failure: A replication with a labelled LD sample. *Learning Disability Quarterly, 5,* 173-176.

Pearl, R., Bryan, T., & Donahue, M. (1980). Learning disabled children's attributions for success and failure. *Learning Disability Quarterly, 3,* 3-9.

Pelletier, L. G., Brière, N. M., Blais, M. R., & Vallerand, R. J. (1988). Persisting vs dropping out: A test of Deci and Ryan's theory. *Canadian Psychology, 29*(2a), (abstract, 600).

Pelletier, L. G., & Vallerand, R. J. (1985, October). *Effects of coaches' interpersonal behavior on athletes' motivation level.* Paper presented at the annual conference of the Canadian Society for psychomotor Learning and Sport Psychology, Montreal, Quebec.

Pelletier, L. G., & Vallerand, R. J. (1989). Behaviorial confirmation in social interaction: Effects of teachers'expectancies on students' intrinsic motivation. *Canadian Psychology, 30*(2a), (abstract, 404).

Peterson, C., & Seligman, M. E. P. (1984). Causal explanations as a risk factor for depression: Theory and evidence. *Psychological Review, 94,* 347-374.

Petri, H. L. (1981). *Motivation: Theory and research.* Belmont, CA: Wadsworth.

Pratton, J., & Hales, L. W. (1986). The effects of active participation on student learning. *Journal of Educational Research, 79,* 210-215.

Rarick, G. L., Dobbins, D. A., & Broadhead, G. D. (1976). *The motor domain and its correlates in educational handicapped children.* Englewood Cliffs, NJ: Prentice-Hall, Inc.

Reeve, J., Olson, B. C., & Cole, S. G. (1985). Motivation and performance: Two consequences of winning and losing in competition. *Motivation and Emotion, 9,* 291-298.

Reid, G. (1987). Motor behavior and psychosocial correlates in young handicapped performers. In D. Gould & M. R. Weiss (Eds.), *Advances in pediatric sport sciences: Vol. 2. Behaviorial Issues* (pp. 235-258). Champaign, IL: Human Kinetics.

Rejeski, W., Daracott, C., & Hutslar, S. (1979). Pygmalion in youth sport: A field study. *Journal of Sport Psychology, 1,* 311-319.

Roberts, G. C. (1984). Toward a new theory of motivation in sport: The role of perceived ability. In J. Silva & R. Weinberg (Eds.), *Psychological foundations of sport* (pp. 214-228). Champaign, IL: Human Kinetics.

Rosenthal, R., & Jacobson, L. (1968). *Pygmalion in the classroom: Teacher expectation and pupils' intellectual development.* New York, NY: Holt, Rinehart, & Winston.

Rosenthal, R., & Rubin, D. B. (1978). Interpersonal expectancy effects: The first 345 studies. *Behaviorial and Brain Sciences, 3,* 377-386.

Ross, M. (1975). Salience of reward and intrinsic motivation. *Journal of Personality and Social Psychology, 32,* 245-254.

Rotter, J. B. (1966). Generalized expectencies for internal versus external control of reinforcement. *Psychological Monographs, 80,* (1, Whole No. 609).

Ruble, D. N., & Boggiano, A. K. (1980). Optimizing motivation in an achievement context. In B. K. Keogh (Ed.), *Advances in special education* (Vol. 1, pp. 183-238). Greenwich, CT: JAI Press.

Ryan, R. M. (1982). Control and information in the intrapersonal sphere: An extension of cognitive evaluation theory. *Journal of Personality and Social Psychology, 43,* 450-461.

Ryan, R. M., Connell, J. P., & Deci, E. L. (1985). A motivational analysis of self-determination and self-regulation in education. In C. Ames & R. E. Ames (Eds.), *Research on motivation in education: Vol. 2. The classroom milieu* (pp. 13-51). New York, NY: Academic Press.

Ryan, R. M., Connell, J. P., & Grolnick, W. S. (in press). When achievement is not intrinsically motivated: A theory and assessment of self-regulation in school. In A. K. Boggiano & T. S. Pittman (Eds.), *Achievement and motivation: A social-developmental perspective.* Cambridge: Cambridge University Press.

Ryan, R. M., & Grolnick, W. S. (1986). Origins and pawns in the classroom: Self-report and projective assessments of individual differences in children's perceptions. *Journal of Personality and Social Psychology, 50,* 550-558.

Ryan, R. M., Vallerand, R. J., & Deci, E. L. (1984). Intrinsic motivation in sport: A cognitive evaluation theory interpretation. In W. Straub & J. Williams (Eds.), *Cognitive sport psychology* (pp. 231-242). Lansing, NY: Sport Science Associates.

Sansone, C. (1986). A question of competence: The effects of competence and task feedback on intrinsic interest. *Journal of Personality and Social Psychology, 51,* 918-931.

Schunk, D. H. (1989). Self-efficacy and cognitive achievement: Implications for students with learning problems. *Journal of Learning Disabilities, 22,* 14-22.

Schunk, D. H., & Cox, P. D. (1986). Strategy training and attributional feedback with learning disabled students. *Journal of Educational Psychology, 78,* 201-209.

Skinner, B. F. (1953). *Science and human behavior.* New York, NY: Macmillan.

Slavin, R. E. (1986). Cooperative learning: Engineering social psychology in the classroom. In R. S. Feldman (Ed.), *The social psychology of education: Current research and theory* (pp. 153-171). New York, NY: Cambridge.

Smith., C. R. (1986). The future of the LD field: Intervention approaches. *Journal of Learning Disabilities, 19,* 473-476.

Smith, D. C., Adelman, H. S., Nelson, P., Taylor, L., & Phares, V. (1987). Students' perceptions of control at school and problem behavior and attitudes. *Journal of School Psychology, 25,* 167-176.

Snyder, M. (1984). When beliefs create reality. In L. Berkowitz (Ed.), *Advances in experimental social psychology* (Vol. 18, pp. 257-305). New York, NY: Academic Press.

Snyder, M., Tanke, E. D., & Berscheid, E. (1977). Social perception and interpersonal behavior: On the self-fulfilling nature of social stereotypes. *Journal of Personality and Social Psychology, 35,* 656-666.

Swann, W. B., & Pittman, T. S. (1977). Initiating play activity of children: The moderating influence of verbal cues on intrinsic motivation. *Child Development, 48,* 1128-1132.

Switzky, H. N., & Haywood, H. C. (1974). Motivational orientation and the relative efficacy of self-monitored and externally imposed reinforcement schedules. *Journal of Personality and Social Psychology, 30,* 360-366.

Taylor, M. J. (1987, Sept/Oct.). Leisure counselling as an integral part of program development. *CAHPER Journal,* 21-24.

Taylor, C. B., Sallis, J. F., & Needle, R. (1985). The relation of physical activity and exercise to mental health. *Public Health Reports, 100,* 195-201.

Thomas, A., & Pahely, B. (1982). Effects of classroom training on LD students' task persistence and attributions. *Learning Disability Quarterly, 5,* 133-144.

Thomas, J. R., & Tennant, L. K. (1978). Effects of rewards on children's motivation for an athletic task. In F. Smoll & R. Smith (Eds.), *Psychological perspectives in youth sports* (pp. 123-144). Washington, DC: Hemisphere Pubs.

Thompson, C. E., & Wankel, L. M. (1980). The effect of perceived activity choice upon frequency of exercise behavior. *Journal of Applied Social Psychology, 10,* 436-443.

Torgesen, J. K. (1986). Learning disabilities theory: Its current state and future prospects. *Journal of Learning Disabilities, 19,* 461-472.

Tzuriel, D., & Haywood, H. C. (1985). Locus of control and child-rearing practices in intrinsically motivated and extrinsically motivated children. *Psychological Reports, 57,* 887-894.

Vallerand, R. J. (1981). Intrinsic motivation and adapted physical activity. In S. Krotsky, F. Caron, L. Jankowski, & G. Reid (Eds.), *Current research in adapted physical activity* (pp. 137-153). Montreal: Presses de l'Université de Montréal.

Vallerand, R. J. (1983). Effect of differential amounts of positive verbal feedback on the intrinsic motivation of male hockey players. *Journal of Sport Psychology, 5*, 100-107.

Vallerand, R. J., & Bissonnette, R. (1988). *On the predictive effects of intrinsic, extrinsic, and amotivational styles on behavior: A prospective study.* Manuscript submitted for publication.

Vallerand, R. J., & Blais, M. R. (1986). *A cognition-affect-intrinsic motivation model: An extension to cognitive evaluation theory's perceived competence process.* Unpublished manuscript, Université du Québec à Montréal.

Vallerand, R. J., Blais, M. R., Brière, N. M., & Pelletier, L. G. (1989). Construction et validation de l'Echelle de Motivation en Education (EME). *Revue Canadienne des Sciences du Comportement, 21*, 323-349.

Vallerand, R. J., Deci, E. L., & Ryan, R. M. (1987). Intrinsic motivation in sport. In K. Pandolf (Ed.), *Exercise and sport science reviews* (Vol. 15, pp. 389-425). New York, NY: MacMillan Pub.

Vallerand, R. J., Gauvin, L. I., & Halliwell, W. R. (1986a). Negative effects of competition on children's intrinsic motivation. *Journal of Social Psychology, 126*, 649-657.

Vallerand, R. J., Gauvin, L. I., & Halliwell, W. R. (1986b). Effects of zero-sum competition on children's intrinsic motivation and perceived competence. *Journal of Social Psychology, 126*, 365-472.

Vallerand, R. J., & Halliwell, W. R. (1983). Formulations théoriques contemporaines en motivation intrinsèque: Revue et critique. *Psychologie Canadienne, 24*, 243-256.

Vallerand, R. J., & O'Connor, B. P. (1989). Motivation in the elderly: A theoretical framework and some promising findings. *Canadian Psychology, 30*, 662-680.

Vallerand, R. J., & Pelletier, L. G. (1985, October). *Coaches' interpersonal styles, athletes' perceptions of their coaches' styles, and athletes' intrinsic motivation and perceived competence: Generalization of the world of swimming.* Paper presented at the annual conference of the Canadian Society for Psychomotor Learning and Sport Psychology, Montreal, Quebec.

Vallerand, R. J., & Reid, G. (1984). On the causal effects of perceived competence on intrinsic motivation: A test of cognitive evaluation theory. *Journal of Sport Psychology, 6*, 94-102.

Vallerand, R. J., & Reid, G. (1988). On the relative effects of positive and negative verbal feedback on males and females' intrinsic motivation. *Canadian Journal of Behavioral Sciences, 20,* 239-250.

Watkinson, E. J., & Wall, A. E. (1982). *The PREP play program: Play skill instruction for mentally handicapped children.* Ottawa, ON: Canadian Association for Health, Physical Education and Recreation.

Weinberg, R. S., & Jackson, A. (1979). Competition and extrinsic rewards: Effect on intrinsic motivation and attribution. *Research Quarterly, 50,* 494-502.

Weiner, B. (1985). An attributional theory of achievement motivation and emotion. *Psychological Review, 92,* 548-573.

Weiss, M. R., Bredemeier, B. J., & Shewchuk, R. M. (1985). An intrinsic/extrinsic motivation scale for the youth sport setting: A confirmatory factor analysis. *Journal of Sport Psychology, 7,* 75-91.

White, R. W. (1959). Motivation reconsidered: The concept of competence. *Psychological Review, 66,* 297-333.

Zuckerman, M., Porac, J., Lathin, D., Smith, R., & Deci, E. L. (1978). On the importance of self-determination for intrinsically motivated behavior. *Personality and Social Psychology Bulletin, 4,* 443-446.

SECTION III:

SPECIAL POPULATIONS

Problems in Movement Control
G. Reid (editor)

MOVEMENT CONTROL AND DOWN'S SYNDROME: A NEUROPSYCHOLOGICAL APPROACH

Digby Elliott
School of Physical Education and Athletics
McMaster University

Over the last two decades, process-oriented researchers with an interest in mental retardation have attempted to determine how perceptual, cognitive and motor deficiencies in this population can best be characterized. Drawing on early information processing models (e.g., Atkinson & Shiffrin, 1968), investigators interested in mental retardation have distinguished between performance deficiencies that are due to differences in some structural feature of the processing system and differences that might arise due to control processes. Since control processes are viewed as optional strategies that an individual may or may not bring to bear on a task, control process deficiencies are seen as being amenable to training while structural deficiencies are not.

Generally, research indicating that performance deficiencies in mentally retarded persons are due to strategic shortcomings has been identified with a developmental lag approach to mental retardation. In this approach, mental retardation is characterized by a slow rate of learning on a wide variety of tasks. Although distinct learning histories may result in motivational and attentional differences between mentally retarded and nonretarded persons (Zigler, 1967) performance dissimilarities are expected to be more quantitative than qualitative. That is, mentally retarded persons are expected to perform perceptual, cognitive and motor tasks in ways similar to nonretarded persons of the same developmental or mental age.

The developmental approach has been dominant in recent years because of the general optimism it entails. Specifically, development is viewed as a life-long process, and while some aspects of development (e.g., motor development) may be slow in mentally retarded persons, development proceeds none the less. The difference or deficit approach on the other hand is seen as a more stagnant model, since deficiencies are associated with the breakdown of specific structural systems and development is deemed likely to proceed only to some limited point.

In this chapter it will be argued that while the control processes - structural difference distinction is useful to researchers attempting to understand how mentally retarded people learn and organize movements, both the developmental and difference approach to mental retardation are problematic; the former approach because it ignores individual differences, and the latter approach because it ignores developmental similarities. The focus of the chapter will be on research my colleagues and I have conducted over the last several years with Down's Syndrome persons in which we have drawn on neuropsychological models of cerebral organization to attempt to understand some of the general and specific perceptual-motor problems experienced by these people. What I intend to argue, using research with Down's Syndrome persons as an example, is that *specific* difference models can prove fruitful when they are nested in an overall developmental approach to mental retardation.

Down's Syndrome - General

Functionally, Down's Syndrome persons can range from the mild to profound levels of mental retardation. Within a functional category Down's Syndrome persons can be expected to perform various cognitive and motor tasks in a manner more similar to other retarded persons within that category than to Down's Syndrome persons who are outside that particular category. Despite this general rule, Down's Syndrome individuals within a functional category exhibit differences from other persons at the same general intellectual level. Studies for example, indicate that Down's Syndrome persons perform relatively poorly on tasks involving sequential language processing (Hartley, 1986), vocal imitation (Mahoney, Glover & Finger, 1981) and auditory sequential memory (Marcell & Armstrong, 1982). In the motor domain, it has been suggested that persons with Down's Syndrome have difficulty structuring and utilizing motor programs (Anwar, 1981; Frith & Frith, 1974). In contrast, individuals with Down's Syndrome tend to exhibit performance advantages when compared to subjects of a similar mental age on tasks that involve visual-motor ability (Edwards, Elliott & Lee, 1986) and visual pattern discrimination (Silverstein, Legutki, Friedman & Takayama, 1982).

Recently my colleagues and I (Elliott & Weeks, in press; Elliott, Weeks & Elliott, 1987b) have proposed a neuropsychological model of cerebral organization for Down's Syndrome persons that attempts to explain this pattern of specific function/dysfunction. The main feature of this model is the proposed biological dissociation between the cerebral areas responsible for speech perception and the areas responsible for the production of complex movement including speech. This dissociation occurs because Down's Syndrome persons exhibit an atypical pattern of cerebral specialization. Evidence regarding cerebral specialization in Down's Syndrome persons comes from studies examining ear advantages for dichotic listening and manual asymmetries in movement control. In subsequent sections of this chapter I will review the research pertaining to cerebral specialization in Down's Syndrome persons, outline the model and report some preliminary studies that support the model. In a final section of the paper I will suggest how the approach we have taken can be used to guide future research with Down's Syndrome persons as well as research with other subgroups of mentally retarded individuals.

Down's Syndrome - Evidence for Atypical Cerebral Specialization

Initial reports of atypical cerebral specialization in Down's Syndrome persons came from studies employing the dichotic listening technique. While most right-handed individuals display a right ear (left hemisphere) advantage for the perception of speech sounds, experiments with Down's Syndrome persons evidenced either no ear advantage (Sommers & Starkey, 1977; Tannock, Kershner & Oliver, 1984) or a left ear (right hemisphere) advantage (Hartley, 1981; Pipe, 1983; Reinhart, 1976; Zekulin-Hartley, 1981, 1982) in these individuals. Studies employing a mentally retarded non-Down's Syndrome control group (Pipe, 1983) have demonstrated that this tendency toward reversed cerebral specialization for speech perception is not a result of mental retardation per se, since other retarded persons display typical right ear advantages. Thus the dichotic listening work suggests that Down's Syndrome persons have syndrome-specific differences in brain organization.

Based primarily on dichotic listening findings, Hartley (1982) hypothesized that some of the specific sequential language problems (e.g., Ashman, 1982) exhibited by Down's Syndrome persons may have a biological origin related to atypical cerebral development. Specifically Down's Syndrome persons may be performing sequential language tasks with a right hemisphere that is either ill-equipped or inefficient in the processing of that type of information. Hartley's (1982) model would certainly be classified as a specific deficit model of dysfunction in this population.

Excited by the dichotic listening findings, researchers in our laboratory (Elliott, 1985; Elliott, Edwards, Weeks, Lindley & Carnahan, 1987a; Elliott & Weeks, in press; Elliott, Weeks & Jones, 1986a) attempted to follow-up this work from two perspectives. First we tried to determine if reversed cerebral specialization in Down's Syndrome individuals was the rule or if reversed specialization for speech perception in these individuals was the exception to the rule. From a second but related perspective we attempted to determine if atypical cerebral specialization in Down's Syndrome persons had any implications for their ability to organize and control simple limb movements.

In our initial experiments, we examined asymmetries in limb movements. Our studies were based on the idea that limb differences in the planning and production of various classes of movement are the result of the efficiency of the contralateral cerebral hemisphere in performing certain types of processing activity (Carnahan & Elliott, 1987; Roy & MacKenzie, 1978; Taylor & Heilman, 1980; Todor, Kyprie & Price, 1982). Specifically, right limb advantages in rapid tapping and sequencing have been attributed to a left cerebral hemisphere superiority for processing and organizing information sequentially. In contrast, left side superiority for spatial positioning and the perception of spatial arrangement (Benton, Varney & deHamsher, 1978; Carnahan & Elliott, 1987; Roy & MacKenzie, 1978; Witelson, 1974) have been suggested to reflect the ability of the right hemisphere to process that type of information.

In an initial experiment (Elliott, 1985 Experiment 1), we examined the ability of 12 Down's Syndrome, 12 undifferentiated retarded and 12 nonretarded adults to finger-tap as rapidly as possible with their right or left index finger for a 15 s interval. All the subjects were right-handed. As expected the non-retarded adults outperformed the other two groups and exhibited the typical right hand advantage for this type of task (mean right hand performance = 99.0 taps, mean left hand performance = 87.0 taps). Both the Down's Syndrome subjects and the mentally retarded control subjects evidenced no hand differences (Down's: right hand = 61.1 taps, left hand = 60.5 taps; Control: right hand = 53.5 taps, left hand = 50.9 taps). Examination of the individual subject data within each group indicated that while subjects in the retarded control group tended to exhibit either a distinct left hand or right hand advantage for this task, Down's Syndrome persons failed to exhibit an advantage. In terms of the original rationale for the study, our results suggested that Down's Syndrome persons may be less specialized than non-Down's Syndrome persons for the organization and control of sequential movement. At least compared to other mentally retarded persons, this did not appear to be a handicap in terms of overall performance. This finding contrasts with the work of Frith and Frith (1974) who found that Down's Syndrome persons performed more slowly on a finger-tapping task than a group of autistic subjects of the same mental age.

In a follow-up study (Elliott et al., 1986a), we again examined right and left hand finger-tapping in right-handed Down's Syndrome adults and a group of nonretarded adults. Our equipment in this second experiment allowed us to partition each finger-tap into a depression and release phase. By examining the within-subject standard deviations of each of these two phases we were able to arrive at indices of finger-tapping variability as well as overall performance. These measures of variability are of interest because hand differences in variability are thought to reflect movement control differences between the two cerebral hemispheres (Peters, 1976; Roy & Elliott, 1986; Todor et al., 1982). Specifically, Todor and Smiley (1985) have suggested that reduced right hand variability in finger-tapping is related to a left hemisphere superiority in the parameterization and timing of force.

As expected the nonretarded subjects outperformed the Down's Syndrome subjects. This advantage was due primarily to the extended time Down's Syndrome persons spent in the release phase of the tapping movement. While the apparatus itself may have helped brake the depression of the key, movement reversal during the release portion of the movement was probably more dependent on the subjects' ability to time when a change in direction was required.

In contrast to the control subjects, our Down's Syndrome subjects again failed to exhibit a clear right hand advantage for finger-tapping. However, the Down's Syndrome subjects exhibited the same pattern of variability for both the release and depression data as the nonretarded subjects, with the left hand in all cases being more variable than the right hand. If the relatively consistent performance of the right hand reflects a left hemisphere advantage for force modulation, this finding might be considered the first evidence that Down's Syndrome persons are left hemisphere specialized for the organization and control of hand movements.

Another neuropsychological paradigm used to examine cerebral specialization for movement organization and control is the interlimb transfer of training paradigm. Typically when an individual learns a movement task with one hand a certain proportion of this learning transfers to the other hand (e.g., Cook 1933a, 1933b, 1934). Interestingly, there is an asymmetry for this type of intermanual transfer of training. Specifically, there is more transfer of training from the left hand to the right hand than vice versa (Edwards & Elliott, 1987; Hicks, 1974; Taylor & Heilman, 1980). This asymmetry is thought to reflect left hemisphere specialization for movement control. That is, when an individual learns a task with the right hand, only the left hemisphere needs to be involved, since it contains specialized left hemisphere mechanisms important for the organization of movement (Kimura & Archibald, 1974) and because the control of distal musculature is primarily contralateral (Kuypers, 1981). However, when the left hand is performing/learning a task both cerebral hemispheres must play a role -- the left hemisphere because of its overall part in movement organization and the right hemisphere because it has the primary role in controlling the distal musculature of the left hand. Thus asymmetries in transfer of training have been hypothesized to reflect the more diffuse organization associated with left hand performance. Our goal in adopting a transfer of training paradigm was to determine if Down's Syndrome people exhibit the same asymmetric transfer of training pattern as right-handed control subjects, thus indicating predominant left hemisphere involvement in movement organization.

In an initial study, we (Elliott, 1985, Experiment 2) had 26 right-handed Down's Syndrome adults and 26 right-handed nonretarded adults practice a finger-tapping task with either the right or left index finger. Based on pretraining and posttraining performance measures taken on both hands we demonstrated that both groups exhibited more transfer of training following left hand practice. Based on explanations of the asymmetry in normal right-handed individuals (Edwards & Elliott, 1987; Taylor & Heilman, 1980), our findings suggest that Down's Syndrome persons are left hemisphere specialized for the control and organization of movement.

Recently, we (Edwards & Elliott, in press) have replicated this finding using a more complicated two finger sequencing task, involving alternate finger-lifting. This study involved 24 male adults with Down's Syndrome and 24 children. As well as exhibiting asymmetric transfer of training, both groups were more variable in their finger-sequencing when performing with the left hand. Again this is evidence for left hemisphere specialization for movement control. In this experiment, we also examined unintended finger movements in the nonperforming hand in order to obtain an index of what has been called contralateral motor overflow. Of interest was the finding that the Down's Syndrome subjects exhibited less overflow than the control group of a similar mental age. Thus while motor overflow is often used to diagnose neurological impairment, it is not a characteristic of all mentally retarded groups.

One area that has been researched extensively with nonretarded people is cerebral specialization for the organization and production of speech. A popular neuropsychological paradigm has been the dual-task paradigm in which subjects are required to perform a unimanual movement task while they are also engaged in a speech production task (see Kinsbourne & Hiscock, 1983 for a review). The general finding has been, that compared to single task control conditions, speech production (see Carnahan, Elliott & Lee, 1986) disrupts right limb performance more than left limb performance. The most popular explanation for this finding (Kinsbourne & Hicks, 1978) is that during right hand (or foot) performance there is within hemisphere interference between the left cerebral areas responsible for speech production and those responsible right limb movement control. For left hand performance, this interference is reduced or eliminated because the cerebral areas responsible for speech production (left hemisphere) are functionally distant from those responsible for left hand (right hemisphere) movement control. Since the evidence suggesting that people with Down's Syndrome have an atypical pattern of cerebral specialization comes mainly from research examining speech perception (Hartley, 1981; Pipe, 1983), we felt that the dual-task paradigm provided an excellent vehicle for examining specialization for speech production in this group. Our logic was that if Down's Syndrome adults have a left hemisphere specialization for speech production, they would be expected to demonstrate the same dual task effects as nonretarded right-handed adults. However, if speech production is reversed as is speech perception then concurrent speech should "interfere more with left-hand performance than right-, supporting the notion that people with Down's Syndrome rely on right hemisphere speech and language mechanisms" (Elliott et al., 1987a, p. 481).

In this study (Elliott et al., 1987a), 12 right-handed Down's Syndrome adults and 12 right-handed university students performed a unimanual finger-tapping task with both the right and left index finger. Half the subjects in each group were female. The finger-tapping task was performed alone and while subjects were required to sound-shadow high-frequency single syllable words (Thorndike & Lorge, 1944). While Down's Syndrome subjects performed more poorly than control subjects in all conditions, of interest was the finding that Down's Syndrome persons exhibited the same pattern of dual-task interference as control subjects. For male subjects, sound-shadowing disrupted only right hand performance, while for females subjects both right-hand and left-hand performance suffered in the dual-task situation (for discussion of gender differences see Elliott, Weeks, Lindley & Jones, 1986b). Thus at least for males, the results of this experiment suggest left hemisphere specialization for speech production. Regardless of group, gender or condition, all subjects exhibited more finger-tapping variability with their left-hand than their right hand again indicating that the left cerebral hemisphere may have a special role to play in the parameterization of force in finger movements (see Todor & Smiley, 1985).

A Neuropsychological Model: Initial Findings and Implications

While there certainly is no consensus on the issue (e.g., Tannock et al., 1984), the majority of dichotic listening studies (Hartley, 1981; Pipe, 1983; Zekulin-Hartley, 1981, 1982) indicate that people with Down's Syndrome exhibit an atypical right hemisphere specialization for the perception of speech. In contrast, research from our laboratory suggests that left hemisphere mechanisms play a special role in the organization and control of complex movement, including speech production. My colleagues and I (Elliott & Weeks, in press; Elliott et al., 1987b) have recently proposed that this biological dissociation between mechanisms that normally overlap may be responsible for some of the specific deficits exhibited by this group. For example, some of the language based problems exhibited by Down's Syndrome persons (Ashman, 1982; Hartley, 1982) may be the result of a "left-right structural dissociation" that "disrupts the interaction between cerebral mechanisms responsible for speech perception and speech production" (Elliott et al., 1987b, p. 268). In fact our model predicts that because of this dissociation, people with Down's Syndrome will have difficulty with any task requiring both speech perception and the production of complex movements, including speech. Thus our model explains why people with Down's Syndrome exhibit specific deficits in tasks involving sequential language processing (Ashman, 1982; Hartley, 1982), vocal imitation (Mahoney et al., 1981) and auditory sequential memory (Marcell & Armstrong, 1982), but not on tasks involving visual and visual-motor abilities (e.g., Edwards et al., 1986; Silverstein et al., 1982). Moreover in three recent studies, we (Elliott & Weeks, in press) have been able to demonstrate that

Down's Syndrome persons have problems performing tasks that require both speech perception and the production of nonspeech movements.

In a preliminary study, we (Elliott & Weeks, in press) employed an apraxia battery (Kools, Williams, Vickers & Caell, 1971) in order to compare ability of Down's Syndrome persons (n=19) and non-Down's Syndrome persons (n=18) to perform simple limb and oral movements to either a verbal or visual cue. The battery involves subjects producing 10 oral (e.g., stick out your tongue) and 10 limb (e.g., put your finger in your ear) movements to a verbal command and following a demonstration. Zero, one or two points can be awarded for each response and thus an overall score out of twenty is possible for each of the four categories (e.g., oral-visual). Of interest, for purposes of our model, was that Down's Syndrome subjects performed more poorly following a verbal cue than following a visual cue regardless of whether the movement was manual or oral. The undifferentiated mentally retarded control subjects however performed equally well to verbal and visual cues. Thus as our model (Elliott & Weeks, in press; Elliott et al., 1987b) predicted, Down's Syndrome persons displayed specific dysfunction when they were required to perform a task that required both speech perception and movement production.

Following the apraxia study, we examined our model with two studies in which we employed more controlled, experimental procedures. In both studies subjects were required to perform a sequencing task that involved three distinct hand movements (shift a lever, pull a switch, turn a dial) which could be specified in any order. The subjects' task was to complete the sequence as rapidly as possible with either the right or left hand, and of primary interest was whether the order was specified visually or verbally. On visual trials small light emitting diodes located next to each manipulandum (i.e., lever, switch, dial) defined the order. In our first experiment the verbal cue specified the position of the manipulandum on our sequencing apparatus (e.g., middle, top, bottom). As predicted, the nonretarded control subjects in this experiment performed the sequencing task equally well (movement time) with a verbal (1305 ms) and visual (1348 ms) cue, while Down's Syndrome subjects exhibited relatively poorer performance in the verbal (3740 ms) as opposed to visual (3426 ms) condition.

In a second experiment using the same apparatus, we specified the action to be performed with our verbal cue (shift, pull, turn) rather than the position of the manipulandum on the sequencing board. For this situation our group by movement cue interaction for movement time was even more pronounced (Nonretarded: visual = 1210 ms, verbal = 1201 ms; Down's Syndrome: visual = 2960 ms verbal = 3574 ms). Thus regardless of the type of verbal cue, Down's Syndrome subjects exhibit problems compared to situations in which their movements can be organized on the basis of visual information. Once again, it is our position that this specific pattern of deficit results from a biological dissociation between the cerebral areas responsible for speech perception and those responsible for the organization and execution of movement.

Although our model is definitely a specific deficit model of dysfunction, we do not believe our findings necessitate an attitude of pessimism. Rather research like ours can be used to guide how remedial and instructional programs can best be organized. For example if Down's Syndrome persons have difficulty producing movement to verbal instructions then a more visual instructional strategy might be employed with these individuals. What we need to do in our research with mentally retarded persons is go beyond the simple identification of a performance deficit, and ask questions about the psychological and biological processes contributing to the deficit. Based on our understanding of these processes we can devise task strategies that diminish the importance of specific information processing problems.

Certainly neuropsychologists working with brain-injured adults have long recognized how specific many information processing problems can be, and that poor performance on a task can arise for a variety of different reasons (Kinsbourne, 1971). In the area of mental retardation, the major stumbling block to an experimental neuropsychological approach has been the notion that one deficit, common to all mentally retarded persons, can be isolated (e.g., Ellis, 1963; Spitz, 1963). While there are certainly subgroups of mentally retarded persons that can be expected to have some similarities, the majority of mentally retarded persons can be expected to show their own distinct pattern of function/dysfunction. It is time that researchers interested in mental retardation stopped allowing the general pattern of dysfunction, that by definition is associated with mental deficiency, to mask individual differences (Roy, Elliott, Dewey & Square-Storer, in press).

Future Directions

Although we are not naive enough to suggest our model of cerebral specialization for Down's Syndrome persons provides any final solutions, we do believe that the model provides a starting point for a number of research approaches. For our own part we plan to examine cerebral asymmetries in this population using a number of other paradigms. To date we have attempted to examine specialization for spatial-tactile perception with tasks for which other investigators have found left hand (right hemisphere) advantages. For example, Witelson (1974) has shown that right-handed children are better able to match felt nonsense shapes to their visual analogue when the tactile exploration is done with the left as opposed to the right hand. As well, Benton et al. (1978) have demonstrated that the left hand is better than the right hand at judging the spatial orientation of a series of metal rods. The results of studies we have performed using these two paradigms (Elliott & Weeks, in press; Elliott et al.,

1987b) have been disappointing, since we not only failed to find hand advantages for our own Down's Syndrome subjects but also for our nonretarded control subjects (cf. Benton et al., 1978; Witelson, 1974). Part of the problem is that the phenomena under consideration are just not very robust (Hannay & Smith, 1979; Jones & Elliott, 1988). Added to this is the problem of being certain that the Down's Syndrome subjects and mental age control subjects understand the rather complicated nature of the judgments they are required to perform. For this latter reason, and because it is difficult to insure that mentally retarded people maintain fixation in a tachistospocic study we have not examined visual field asymmetries. Recently however, Smith, Cash, Barr and Putney (1986) have developed a procedure that while time demanding, will work with this population. The technique involves training subjects to visually fixate and then to initiate their own trials. It does not require verbal instruction. The visual field studies with Down's Syndrome persons remain to be done.

With respect to other approaches, the use of regional cerebral blood flow, sodium amytal and evoked potential techniques would add to our understanding of the relationship between cerebral and behaviourial events in this population (see Bryden, 1982). Certainly it would be nice to have some confirmation of the speech perception-speech production dissociation from more direct approaches.

Another area for potential investigation is handedness in Down's Syndrome persons. In our work to date, we have usually restricted ourselves to right-handed Down's Syndrome persons. While we have made no attempt to sample proportionally from all functional categories, approximately 85% of the Down's Syndrome persons available to us at workshops and in educational settings have been right-handed, as determined by our simple preference measures. Thus, the incidence of right-handedness appears to be only slightly lower than in a normal North American population (Hicks & Kinsbourne, 1976). Perhaps by examining left-handed Down's Syndrome persons, and the relationship between performance and preference in this atypical group we may gain some insights into the origins of handedness and the relationship of handedness to cerebral specialization.

As an individual who works in a physical education department, one of my interests is with the implications of our model of cerebral specialization and manual performance for skill instruction. While we have demonstrated that Down's Syndrome persons *perform* better in a visual-motor than a verbal-motor situation, it does not necessarily follow that a visual approach to instruction will prove better for long-term retention and *learning*. Learning studies need to be conducted both in the laboratory and the field. It is perhaps in this area that our model has some potential practical implications.

While research such as ours should give us more insight into the general and specific information processing problems experienced by Down's Syndrome persons, it may also feed back and have some impact on more general psychological theory. For example, by conducting studies to examine the dissociation of speech perception and movement production in persons with Down's Syndrome, insight into the functional overlap of these two important systems in normals may be obtained. At a more biological level, research on cerebral asymmetry with genetically atypical groups such as Down's Syndrome persons, may add to our understanding of the genetic basis for cerebral specialization.

Summary

In this chapter, I have reviewed research which indicates that persons with Down's Syndrome have specific problems with tasks that require both the perception of speech and movement production. As well, I have presented a neuropsychological model that was developed to explain this specific deficit. Thus while Down's Syndrome persons share the general intellectual difficulties of other mentally retarded persons, understanding their specific patterns of function/dysfunction may be useful for persons engaged in motor skill instruction.

Moreover, if specific deficits can be identified and explained in Down's Syndrome persons, they undoubtedly exist in other subgroups of mentally retarded persons. Perhaps it is time for researchers to step beyond the development vs. difference controversy, and concede that both approaches have something to offer to our understanding of mental retardation.

Author Notes

1. Send requests for reprints to Digby Elliott, School of Physical Education and Athletics, McMaster University, Hamilton, Ontario, Canada, L8S 4K1.

References

Anwar, F. (1981). Motor function in Down's syndrome. In N. R. Ellis (Ed.), *International review of research in mental retardation,* (Vol. 10, pp. 107-138). New York, NY: Academic Press.

Ashman, A. F. (1982). Coding, strategic behavior and language performance of institutionalized mentally retarded young adults. *American Journal of Mental Deficiency, 86,* 627-636.

Atkinson, R. C. & Shiffrin, R. M.(1968). Human memory: A proposed system and its control processes. In K. W. Spence & J. T. Spence (Eds.), *The psychology of learning and motivation* (Vol. 2, pp. 89-197). New York, NY: Academic Press.

Benton, A. L., Varney, N. R., & deHamsher, K. S. (1978). Lateral differences in tactile directional perception. *Neuropsychologia, 16,* 109-114.

Bryden, M. P. (1982). *Laterality. Functional asymmetry in the intact brain.* New York, NY: Academic Press.

Carnahan, H., Elliott, D., & Lee, T.D. (1986). Dual-task interference between speaking and listening and a unipedal force production task. *Neuropsychologia, 24,* 583-586.

Carnahan, H., & Elliott, D. (1987). Pedal asymmetry in the reproduction of spatial locations. *Cortex, 23,* 157-159.

Cook, T. W. (1933a). Studies in cross education: Mirror tracing the star-shaped maze. *Journal of Experimental Psychology, 16,* 144-160.

Cook, T. W. (1933b). Studies in cross education: Further experiments in mirror tracing the star-shaped maze. *Journal of Experimental Psychology, 16,* 679-700.

Cook, T. W. (1934). Studies in cross education: Kinesthetic learning of an irregular pattern. *Journal of Experimental Psychology, 17,* 749-762.

Edwards, J. M., Elliott, D., & Lee, T. D. (1986). Contextual interference effects during skill acquisition and transfer in Down's syndrome adolescents. *Adapted Physical Activity Quarterly, 3,* 250-258.

Edwards, J. M., & Elliott, D. (1987). Effect of unimanual training on contralateral motor overflow in children and adults. *Developmental Neuropsychology, 3,* 299-309.

Edwards, J. M., & Elliott, D. (in press). Asymmetries in intermanual transfer of training and motor overflow in adults with Down's syndrome and nonhandicapped children. *Journal of Clinical and Experimental Neuropsychology.*

Elliott, D. (1985). Manual asymmetries in the performance of sequential movement by adolescents with Down syndrome. *American Journal of Mental Deficiency, 90,* 90-97.

Elliott, D., Weeks, D. J., & Jones, R. (1986a). Lateral asymmetries in finger tapping by adolescents and young adults with Down syndrome. *American Journal of Mental Deficiency, 90*, 472-475.

Elliott, D., Weeks, D. J., Lindley, S., & Jones, R. (1986b). Sex differences in dual-task interference between speaking and a manual force-production task. *Perceptual and Motor Skills, 62*, 3-8.

Elliott, D., Edwards, J. M., Weeks, D. J., Lindley, S., & Carnahan, H. (1987a). Cerebral specialization in young adults with Down syndrome. *American Journal of Mental Deficiency, 91*, 480-485.

Elliott, D., Weeks, D. J., & Elliott, C. L. (1987b). Cerebral specialization in individuals with Down syndrome. *American Journal of Mental Retardation, 92*, 263-271.

Elliott, D., & Weeks, D. J. (in press). Cerebral specialization and the control of oral and limb movements for individuals with Down's syndrome. *Journal of Motor Behavior.*

Ellis N. R. (1963). The stimulus trace and behaviorial inadequacy. In N. R. Ellis (Ed.), *Handbook of mental deficiency* (pp. 134-158). New York, NY: McGraw-Hill.

Frith, U., & Frith, C. D. (1974). Specific motor disabilities in Down's syndrome. *Journal of Child Psychology and Psychiatry, 15*, 293-301.

Hannay, H. J. & Smith, A. C. (1979). Dichhaptic perception of forms by normal adults. *Perceptual and Motor Skills, 49*, 991-1000.

Hartley, X. Y. (1981). Lateralisation of speech stimuli in young Down's syndrome children. *Cortex, 17*, 241-248.

Hartley, X. Y. (1982). Receptive language processing of Down's syndrome children. *Journal of Mental Deficiency Research, 26*, 263-269.

Hartley, X. Y. (1986). A summary of recent research into the development of children with Down's syndrome. *Journal of Mental Deficiency Research, 30*, 1-14.

Hicks, R. E. (1974). Asymmetry of bilateral transfer. *American Journal of Psychology, 87*, 667-674.

Hicks, R. E., & Kinsbourne, M. (1976). On the genesis of human handedness: A review. *Journal of Motor Behavior, 8*, 257-266.

Jones, R., & Elliott, D. (1988). Intra- and interhemispheric integration of tactual and visual spatial information. *Bulletin of the Psychonomic Society, 26*, 229-231.

Kimura, D., & Archibald, Y. (1974). Motor functions of the left hemisphere. *Brain, 97*, 337-350.

Kinsbourne, M. (1971). Cognitive deficit: Experimental analysis. In J. L. McGaugh (Ed.), *Psychobiology* (pp. 285-348). New York, NY: Academic Press.

Kinsbourne, M., & Hicks, R. E. (1978). Functional cerebral space: A model for overflow, transfer and interference effects in human performance. In J. Requin (Ed.), *Attention and performance VII.* (pp. 345-362). New York, NY: Academic Press.

Kinsbourne, M., & Hiscock, M. (1983). Asymmetries of dual task performance. In J. B. Hellige (Ed.), *Cerebral hemisphere asymmetry: Method, theory and application* (pp. 255-334). New York, NY: Praeger.

Kuypers, H. G. J. M. (1981). Anatomy of the descending pathways. In V. E. Brooks (Ed.), *Handbook of physiology: Sec. 1. The nervous system: Vol. 2. Motor control* (pp. 597-666), Baltimore, MD: American Physiological Society.

Kools, J. A., Williams, A. F., Vickers, M. J., & Caell, A. (1971). Oral and limb apraxia in mentally retarded children with deviant articulation. *Cortex, 7*, 387-400.

Mahoney, G., Glover, A., & Finger, I. (1981). Relationship between language and sensorimotor development of Down syndrome and nonretarded children. *American Journal of Mental Deficiency, 86*, 21-27.

Marcell, M. M., & Armstrong, V. (1982). Auditory and visual sequential memory of Down syndrome and nonretarded children. *American Journal of Mental Deficiency, 87*, 86-95.

Peters, M. (1976). Prolonged practice of a simple motor task by preferred and non-preferred hands. *Perceptual and Motor Skills, 43*, 447-450.

Pipe, M. E. (1983). Dichotic-listening performance following auditory discrimination training in Down's syndrome and developmentally retarded children. *Cortex, 19*, 481-491.

Reinhart, C. (1976). *The cerebral lateralization of speech processes in Down's syndrome and normal individuals.* Unpublished master's thesis, University of Saskatchewan, Saskatoon, Sask.

Roy, E. A., & MacKenzie, C. L. (1978). Handedness effects on kinesthetic spatial judgments. *Cortex, 14*, 250-258.

Roy, E. A., & Elliott, D. (1986). Manual asymmetries in visually directed aiming. *Canadian Journal of Psychology, 40*, 109-121.

Roy, E. A., Elliott, D., Dewey, D., & Square-Storer, P. (in press). Impairments to praxis and sequencing in adult and developmental disorders. In C. Bard, M. Fleury & L. Hays (Eds.), *Physical activity, growth and motor development across the lifespan: Vol. 2. Development of eye-hand coordination across the lifespan.* University of South Carolina Press.

Silverstein, A. B., Legutki, G., Friedman, S. L., & Takayama, D. L. (1982). Performance of Down syndrome individuals on the Stanford-Binet intelligence scale. *American Journal of Mental Deficiency, 86*, 548-551.

Smith, S. T., Cash, C., Barr, S. E., & Putney, R. T. (1986). The nonspeech assessment of hemispheric specialization in retarded children. *Neuropsychologia, 24*, 293-296.

Sommers, R. K., & Starkey, K. L. (1977). Dichotic verbal processing in Down's syndrome children having qualitatively different speech and language skills. *American Journal of Mental Deficiency, 82*, 44-53.

Spitz, H. H. (1963). Field theory in mental deficiency. In N. R. Ellis (Ed.), *Handbook of mental deficiency* (pp. 11-40). New York, NY: McGraw-Hill.

Tannock, R., Kershner, J. R., & Oliver, J. (1984). Do individuals with Down's syndrome possess right hemisphere language dominance? *Cortex, 20*, 221-231.

Taylor, H. G., & Heilman, K. M. (1980). Left-hemisphere motor dominance in right-handers. *Cortex, 16*, 587-603.

Thorndike, E. L., & Lorge, I. (1944). *The teacher's workbook of 30,000 words.* New York, NY: Columbia University.

Todor, J. I., Kyprie, P. M., & Price, H. L. (1982). Lateral asymmetries in arm, wrist and finger movements. *Cortex, 18*, 515-523.

Todor, J. I., & Smiley, A. L. (1985). Performance differences between the hands: Implications for studying disruption to limb praxis. In E. A. Roy (Ed.), *Neuropsychological studies of apraxia and related disorders* (pp. 309-344). Amsterdam: North-Holland.

Witelson, S. F. (1974). Non linguistic tactual perception using a dichotomous stimulation technique. *Cortex, 10,* 3-17.

Zekulin-Hartley, X. Y. (1981). Hemispheric asymmetry in Down's syndrome children. *Canadian Journal of Behavioural Science, 13,* 210-217.

Zekulin-Hartley, X. Y. (1982). Selective attention to dichotic input of retarded children. *Cortex, 18,* 311-316.

Zigler, E. (1967). Familial mental retardation: A continuing dilemma. *Science, 155,* 292-298.

Problems in Movement Control
G. Reid (editor)

SHORT-TERM MEMORY FOR MOTOR SKILLS IN MENTALLY RETARDED PERSONS: TRAINING AND RESEARCH ISSUES

John H. Hoover
University of South Dakota

and

James S. Horgan
College of Health, Physical Education and Recreation
University of Illinois - Chicago

Individual differences in memory have been recognized since the classical period of Plato (Marshall & Fryer, 1978). It has been the prevalent belief that certain individuals consistently recalled more information than others. Additionally ploys used to enhance memory also date to the classical era. From Plato to the present century, the predominant metaphor for understanding memory was the wax tablet. This "geographical" perspective (memory as a place) would have teachers imprint or etch items into a storage facility or library. Until recently there was very little known about the processes by which information made its entrance into the system other than the observation that material could be made memorable by purposefully relating it to past experience.

This view contrasts sharply with the emphasis now placed on the actions taken by memorizers as new material is learned. These actions are viewed as skills which learners bring to bear on tasks and in their aggregate may be considered a *policy* designed to produce maximum recall. Put another way, there has been a trend from emphasis on "memory" the noun to "memorize" the verb. This view is not new (Bartlett, 1932) but has led to a great deal of empirical investigation over the past twenty years. Much of this work has been directed toward understanding the processes implicated in the consistently poor memory performance of mentally retarded persons (Detterman, 1979). An argument can be made that the primary difference between mentally retarded memorizers and their nonretarded counterparts, lies not in the neural apparatus, which would be implicated in long-term memory deficits, but in the organization of "actions" taken by retarded learners which are believed to be associated with short-term memory. This idea will be further developed below and related to the acquisition of motor skills by mentally retarded persons.

Viewing memory as a series of putatively controllable skills, rather than as an immutable trait implies that mentally retarded persons' memory shortcomings are a component of behaviour that is sensitive to intervention. In fact, a body of literature has been dedicated to this question (cf., Ashcraft & Kellas, 1974; Brown, Campione, Bray & Wilcox, 1973; Butterfield, Wambold & Belmont, 1973; Hagen, Streeter & Raker,1974). In addition, application of the cognitive memory paradigm has been extended to the domain of motor skills in retarded persons (Horgan, 1983a, 1983b; Kelso, Goodman, Stamm & Hayes, 1979; Reid, 1980a, 1980b). A generalization that will also be developed is that, as a group, mentally retarded persons are more variable in their propensity for adopting appropriate memory (mnemonic) strategies than are their nonretarded peers. The fact that this occurs, both in learning symbolic material and in the maintenance of proprioceptive and kinaesthetic information, has significant implications for retarded learners and their teachers. Each day a mentally retarded person's memory is taxed by demands such as learning the sequence of movements in a job routine or requirements to precisely reproduce limb or body positions in recreation or sport. Failure to develop or adopt a reasonable policy for driving the memory system will most certainly result in diminishing the potential of mentally retarded individuals. The negative implications of the latter can have a far-reaching effect. For example, Fisher and Zeaman (1973) demonstrated that short-term memory deficits produce problems during the acquisition phase of discrimination learning.

The remainder of this chapter is divided into three major sections. The first is devoted to the study of memory from the cognitive tradition, including a brief presentation of a generic and widely accepted model, followed by a brief explanation of methods used by researchers to investigate short-term memory. Second, a brief review of short-term memory in mentally retarded persons is presented. Studies in which the mentally retarded were trained to use memory strategies (mnemonics) are emphasized here as well. The final section consists of a proposal for application of memory strategies in training as well as directions for research.

The Study of Memory: How is it Undertaken

An Information Processing Model

A typical stage information processing theory (e.g. Atkinson & Shiffrin, 1968), allows researchers to use timing and other experimental methods to determine the manner in which the memory system operates (see also Baddeley & Hitch, 1974; Neisser, 1976). Information, passes through the system in a serial or sequential fashion; this process consumes a small, but quantifiable period of time. The elements of the system which bear attention in the discussion of memory are: a) a very short-term sensory store, i.e., sensory register, b) a relatively longer information storage component that is variable referred to as, working (active) or short-term memory, and c) long-term memory. Both the sensory register and short-term memory must act upon information quickly or the information will decay rapidly. Long-term memory is nearly unlimited in capacity and information decay is very slow. Storage in long-term store is dependent upon repetitive cycling through active memory.

An important aspect of Atkinson and Shiffrin's model, particularly for the study of mental retardation, is the distinction between "control" and "structural" features of the memory system. Control features of performance are those processes which can be altered or changed to meet information handling requirements. Control features by definition can be altered through training or incidental interactions and result in more efficient responses to the environment. Structural parameters are those limitations on the system which training and environmental interaction cannot modify. For example, each individual has capacity limitations or an absolute limit to the amount of raw information that can be processed within a given time period; a structural feature. Conversely, in those instances where "control" *can* be exerted, memorizers can select from several strategies when confronted with the need to remember; these can markedly improve efficiency in information handling. For example, naming memorial stimuli (an inefficient strategy, but better than passive reception) or rehearsing items cumulatively (a better strategy) could be adopted (Brown, Campione & Murphy, 1974). What makes strategy selection a control parameter is the nature of the information available to the learner and whether it is sensitive to subject-initiated action. In addition, it is apparent that specific strategies can be taught to those who do not ordinarily use them spontaneously (Brown et al., 1974). In almost every instance, strategy usage increases the efficiency with which information is passed through the neural structure, and adds to the capacity of the memorizer to handle additional information (Spitz, 1979).

The relevance of cognitive models in the study of mental retardation is obvious. For example, a dilemma faced by educators of mentally retarded persons is to decide at what point in an instructional sequence to modify a task due to excessive cognitive demands. In the area of motor skills, it has been suggested that research efforts be directed toward delineation of tasks that will likely represent structural barriers in the learning of mildly retarded persons and those which are sensitive to modification through training (Hogg, 1986; Reid, 1986, Wade, Hoover & Newell, 1983). As it is presently understood the short-term memory deficiency identified among mentally retarded persons seems to be primarily a control dimension of performance. Studies (to be reviewed later) from both the cognitive and motor domains have shown that mentally retarded persons are poor memorizers because they fail to spontaneously adopt useful strategies, the most obvious and effective of which is rehearsal. Furthermore, once the relevance of these strategies are taught to mentally retarded learners their performance improves on the recall of both lists (Brown et al., 1974) and arm-movements (Horgan, 1983b; Reid, 1980a). Short-term memory, or working memory (Baddeley & Hitch, 1974) appears to be the locus of memory problems in mildly retarded persons. Once information is deposited in the long-term memory store, only minimal differences between mentally retarded and nonretarded persons are observed (Fagan, 1966; Hayes & Routh, 1972). The remainder of this chapter will be devoted to the short-term memory characteristics of mentally retarded persons.

Short-term memory is invoked when information must be kept active in the storage facility for a relatively brief period of time. For example, a researcher might present a series of numbers (digit span) and direct subjects to memorize them in order. Following this presentation, a period of time passes where the digits are not available visually, followed by a request to reproduce them in their order of presentation. If this period, called the "recall interval", is between 2-30 seconds short-term memory is typically operating.

In 1963 Ellis published an influential paper in which it was hypothesized that mentally retarded persons displayed deficient short-term memory because of a biological (i.e., structural) defect. Ellis argued that the trace of sensory data in the neural apparatus decays more rapidly in mentally retarded persons. This concept was based on the consistent findings that in mentally retarded learners, digit span decreased as a function of recall interval. The longer subjects were asked to wait before initiating a response, the more information they "lost" (within the time limits of the short-term memory interval). This can be contrasted with the performance of nonretarded subjects who, when there are no extraneous demands placed on central processing, show no such decline with increases in the recall interval. However, as Ellis (1970) later pointed out, this early view was fundamentally flawed. What had not been controlled was the propensity of nonretarded memorizers to act strategically on incoming information. Mentally retarded persons, it was later found, failed to spontaneously adopt an effective policy (strategy) to aid in their attempts to remember. This is pointed out to emphasize the complexity of memory research and to make the point that successful retention can best be thought of as a series of related skills or actions and not merely a discrete process (Adams, 1987). In the experiments reviewed by Ellis, the rather simple action presumed to have been adopted by nonretarded learners was cumulative repetition of information during the recall interval (rehearsal). It is now widely held that mentally retarded persons are less likely to rehearse information to be remembered of their own volition than are their nonretarded peers. This control dimension of performance provides a plausible explanation as to the memory difficulties of mentally retarded persons. But how can a so-called rehearsal deficit be quantified?

It is assumed that mildly retarded learners show retention decrements as a result of failure to act effectively (exert "control") on incoming information. One fundamental and obvious action that can be adopted by a memorizer is to repeat a list of items while waiting to recall them. This repetition, be it overt or covert (not observable), is referred to as rehearsal. Obviously, when researchers make inferences about processes other than ones they are able to observe directly, it produces theoretical and methodological difficulties (see Detterman, 1979 for a detailed review). Because the absence of spontaneous, cumulative rehearsal is central to understanding memory deficits in mildly retarded learners, it is worth examining some of the methodological and measurement issues associated with the process. In this way, analogs developed in the domain of motor learning will be easier to understand. While it is not an easy proposition to investigate covert phenomena such as rehearsal, neither is it impossible. Because our understanding of memory is so intimately related to research methodology, some of the procedures used by researchers are explained in the text which follows.

The Study of Rehearsal

Investigators often work from the assumption, based on an analysis of a memory task, that rehearsal would aid performance. The performance of these subject's, essentially a control group, is observed for patterns of error or accuracy in performance. The available rehearsal time can also be manipulated. Scientists can also construct situations where persons who are normally expected to rehearse are prevented from doing so and subsequently observe systematic reduction in recall accuracy. A comparison of this group's performance with a control group yields a quantification of rehearsal.

With a few variations, the above protocols are by far the most conventional for use in the study of rehearsal among mentally retarded persons. For example, Borys and Spitz (1976) asked mentally retarded subjects to memorize common pictures under two conditions. In the first, subject were not impeded during the retention interval (the period between the last stimulus and the request to reproduce the list). In the second condition, subjects were asked to perform an unrelated cognitive activity during the retention interval. This is typically referred to as an "interpolated activity" (Peterson & Peterson, 1959) and can take the form of any mental or physical exercise which the experimenter believes would compete and interfere with the process of rehearsal. The mechanism for the interfering nature of the interpolated activity is called retroactive interference, and probably results from a diversion of attention produced by competition with the primary information to be recalled. In this case, a portion of working memory must be allocated to the performance of the secondary (interpolated) task and, hence, the level of central resource available for rehearsal is reduced (Carr, 1984).

Borys and Spitz (1976) reported that performing an interpolated task resulted in poor performance on the part of mentally retarded memorizers. These data contravene expectations raised by the interpolated activity argument. If mentally retarded subjects were not rehearsing, the interpolated activity should not have effected their performance. As a matter of fact, this finding is rather typical as will be discussed later (cf., Ferretti, 1982).

Butterfield et al. (1973) referred to another method of investigating rehearsal as the task-analytic method. Here, investigators teach a rehearsal strategy to subjects who presumably are not using it in a situation where it would aid recall. Using this technique, Brown and Barclay (1976) compared the recall of mildly retarded young people who had been instructed to rehearse with those who had been asked only to name stimuli. Subjects who had been instructed to rehearse as well as subjects who were asked to anticipate the next picture on a list during the acquisition phase of learning, outperformed subjects who were asked only to name target pictures.

Several other issues related to the use of rehearsal in memory research deserve mention. Many early studies of memory in mentally retarded persons relied on the "recency effect" to make inferences about rehearsal. At this level of analysis, an example of which is digit span, correct recall is plotted against serial position (see Figure 1). Serial position refers to the order position of a stimulus relative to others.

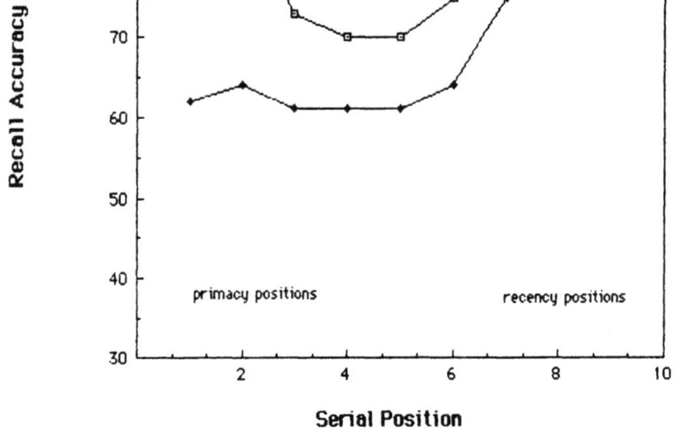

Figure 1: Hypothetical serial position curves for nonretarded and retarded learners.

For example, in the list "block, airplane, cow, hamburger"; block occupies serial position number one, airplane is two, etc. Items appearing early in the list are called "primacy" items; items appearing later in the list are referred to as "recency" items. Depending upon the recall interval and presentation rate, primacy items are thought to require rehearsal while recency items are associated with sensory registration. This is sensible, in that the most recently presented items require less processing through rehearsal. The only way to counteract interference exerted by later items on those presented earlier is to strengthen their maintenance in short-term memory through the adoption of some form of mnemonic strategy, ie., rehearsal. Retroactive interference does not occur for items later in the list because the information load is either very low or non-existent.

In the case of mentally retarded learners, one could reasonably predict that if they did not rehearse, performance would be relatively poor on primacy items when compared to nonretarded memorizers who did rehearse; this appears to be the case (Brown, 1974; Ellis, 1970). Cohen and his colleagues reported an interesting line of research supporting short-term memory deficits on the part of mentally retarded learners. No significant correlation was observed between recall of primacy items and intelligence when subjects of average ability were tested (Cohen & Sandberg, 1977). However, when mildly retarded subjects were included in a subsequent sample, a positive correlation emerged, an indication that the higher the IQ, the more items were recalled.

One criticism of memory research is that much of it uses gross measures of recall to infer the existence of complex neural processes "inside" learners (cf., Baumeister,1984; Borkowski & Cavanaugh, 1979; Campione, 1986; Detterman, 1979). Several methods have been proposed to deal with the measurement of rehearsal effects without sole reliance upon error information.

Flavell, Beach & Chinsky (1966) asked trained lip readers to watch children rehearse. Correct recall was associated with observable lip movements, assumed to be sub-vocal rehearsal. Other researchers have asked subjects to rehearse overtly, that is aloud. Still others have used a temporally-based rehearsal protocol with mentally retarded subjects. When subjects were left to rehearse independently, the time that they dedicated to observing stimuli at varying points in the list were measured (Ashcraft & Kellas, 1974; Butterfield et al., 1973). By contrast, Ferretti (1982) inverted the conventional interpolated activity design. In this study, mentally retarded subjects produced reaction-times while rehearsing which were compared to times when subjects were only attending to the reaction time task. The inference was that if subjects were rehearsing, associated reactions times would be slower.

The above experimental models for the study of short-term memory have been applied to the problems of motor memory in mentally retarded persons. The first problem faced by researchers was to find a motoric analog for the most frequently used dependent variable in memory studies, the percentage of items correctly recalled. Researchers have adopted various measures of reproduction error to quantify the operation of memory for proprioceptive and kinaesthetic information. In a typical study, subjects produce either a preselected movement (determined by the subject) or one determined by the experimenter (constrained) which is delimited to one degree of freedom in order to reduce experimental error. Following a recall interval, the subject attempts to reproduce the movement. In cognitive memory studies permutations of correct recall are used to quantify memory. In the motor domain, the linear error of reproduction between a target movement and a reproduction movement is typically taken as an index of recall accuracy.

Several caveats to the interpretation of these scores have been posited. First, the range of allowable target movements must be controlled because linear metrics are sensitive to range effects (Horgan & Horgan, 1982). Second, there has been a great deal of debate about the correct statistical treatment of derived error scores (cf. Henry, 1974). Signed or constant error scores tend to underestimate error because consecutive trials bracketing on either side of the target criterion, even by a wide margin, may negate one another over trials resulting in artificially low error values. One solution is to employ absolute or unsigned values to error scores. Unfortunately, important information is lost regarding the relative accuracy of recalled arm positions if this method is employed. As a result, most researchers now use a metric suggested by Henry (1974) which he referred to as "total error". Total error is a composite of both constant and variable error (squared to eliminate signs). A third problem with linear error scores as an analog to "percent-correct recall" is that the length of subjects' arms co-varies with error, independent of experimental conditions. Horgan and Horgan (1982) demonstrated that measurement error resulting from intersubject differentials in arm-length can be reduced by converting error scores from linear metrics to their angular analog prior to analysis. In addition, it was argued that angular displacement is a more accurate index of the actual movement made by subjects (which is inherently angular) than is a linear error measure.

Motor Memory in Mentally Retarded Persons

General Findings: An Overview

The short-term memory deficits of mildly retarded learners appear to be associated with variable use of spontaneous rehearsal strategies. Instruction to rehearse pictorial and numeric information reduces variability as well as recall error (e.g., Belmont & Butterfield, 1969; Brown & Barclay, 1976; Kellas, Ashcraft & Johnson, 1973; Turnball, 1974). Conclusions drawn from the primacy studies support the notion that some mentally retarded memorizers are less likely to spontaneously rehearse than their nonretarded counterparts (Brown, 1974; Cohen & Nealon, 1979; Ellis, 1970, and are less aware of the value associated with adoption of a rehearsal strategy (Brown, 1974).

When studies employing the interpolated activity model are examined, the picture becomes confused. The expectancy is that interpolated activity should not inhibit the performance of mentally retarded memorizers because they do not spontaneously use a cumulative rehearsal strategy. However, a typical finding is that the performance of mentally retarded subjects is inhibited under interpolated conditions (Borys & Spitz, 1976; Fagan, 1966). In fact, the only study where the performance of mentally retarded subjects was equal under interpolated activity and non-interpolated activity conditions was one where the to-be-remembered information was proprioceptive and kinaesthetic in nature (Horgan, 1983b). Thus, it cannot be assumed that all mentally retarded subjects fail to rehearse. A more realistic stance is that there is a greater degree of inter- and intra-subject variability in the propensity of mentally retarded persons to employ a cumulative rehearsal strategy, as is generally the case in their expression of motor skills (Hoover & Wade, 1985).

Another explanation for deficits in short-term memory emerges when studies employing a training approach are compared to those employing interpolated activity or retroactive interference. There is a fundamental difficulty on the part of mentally retarded learners to direct attention to salient features of stimulus arrays (Zeaman & House, 1979); maintain vigilance over the duration of a protracted laboratory tasks (Krupski, 1977); and, there is a possibility that mentally retarded persons may allocate resources in a qualitatively different fashion than their nonretarded peers (Carr, 1984). Thus, studies employing a training or task analytical approach may overestimate the influence of rehearsal by directing subjects' attention to the task, while conditions in interpolated activity studies may magnify existing attentional problems. In either case there exists the possibility of a confound between attention and memory which are, nonetheless, highly interdependent processes (Baddeley & Hitch, 1974; Carr, 1984).

Before a specific review of motor memory is undertaken, several points about memory in mentally retarded persons need to be briefly summarized. In a major review of memory studies, Detterman (1979) concluded that no matter what 'locus' for memory deficits were investigated, researchers find deficit performance in mentally retarded subjects. Of late, several caveats to this conclusion have been raised, two of which are highlighted. First, Ellis and his associates, (Ellis & Meador, 1985; Ellis, Meador & Bodfish, 1985) have searched for memory tasks, dependent on so-called automatic processing (Hasher & Zacks, 1979). Presumably, it these tasks showed no differences between mentally retarded and nonretarded learners, support would be provided for the notion that active processing deficits alone inhibit memory performance in mentally retarded learners. This line of work has produced mixed results, but some evidence exists for limited differences between mentally retarded and nonretarded memorizers on such "passive" memory tasks as recognition, memory for number of events and position recall (Ellis, 1988; Ellis et al., 1985). Second, once material is learned equally well by mentally retarded and nonretarded persons, little difference has been found to exist between the long term memory decay of either group. This appears to be true in the case of pictorial (McCartney, 1987) as well as motoric information (Scott, 1971; cited in McCartney).

Though it will not be explored in depth, another source of memory deficits deserves mention. The degree of conscious knowledge one has about memory in general (known as metamemory), and particularly about the idiosyncratic operation of one's own memory system produces systematic differences in recall (Flavell, 1978). There is some indication that retarded persons, as a group, bring an insufficient strategic repertoire to memory tasks (Campione & Brown, 1977). This generalization has not been applied in depth to the motor domain, but both Horgan (1983b) and Reid (1980b) have alluded to this issue. Certainly the role of metamemory in the motor learning of mentally retarded persons needs to be examined; this position is made particularly salient by the possibility that metamemory and strategy adoption may be closely allied with maintenance and generalization of both skills and associated learning strategies (Borkowski & Cavanaugh, 1979; Borkowski, Reid & Kurtz, 1984).

Motor Short-Term Memory in Mentally Retarded Persons

Short-Term Memory Findings: An Overview

Studies of the proprioceptive and kinaesthetic memory of mildly retarded persons are reviewed below along with their instrctional implications. Two issues in short-term memory for limb position are central in this discussion. These are the roles played by; (a) the nature of the to-be-remembered material, and (b) the effect of target preselection.

In a closed-loop theory of motor learning (Adams, 1971), learners are thought to adjust their performance to sensory representations of the target position qualities that are experienced. Thus, variable error tends to decrease as a function of trials. One prediction to follow from this conceptualization is that the "feel" of endpoints is easier to recall than is the extent or magnitude of the distance moved due to a stronger memory trace laid down by the former. This is thought to be the case because end position seems a more stable or concrete cue and, hence, can be more easily coded. In the case of nonretarded persons these theoretical predictions were confirmed experimentally (Keele & Ells, 1972; Laabs, 1973). Interestingly, the degree to which this generalization holds for mentally retarded memorizers is unknown. In deference to Adams (1971) it must be said, that the predictions of closed-loop theory are predicated upon the assumption that the central nervous system is structurally intact. Further, the sparse extant information suggests that any experimenter-provided strategy improves arm-positioning performance, be it instructions to attend to movement extent or location cues (Horgan, 1983b; Reid, 1980a).

In addition to location-cues available to subjects, self-selection of target endpoints also tends to improve recall in nonretarded subjects (Martiniuk, 1973). This generalization appears to be accurate for the memory of mentally retarded persons as well (Kelso et al., 1979). Due to the limited number of studies these results must be considered with caution.

Several investigations have been reported in which the research methodologies outlined here have been used to examine the short-term memory of mentally retarded persons for limb position. Though the studies to be reviewed were designed to investigate divergent aspects of motor memory, they share the use of the linear track way to quantify movement accuracy of mildly retarded subjects in arm-positioning tasks, and the adoption of the cognitive models explicated above.

Sugden (1978) compared the performance of mildly retarded[1] males to those of both mental age and chronological age matched nonretarded subjects. Of interest was evidence of rehearsal strategies used by mentally retarded subjects over 10- and 30-second retention intervals under various demands of movement length (20, 25, 30, 35 cm).

The memory of nonretarded subjects was superior to that of mentally retarded at all criterion distances during retention intervals with no activity demands, but not when an interpolated activity was required. The nature of the differences indicated that performance of nonretarded boys' was markedly impeded by interpolated activity while that of mentally retarded subjects was affected to a lesser degree. This supports the notion of a rehearsal deficit among mentally retarded subjects, but only on a group-wide or average performance basis. Since most or all nonretarded subjects spontaneously rehearsed during non-interpolated activity conditions, their performance was more affected by the interpolated activity since it diverted attention from rehearsal operations. Mentally retarded subjects, on the other hand, were relatively unaffected because, as a group, they did not rehearse during the non-interpolated interval; this interpretation was preferred by Sugden and on the surface is quite reasonable. However, the recall of mentally retarded males at 30-seconds (across all movement lengths) was reliably superior under non-interpolated

---

1 Sugden used the British terminology "Educationally subnormal". Subjects in the study, generally had IQ's in the mildly retarded range.

conditions, suggesting that at least some retarded subjects were prevented from rehearsing by the interpolated activity.

There are other plausible explanations for the poor performance of mentally retarded learners under interpolated activity that do not imply a rehearsal deficit. For example, Duncan (1980) pointed out that decrements in performance under a divided attention protocol can be explained via performance-accuracy tradeoffs. In addition, drawing attention from the task with interpolated activity, perhaps affects mentally retarded persons differentially on the basis that their attentional resources are inefficiently allocated (Carr, 1984). Nonetheless, the most parsimonious explanation of Sugden's results is that, as a group, mentally retarded persons rehearsal performance is more variable but that some of them do, indeed, rehearse proprioceptive information when asked to recall arm movements. This data coincides nicely with interpolated activity studies employing pictorial material. Though expectations are that interpolated activity will *not* affect the recall of mentally retarded subjects, a more typical finding is that it does decrease their recall (cf., Borys & Spitz, 1976). Certainly, however, the preponderance of data support the notion that interpolated activity negatively impacts the performance of nonretarded subjects to a greater extent that it does mildly retarded learners.

Mildly retarded subjects were shown to rehearse limb positions spontaneously in a series of experiments undertaken by Kelso et al. (1979). Subjects were asked to code kinaesthetic information (endpoints) in a blindfolded condition. Participants recalled self-selected endpoints more precisely and consistently than experimenter-constrained endpoints. In addition, lower reproduction errors were associated with the non-interpolated condition; this was the case at both 7- and 15-second retention intervals. The rehearsal performance of mildly retarded subjects was more variable than that of their nonretarded counterparts. For example, no decrement in performance over time would be expected (during short-term memory intervals) if subjects rehearse. Kelso et al. (1979) reported that nonretarded subjects suffered no decrement at 15-second (in non-interpolated activity conditions) compared with their 7-second condition; while mentally retarded participants' recall was substantially inferior at 15-seconds as compared to the 7-second interval. Again, the obvious conjecture would be to assign the differences to intersubject variability. First, since the mentally retarded group performed better under non-interpolated conditions, there is some evidence that at least a portion of the subjects spontaneously rehearsed. Since the mentally retarded group's performance represented a decrement in recall between 7- and 15-seconds recall interval, however, it appears that some mentally retarded participants did not rehearse. Reduction in correct recall as a function of time is associated with a failure to rehearse; and, of course, is artificially achieved when subjects are prevented from doing so.

The findings of Kelso and associates (1979), like that of Sugden can also be explained by attentional factors. It is logical to assume that rehearsal requires the allocation of attentional resources (Kahneman, 1973). It then follows that if mentally retarded subjects are less able to maintain the required level of attention, it is possible that they would lose some information between 7- and 15-seconds even under non-interpolated activity conditions (Carr, 1984).

Another possibility suggested by Reid (1980a) is that Kelso et al.'s (1979) mentally retarded subjects were not in fact rehearsing spontaneously. Reid pointed out that by directing subjects to "remember the endpoint" of self-selected movements, they might have been subtly encouraged to rehearse. It might be added that these instructions also might have directed attentional resources to the task, thus enhancing performance independently of rehearsal.

There are two important parallels between research findings from what might be termed the traditional cognitive domain and studies in which short-term memory for proprioceptive/kinaesthetic information was examined. First, it is difficult to escape the conclusions from the information processing orientation, particularly with the idea of a control deficit in short-term memory, that a rehearsal deficit exists in retarded learners. Second, findings from research utilizing the interpolated activity design are ambiguous. Mentally retarded persons are comparatively less affected by interpolated activity requirements than their nonretarded counterparts. Both Sugden (1978) and Kelso et al. (1979), however, found that retarded subjects performed significantly poorer under dual-task conditions. There appears to be a rehearsal deficit, so *some* subjects probably did rehearse. As will be shown in the next section, findings reported in studies where task-analytic or "training" methodology was employed are far less ambiguous.

Short-Term Memory Training Studies

Reid (1980a) extended the rehearsal concept a step further and asked whether directly training mentally retarded subjects to rehearse would enhance recall performance on the same task employed by Sugden (1978) and Kelso et al. (1979). Reid instructed subjects to remember the "feel" of self-selected movements and where they stopped in relation to their body (p. 223). Subjects instructed in the use of a rehearsal mnemonic reliably outperformed their non-instructed counterparts over the 15-second, but not over the 7-second intervals. This proved to be the first empirical evidence that a rehearsal strategy operates effectively on proprioceptive/kinaesthetic information and that it can be taught to mentally retarded subjects as is the case with other types of memorial stimuli. The least that can be concluded is that instructions to rehearse standardized task-approach strategies were employed by subjects.

This line of inquiry was next taken up by Horgan (1983b), who employed the arm-positioning paradigm to compare instructions favouring either movement location or extent-of-movement cues. Movement location cues produce superior recall in nonretarded subjects, presumably because the feel of endpoints produces a stronger memory trace, in effect giving subjects something concrete to rehearse during the recall interval (Keele & Ells, 1972; Laabs, 1973). Interestingly, both location (experiment 1) and extent cues (experiment 2) aided the recall of mentally retarded subjects. Though not directly compared, both extent cues and location cues produced an effect size of about 1 standard deviation (expressed in "uninstructed" units).

Although not directly intended, Horgan's data (1983b) may be the most persuasive evidence for the role of attention of the papers reviewed. Since nonretarded subjects are consistently better able to rehearse endpoints, it is hard to invoke the rehearsal explanation in the Horgan data. Rather, a more parsimonious explanation may be that any set of specific instructions focus attentional resources of mentally retarded subjects on the task, thus improving performance, perhaps independently of rehearsal. It is difficult indeed to explain, why it is somehow relatively easier for mentally retarded subjects to rehearse extent-of-movement data than their nonretarded counterparts.

To summarize, it seems that the process of infusing memorial information on an attentive sensory apparatus may be sufficient to hold proprioceptive information in memory for approximately 7- to 10-seconds. After 7-seconds, information decays rapidly unless subjects adopt an effective processing strategy. An instructive analog for the operation of an ecological system may be drawn from the volume fill-empty differential of a common funnel. Where the funnel reservoir can be filled to capacity with fluid (analogous to memorial stimuli) virtually instantaneously, the narrow funnel neck drains the reservoir (information decay) at a proportionally slower but constant rate until emptied. As with information in short-term memory, unless acted upon, the fluid reservoir of the funnel[2] will be emptied of all its original volume in a predictable time period (for a given volume). In the case of human memory, the rate of decay of the 'information reservoir' (i.e., short-term store), can be dramatically delayed by employing any one of a variety of strategies, the most common of which is rehearsal. Memory for arm-movements among mentally retarded learners seems to operate in a manner quite parallel to verbal or visual information cues. However, as time passes, the ability of mentally retarded and nonretarded subjects to retain proprioceptive/kinaesthetic information diverges. Evidently, the propensity of mentally retarded subjects to rehearse

---

2 Air-tight sealing across the upper rim to the funnel reservoir will significantly reduce the flow rate at the funnel's neck (drain), maintaining the volume in the reservoir for a relatively longer period of time. In other words, the emptying rate will be reduced but not stopped completely.

spontaneously is far more variable than is true for groups of intellectually average subjects.

Instructions to rehearse arm movements either as an image, that is to say covertly (Horgan, 1983b),or overtly (Reid, 1980b) improves the recall performance of mentally retarded subjects. The most parsimonious explanation is that subjects, formerly not rehearsing, came to employ the strategy when so instructed. Nothing in the experimental methodology, however, precludes an explanation for improved performance based on the marshalling of available attentional resources; in fact, Horgan's experiments lends some support to this notion.

Future Directions

In line with Baumeister's (1984) call for ecological validity in research conducted in the field of mental retardation, there is a need to move mnemonic training from the laboratory into applied settings. The applicability of information processing research in industrial, sport and recreational settings remains to be demonstrated. For example, it is not known whether rehearsal-based improvements in recall can be shown for movements more complex than the one degree of freedom linear arm movement; the research reviewed here has been criticized along these lines:

> ... of specific concern to the consideration of skill acquisition in the mentally retarded, is the realization that a very small range of motor skills have been utilized for analysis (often a key press or a simple unidimensional movement) ...
> (Newell, 1985, p. 106)

A move from delineating comparative rehearsal and processing deficits on the part of retarded persons to a training and developmental stance will likely be another research trend. Several writers have suggested that this will entail a cognitive-behaviourial rapprochement (Hogg, 1986; Hoover & Wade, 1985; Wade, Hoover & Newell, 1983). Hogg referred to this trend as a "human factors" approach to the training of mentally retarded persons.

Researchers and practitioners adopting the behaviourial tradition have put together an impressive literature demonstrating gains in motor performance by mentally retarded persons (Hoover & Wade, 1985). It is quite possible that incorporating findings from information processing research may increase the efficiency of behaviourial training. In such a human factors approach, teachers attend both to the learning characteristics of mentally retarded persons as they interact with educational tasks and instructional design. In this way, limitations in memory may be circumvented by changing the stimulus configuration or response demands of tasks.

The process of application may be initiated by incorporating instructions favouring the rehearsal of proprioceptive/kinaesthetic information into training sequences with a behaviourial orientation. In addition, it will probably benefit retarded learners to regularly be provided memory and learning strategies along with primary instruction, though this remains to be demonstrated (Kendall, Borkowski & Cavanaugh, 1980).

No matter how promising the initial data, if rehearsal-based techniques are to impact on practice in mental retardation, maintenance and generalization must be clearly demonstrated. Unfortunately, research has shown that the maintenance and generalization of cognitive strategies is not sanguine at this point (Blackman & Lin, 1984; Borkowski & Cavanaugh, 1979). There is no point inculcating a learning strategy until methods are found to enhance the maintenance of this strategy over time. In addition, motor learning strategies are useful to the extent that they can be used by learners to solve isomorphic motor problems in the same classification of tasks on which they are trained. Neither maintenance nor generalizations of kinaesthetic/proprioceptive information has been demonstrated. Presently, researchers are still showing that a rehearsal strategy can be acquired.

Another problem is to delineate the nature of coded and codable information for the case of mentally retarded memorizers. Proprioceptive information, best represented by location cues, is easier for nonretarded subjects to code for use in short-term memory; is more readily rehearsed, and consequently more susceptible to interference from interpolated activity (Keele & Ells, 1972; Laabs, 1973). As mentioned, the one comparable study undertaken with mentally retarded subjects generated equivocal results favouring neither location nor movement extent cues (Horgan, 1983b). Certainly this is a training issue, the solution to which must be expedited. It is important to identify the nature of rehearsal instructions which have the greatest potential to enhance motor learning in this population.

Researchers may wish to adapt a traditional method for investigating the problem of the nature of rehearsable information. Baddeley (1988) argued for the existence of separate iconic and phonological short-term stores. He based this model on the consistent finding that a pair of visual short-term memory tasks, for example, exert more interference on one-another than two tasks of differing modalities. Thus, the degree of interference between memory for movement information and ones associated with other modalities may provide clues as to whether mentally retarded persons directly rehearse kinesthetic information or first transform it into a form more compatible with visual or auditory short-term stores. Further, mentally retarded learners may differ from their nonretarded counterparts on this dimension of memory.

A final issue is one raised by Campione (1986). He argued that some memory findings may be excessively "task specific." Thus, one responsibility of research workers must be to determine the degree to which cognitive structures operate systematically in mentally retarded subjects across cognitive and motor domains. The lack of knowledge in this area is inexplicable. For example, it is not even known at this time, whether a rehearsal deficit displayed with symbolic (pictorial, numeric) material will also be shown when subjects are asked to recall arm positions. The answers to questions like these will ultimately determine the extent to which the cognitive model is robust regarding the motor learning of mentally retarded persons.

Author Notes

1. Request for reprints should be addressed to John H. Hoover, School of Education, University of South Dakota, Vermillion, South Dakota, USA, 57069.

References

Adams, J. A. (1971). A closed-loop theory of motor learning. *Journal of Motor Behavior, 3*, 111-115.

Adams, J. A. (1987). Historical review and appraisal of research on learning, retention, and transfer of human motor skills. *Psychological Bulletin, 101*, 41-74.

Ashcraft, M. H., & Kellas, G. (1974). Organization in normal and retarded children: Temporal aspects of storage and retrieval. *Journal of Experimental Psychology, 103*, 502-508.

Atkinson, R. E., & Shiffrin, R. M. (1968). Human memory: A proposed system and its control processes. In K. W. Spence & J. T. Spence (Eds.), *The psychology of learning and motivation* (Vol. 2, pp. 89-195). New York, NY: Academic Press.

Baddeley, A. D., & Hitch, G. (1974). Working memory. In G.H. Bower (Ed.), *The psychology of learning and motivation* (Vol. 8, pp. 47-89). London: Academic Press.

Baddeley, A.D. (1988). Working memory and learning disabilities. Paper presented at the twenty-first Gatlinburg Conference on Research and Theory in Mental Retardation and Developmental Disabilities, Gatlinburg, TN, March 1988.

Bartlett, B. J. (1932). *Remembering: A study in experimental and social psychology.* Cambridge, England: Cambridge University Press.

Baumeister, A. A. (1984). Some methodological and conceptual issues in the study of cognitive processes with retarded people. In P. H. Brooks, R. Sperber & C. McCauley (Eds.), *Learning and cognition in the mentally retarded* (pp. 1-38). Hillsdale, NJ: Lawrence Erlbaum.

Belmont, J. M., & Butterfield, E. C. (1969). The relationship of short-term memory to development and intelligence. In L. Lipsett & H. Reese (Eds.), *Advances in child development and behavior* (Vol. 4, pp. 30-82). New York, NY: Academic Press.

Blackman, L. S., & Lin, A. (1984). Generalization training in the educable mentally retarded: Intelligence and its educability revisited. In P. H. Brooks, R. Sperber & L. McCauley (Eds.), *Learning and cognition in the mentally retarded* (pp. 237-263). Hillsdale, NJ: Lawrence Erlbaum.

Borkowski, J. G., & Cavanaugh, J. (1979). Maintenance and generalization of skills and strategies by the retarded. In N. R. Ellis (Ed.), *Handbook of mental deficiency* (2nd, ed., pp. 569-617). Hillsdale, NJ: Lawrence Erlbaum.

Borkowski, J. G., Reid, M. K., & Kurtz, B. E. (1984). Metacognition and retardation: Paradigmatic, theoretical, and applied perspectives. In P. H. Brooks, R. Sperber & C. McCauley (Eds.), *Learning and cognition in the mentally retarded* (pp. 55-75). Hillsdale, NJ: Lawrence Erlbaum.

Borys, S. V., & Spitz, H. H. (1976). Short-term retention in retarded adolescents as a function of load, delay, and interpolated activity. *The Journal of Psychology, 94,* 207-216.

Brown, A. L. (1974). The role of strategic behavior in retarded memory. In N. R. Ellis (Ed.), *International review of research in mental retardation* (Vol.7, pp. 55-111). New York, NY: Academic Press.

Brown, A. L., & Barclay, C. R. (1976). The effects of training specific mnemonics on the metamnemonic efficiency of retarded children. *Child Development, 47,* 71-80.

Brown, A. L., Campione, J. C., Bray, N. W., & Wilcox, B. L. (1973). Keeping track of changing variables: Effects of rehearsal training and rehearsal prevention in normal and retarded adolescents. *Journal of Experimental Psychology, 101,* 123-131.

Brown, A. L., Campione, J. C., & Murphy, M. D. (1974). Keeping track of changing variables: Long-term retention of a trained rehearsal strategy by retarded adolescents. *American Journal of Mental Deficiency, 78*, 446-453.

Butterfield, E. C., Wambold, C., & Belmont, J. M. (1973). On the theory and practice of improving short-term memory. *American Journal of Mental Deficiency, 77*, 654-669.

Campione, J. C. (1986). Reaction time and the study of intelligence. In M. G. Wade (Ed.), *Motor skill acquisition of the mentally handicapped: Issues in research and training* (pp. 155-163). New York, NY: North Holland.

Campione, J. C., & Brown, A. L. (1977) Memory and metamemory development in educable retarded children. In R. V. Kail & J. W. Hagen (Eds.), *Perspectives on the development of memory and cognition* (pp. 367-406). Hillsdale, NJ: Lawrence Erlbaum.

Carr, T. H. (1984). Attention, skill, and intelligence: Some speculations on extreme individual differences in human performance. In P. H. Brooks, R. Sperber & C. McCauley (Eds.), *Learning and cognition in the mentally retarded* (pp. 189-215). Hillsdale, NJ: Lawrence Erlbaum.

Cohen, R. L., & Nealon, J. (1979). An analysis of short-term memory differences between retardates and nonretardates. *Intelligence, 3*, 65-72.

Cohen, R. L., & Sandberg, T. (1977). The relationship between intelligence and short-term memory. *Cognitive Psychology, 9*, 534-554.

Detterman, D. K. (1979). Memory in the mentally retarded. In N. R. Ellis (Ed.), *Handbook on mental deficiency* (2nd, ed., pp. 727-780). Hillsdale, NJ: Lawrence Erlbaum.

Duncan, J. (1980). The demonstration of capacity limitation. *Cognitive Psychology, 12*, 75-96.

Ellis, N. R. (1963). The stimulus trace and behaviorial adequacy. In N. R. Ellis (Ed.), *Handbook of mental deficiency* (pp. 134-158). New York, NY: McGraw-Hill Book Co.

Ellis, N. R. (1970). Memory processes in retardates and normals. In N. R. Ellis (Ed.), *International review of research in mental retardation* (Vol. 4, pp. 1-32). New York, NY: Academic Press.

Ellis, N. R. (1988/ March). Automatic-effortful processing and intelligence level. Invited Address: Twenty-first Gatlinburg Conference on Research and Theory in Mental Retardation and Developmental Disabilities. Gatlinburg, TN.

Ellis, N. R., & Meador, D. M. (1985). Forgetting in retarded and nonretarded persons under conditions of minimal strategy use. *Intelligence, 9,* 87-96.

Ellis, N. R., Meador, D. M., & Bodfish, J. W. (1985). Differences in intelligence and automatic memory processes. *Intelligence, 9,* 265-273.

Fagan, J. F. (1966). Short-term retention in normal and retarded children. *Psychonomic Science, 6,* 303-304.

Ferretti, R. P. (1982). An analysis of passive memory in normal and mentally retarded persons. *Intelligence, 6,* 69-87.

Fisher, M. A., & Zeaman, D. (1973). An attention-retention theory of retardates' discrimination learning. In N. R. Ellis (Ed.), *International review of research in mental retardation* (Vol. 6, pp. 171-257). New York, NY: Academic Press.

Flavell, J. H. (1978). Metacognitive development. In J. M. Scandura & C. J. Brainerd (Eds.), *Structural/process theories of complex human behavior* (pp. 213-245). Alphess g.q. Riin, The Netherlands: Sijtoff & Noordhoff.

Flavell, J. H., Beach, D. R., & Chinsky, J. M. (1966). Spontaneous verbal rehearsal in memory task as a function of age. *Child Development, 37,* 283-299.

Hagen, J. W., Streeter, L. A., & Raker R. (1974). Labeling, rehearsal, and short-term memory in retarded children. *Journal of Experimental Child Psychology, 18,* 259-268.

Hasher L., & Zacks, R. T. (1979). Automatic and effortful processes in memory. *Journal of Experimental Psychology: General, 108,* 356-388.

Hayes, C. S., & Routh, D. K. (1972). Short-term memory in normals and retardates as a function of stimulus intensity and recall interval: A test of Ellis' theory. *Psychological Reports, 30,* 831-836.

Henry, F. M. (1974). Variable and constant performance errors within a group of individuals. *Journal of Motor Behavior, 6,* 149-154.

Hogg, J. (1986). Process and context in ensuring competent motor behavior by mentally retarded people. In M. G. Wade (Ed.), *Motor skill acquisition of the mentally handicapped: Issues in research and training* (pp. 227-241). New York, NY: North-Holland.

Hoover, J. H., & Wade, M. G. (1985). Motor learning theory and mentally retarded individuals: A historical review. *Adapted Physical Activity Quarterly, 3,* 228-252.

Horgan, J. S. (1983a). Measurement bias in memory for movement by mentally retarded and nonretarded children. *Perceptual and Motor Skills, 57,* 663-670.

Horgan, J. S. (1983b). Mnemonic strategy instruction in coding, processing, and recall of movement-related cues by mentally retarded children. *Perceptual and Motor Skills, 57,* 547-557.

Horgan, J. S. & Horgan, J. (1982). Measurement bias in representation of accuracy on linear positioning tasks. *Perceptual and Motor Skills, 55,* 971-981.

Kahneman, D. (1973). *Attention and effort.* Englewood Cliffs, NJ: Prentice Hall.

Keele, S., & Ells, J. (1972). Memory characteristics and kinaesthetic information. *Journal of Motor Behavior, 4,* 127-134.

Kellas, G., Ashcraft, M. H., & Johnson, N. S. (1973). Rehearsal processes in the short-term memory performance of mildly retarded adolescents. *American Journal of Mental Deficiency, 77,* 670-679.

Kelso, J. A. S., Goodman, D., Stamm, C. L., & Hayes, C. (1979). Movement coding and memory in retarded children. *American Journal of Mental Deficiency, 83,* 601-611.

Kendall, C. R., Borkowski, J. G., & Cavanaugh, J. C. (1980). Maintenance and generalization of an interrogative strategy by EMR children. *Intelligence, 4,* 255-270.

Krupski, A. (1977). Role of attention in the reaction time performance of mentally retarded adolescents. *American Journal of Mental Deficiency, 82,* 79-83.

Laabs, G. J. (1973). Retention characteristics of different reproduction cues in motor short-term memory. *Journal of Experimental Psychology, 100,* 168-177.

Marshall, J. C., & Fryer, D. M. (1978). Speak, memory: An introduction to some historic studies of remembering and forgetting. In M. M. Gruenberg & P. Morris (Eds.), *Aspects of memory* (pp. 1-25). London: Methuen.

Marteniuk, R. G. (1973). Retention characteristics of motor short-term memory cues. *Journal of Motor Behavior, 5,* 249-259.

Neisser, U. (1976). *Cognition and reality.* San Francisco, CA: Freeman.

Newell, K. M. (1985). Motor skill acquisition and current orientations. In J. H. Humphreys & J. E. Clarke (Eds.), *Motor development: Current selected research* (Vol. 1, pp. 183-192).

Peterson, L. R., & Peterson, M. (1959). Short-term retention of individual items. *Journal of Experimental Psychology, 58,* 193-198.

Reid, G. (1980a). The effects of memory strategy instruction in the short-term memory of the mentally retarded. *Journal of Motor Behavior, 12,* 221-227.

Reid, G. (1980b). Overt and covert rehearsal in short-term motor memory of mentally retarded and nonretarded persons. *American Journal of Mental Deficiency, 85,* 69-75.

Reid, G. (1986). The trainability of motor processing strategies with developmentally delayed performers. In. H.T.A. Whiting & M.G. Wade (Eds.), *Themes in Motor Development* (pp. 93-107). Dordrecht: Martinus Nijhoff.

Scott, R. S. (1971). Acquisition, retention, and relearning of a gross motor skill with normal and retarded children (Doctoral dissertation, Indiana University, 1971). *Dissertation Abstracts International, 32,* 224A.

Spitz, H. A. (1979). Beyond field theory in the study of mental deficiency. In N. R. Ellis (Ed.), *Handbook of mental deficiency* (2nd ed., pp. 121-141). Hillsdale, NJ: Lawrence Erlbaum.

Sugden, D. A. (1978). Visual motor short term memory in educationally subnormal boys. *British Journal of Educational Psychology, 48,* 330-339.

Torgesen, J., & Kail, R. V. (1980). Memory processes in exceptional children. In B. K. Keogh (Ed.), *Advances in special education* (Vol.1, pp. 55-99). Greenwich, CT: JAI Press.

Turnball, A. P. (1974). Teaching retarded persons to rehearse through cumulative overt labeling. *American Journal of Mental Deficiency, 79,* 331-337.

Wade, M. G., Hoover, J. H., & Newell, K. M. (1983). Training and trainability in motor skills performance of mentally retarded persons. In J. Hogg & P. Mittler (Eds.), *Advances in mental handicap research* (Vol. 2, pp. 175-200). New York, NY: John Wiley & Sons.

Zeaman, D., & House, B. (1979). A review of attention theory. In N. R. Ellis (Ed.), *Handbook of mental deficiency* (2nd ed., pp. 63-120). Hillsdale, NJ: Lawrence Erlbaum.

Problems in Movement Control
G. Reid (editor)
Elsevier Science Publishers B.V. (North-Holland), 1990

FACTORS UNDERLYING INEFFICIENT MOVEMENT IN LEARNING DISABLED CHILDREN

Jo-Anne C. Lazarus
Department of Physical Education and Dance
University of Wisconsin - Madison

A subgroup of the intellectually-normal population of children have been identified as having learning and/or performance difficulties with school-related tasks. Attempts to label, define and understand this problem (i. e. minimal brain dysfunction, attentional deficit disorder, learning disability) have been difficult because the group is extremely heterogenous in terms of behaviourial symptoms. Characteristic of many learning disabled children (the term used throughout the chapter) is their inefficient control of movement.

Evidence will be presented in this chapter to support the view that several mechanisms or processes underlie the poor motor performance of learning disabled children and that through the investigation of their performance on specific motor tasks, these factors can be elucidated and placed within a framework from which to view this disability. The advantage of investigating motor tasks is that they can be made relatively free of the influence of prior experience and thus cut across language and cultural barriers.

Due to the heterogenous nature of this population, it becomes necessary to limit the discussion to identifiable subgroups of learning disabled (LD) children. A large percentage of these children appear to have a functional language impairment manifested in such skills as reading, writing, and spelling (Boder, 1973; Mattis, 1978; Petrauskas & Rourke, 1979). For this reason, the major clinical focus in both assessment and treatment has been on language skills. As a result, many practitioners have come to view learning disabilities primarily as a language deficit that causes concomitant problems in other domains. This subgroup of children often display subtle motor difficulties that do not appear to be a function of the neuromuscular apparatus per se (i. e. a motor output problem) but rather appear to be a function of motor planning. This is evident by their reasonably adequate performance at low levels of information processing, but whose performance declines when the planning or cognitive demands of the motor task are high. Included in this group are children identified as reading-disabled and dyslexic.

There is another cluster of children within the LD population who exhibit visual-spatial-motor difficulties and who are usually considered to be "clumsy" or "awkward" (Denckla, 1972; Haubenstricker, 1982) These children are characterized by poor co-ordination, poor balance and often poor postural control and decreased muscle tone. It is not uncommon for these children to have language-related difficulties as well, particularly in the areas of pronunciation and comprehension. This manifestation of a learning disability hints at a neurological deficit of some sort, albeit "soft" neurological signs, and has been referred to as a "non-verbal learning disability" (Strang, 1979).

The two subgroups described above will be included in this essay, although it is recognized that the various mechanisms underlying their inefficient performance may differ. Children who have a learning disability attributable to other factors (i. e. emotional, behaviourial, motivational) and who exhibit no motor incompetence will not be included in this review.

Theoretical Perspectives

Theories of learning disability have not succeeded in identifying factors responsible for the various patterns of behaviour exhibited by LD children. Just as learning and cognition are conceptualized differently depending on the theoretical orientation of the investigator, so too is the notion of a learning disability. In fact, due to the heterogeneous nature of the population, the behaviourial pattern or patterns themselves have not yet been clearly elucidated.

Some early theorists proposed unidimensional conceptions of learning disabilities which were extremely narrow in scope. They usually focused on a specific type or source of disability. Delacato proposed a theory of neurological organization in which "patterning" of body movements would develop neural connections necessary for uniform dominance or sidedness and in turn "cure" various learning problems and behaviour disorders (Delacato, 1959). Orton proposed a theory of mixed dominance in which mirror images of all incoming stimuli were not suppressed by the dominant hemisphere resulting in specific language disabilities or developmental dyslexia. The central remediation technique involved a visual-auditory-kinaesthetic-tactile approach to learning (Orton, 1937). Perceptual-deficit and psycholinguistic-deficit hypotheses identified specific problem areas and assumed that if you focus attention on alleviating the deficit, learning should result (Bender, 1958; Cruickshank, 1967; Frostig, 1964; Kirk & Kirk, 1971; Wepman, 1960). Such process-oriented approaches resulted in the development of various assessment techniques designed to identify the specific deficit and offer remediation techniques (i. e. Bender-Gestalt Test, Frostig Test of Visual Perceptual Development, Illinois Test of Psycholinguistic Ability).

The preceding single factor theories, although narrow in scope, were pursued by researchers in an attempt to account for the various behaviours manifested by LD children. However, since individuals classified as LD are not homogeneous in symptoms, this method failed to provide a systematic and encompassing view of learning disabilities.

Both Gestalt psychologists (Strauss, Werner) and cognitive structuralists (Piaget) provided models of cognition upon which many LD researchers framed their questions. In dealing with the symptom of distractibility, for example, Cruickshank (1967) was a proponent of the elimination of extraneous sights and sounds in the learning environment. The presence of study cubicles and sparsely decorated rooms evolved out of this notion in an attempt to assist the child in distinguishing figure from ground or pertinent from extraneous stimuli. Other applications of Gestalt psychology include colour coding of specific areas of materials to attract attention to salient features, outlining the "figure" area of material, and delineating margins to indicate the beginning and ending of a line in reading.

Piagetian developmental notions were evident in the works of clinicians such as Marianne Frostig and Carl Delacato. Frostig's Developmental Test of Visual Perception (Frostig, 1964) included tasks such as the constancy of shape, a notion derived largely from Piaget's work on conservation, while proponents of Delacato's neural organization theory (Delacato, 1959) stressed the invariant order of stages in neuro-physiological development, not that unlike Piaget's notion of the invariant order of stages in cognitive development. In borrowing from models of cognition that seemed to fit the symptoms they were dealing with, clinicians in learning disabilities held a narrow view of the psychological organism, focusing on one particular process and failing to view the whole model.

More recently, the popularity of both the artificial intelligence or computer model and the information processing approach in psychology influenced the orientation of many LD theorists (Farnham-Diggory, 1978, 1980; Ross, 1976; Satz & Van Nostrand, 1973; Senf, 1972; Torgeson, 1977; Vellutino, 1978; Wong, 1979a, b). Drawing from the computer model, Torgeson (1977) and Wong (1979a, b) articulate that LD children lack the necessary strategies or cognitive controls for learning. In this conceptualization, the onus for learning is placed on the teachers who are expected to provide the appropriate crutches necessary for the LD child to learn. In viewing the child as an inactive learner, however, the source or mechanism involved in learning, and in turn, the technique to "activate" the child, is not specified.

From an information processing perspective, explanations for the poor performance of LD children involve the specification of various internal structures responsible for this behaviour. Functional irregularities in the integration of information (Senf, 1972), a developmental delay in either selective attention (Ross, 1976) or perceptual and linguistic abilities (Satz & Van Nostrand, 1973), or a verbal deficit (Vellutino, 1978) represent various information processing explanations for the ineffective performance of LD children.

The approaches in the two preceding paragraphs exemplify mechanistic models of development where the organism is reactive, inherently at rest, and active only as a result of external forces (Overton & Reese, 1973). In contrast, an organismic model of development views the organism as an active whole, in continuous transition from one state to another through progressive activities of differentiation and individuation (Overton & Reese, 1973). In the mechanistic model *behaviour* changes with development, whereas in the organismic model *structures* and *functions* change during development.

The mechanistic approaches fail to provide an explanation for the psychological basis of LD because in focusing on specific deficits and trying to alleviate them, they do not consider potential organismic compensations for these deficits. Certainly, children with selective deficits compensate for their inability to perform in a specific manner. Such compensations make it difficult for a researcher or clinician to identify their problem, since tasks are approached in dramatically different ways. Individuals bring to bear their selective structural and/or functional deficits, to each situation under investigation, adding to the interindividual variability so often observed in the performance of this atypical group.

It is the bias of this author that what is needed in the learning disability literature is an all-encompassing organismic model of learning disabilities that can account not only for the specific structural and/or functional deficits of this population (evidenced in the two subgroups delineated above), but also for the compensations that are made in accommodating these deficits. Such an organismic model would suggest that whatever factors play a role in the development of inefficient movement, they are not similar at all points in the life-span but rather *qualitatively* different, accounting for inter-individual variability and novelty in performance.

To date, such a model does not exist, although a neo-Piagetian theory such as Pascual-Leone's Theory of Constructive Operators (Pascual-Leone & Goodman, 1979) could potentially serve as a conceptual framework from which to develop an organismic model of learning disabilities. This theory simulates the psychological system within which the notion of learning (and thus inefficient learning) exists. Viewing the organism as active rather than reactive, it presents psychological constructs which underlie or cause organized patterns of behaviour. Although the constructs presented are psychological, not biological in nature, they are construed from a biological organism. Such a theory is intuitively appealing in that, as a general psychological theory, it should apply across tasks and situations, and not require radical modification to apply to learning disabilities. As an initial step in setting the groundwork for the development of an organismic theory of learning disabilities, this paper will address several factors believed to underlie inefficient movement.

Factors Underlying Inefficient Movement: An Integrative Perspective

Cognitive Style

Cognitive style is a notion that has been represented by the field dependence/field independence construct (Witkin, Dyk, Faterson, Goodenough & Karp, 1962). Perceptually, the field dependence/field independence construct refers to the extent to which an individual's perception is biased by the surrounding visual field. In this regard, relatively field dependent individuals tend to be biased to a greater extent than those who are relatively field independent. Extremes of this field dependence/field independence dimension are defined as a global mode of field approach and an articulated mode of field approach, respectively, representing an individual's cognitive style or preferred mode of processing. It should be made clear that cognitive style and cognitive capacity are distinct concepts. The latter refers to a structural and/or capacity limitation largely due to maturation, while the former reflects optional modes of adaptation to the environment which are largely (but not exclusively) due to learning and experience and therefore in principle changeable with experience (Pascual-Leone, 1975).

Cognitive style has been measured using tests of perception of the upright such as the Rod and Frame Test (Witkin et al., 1962), tests of cognitive restructuring such as the Embedded Figures Test (Witkin, Oltman, Raskin, & Karp, 1971) and the Children's Embedded Figures Test (Witkin et al., 1971), and tests of horizontality of liquids such as the Water Level Test (DeAvila, Havassy & Pascual-Leone, 1976). Although these tests are all measures of cognitive style, they do not demand the use of exactly the same psychological functions for successful performance. Certainly, overemphasis of visual information that is salient but irrelevant would lead to poor performance on all four tasks, supporting commonality across tasks. Yet, particular tasks such as the Water Level Test require additional skills, such as the ability to generate an appropriate response once the irrelevant visual information is inhibited.

Developmentally, there is a trend towards increasing field independency with age. Pascual-Leone (1975) attributes this trend (field dependence to field independence) to developmental changes in mental energy and in the conceptual knowledge or processes co-ordinated by mental energy. This increase in mental energy permits the development of more complex strategies which would contribute to field independency. Although a developmental trend towards field independence exists, relative differences within an age group appear to be reasonably stable (Witkin, Goodenough & Karp, 1967).

In the population of children referred to as learning disabled, the trend towards field independence is delayed relative to the norms (Friedman, Guyer & Tymchuk, 1976; Guyer & Friedman, 1975; Keogh & Donlon, 1972; Lazarus & Kyprie, 1980). This group of children tend to cluster towards the field dependent end of the continuum. It appears that learning disabled children operate under quite a different style than that evident in the nondisabled population.

A particular style results in preferential use of cognitive strategies that either enhance or deter from task performance dependent on optimal compatibility between task demand and cognitive style. Body articulation, a skill demanding differentiation, as well as a motor integration task (Todor & Lazarus, 1982) are better performed by a field independent person. In contrast, memory for faces, forms, and perception of human emotion, skills of a more divergent nature, are better performed by field dependent subjects, often resulting in greater competence in interpersonal relationships. Body awareness has been targeted as a skill deficient in many learning disabled children (Ayres, 1972), while their sensitivity to the feelings and needs of others has also been noted (Lazarus & Kyprie, 1980).

Although learning may be quite different under one or the other cognitive style, each individual is not likely to be dominated completely by one or the other style, but fall somewhere along the continuum. For the purpose of comparison the ends of the continuum are contrasted. The field independent individual tends to differentiate task instructions from salient features in the available cue set (Thomas & Bender, 1977). With this very active participant approach to learning, input material undergoes cognitive restructuring and a rich repertoire of flexible, logical structures emerge (Goodenough, 1976). This type of learning experience develops rich executive control structures which, in turn, effect positive learning experiences and the ability to perform novel tasks.

In contrast, the field dependent individual tends to be dominated by salient cues in concept attainment problems (Thomas & Bender, 1977) and fails to sample fully from the available cue set (Case & Globerson, 1974). This behaviour typifies a spectator approach to learning, resorting to trial and error strategies and overlearning of content rather than processes and relationships (Goodenough, 1976). This type of learning experience develops inflexible control structures which are not easily applicable to new situations. As a result, field dependent subjects have many negative learning experiences and tend to be rigid in their performance, maintaining poor strategies even when ineffective.

In summary, learning disabled children perform poorly on tasks designed to measure field dependence/independence. Characteristically, they tend to be cue triggered, responding almost automatically to the most salient visual cues of the task. The LD child's behaviour on these tasks lacks "controlled" (Hasher & Zacks, 1979) or "effortful" (Shiffrin & Schneider, 1977) processing.

Sequencing

The sequencing of motor acts consists of the serial ordering and integration of individual components for efficient performance. In addition, rhythmical, repetitive activities also include a temporal control component. From a developmental perspective, a consistent age-related improvement in the ability to temporally organize a series of movements has been documented (Wolff & Hurwitz, 1976). In this study, younger children were less able to maintain a steady alternating tapping beat with their index fingers and were more variable between intervals than older children.

In a motor skill such as ball throwing, the temporal component is less crucial, but the necessity for serial ordering and integrating of the elements of the skill can be demonstrated. Younger children (2-3 years old) use a pattern that consists almost exclusively of arm movement (forearm extension, feet stationary, no body rotation; Roberton, 1977; Wickstrom, 1977). They eliminate the need to sequence several components by reducing the complexity of the task to basically one component. In contrast, older children (7-8 years old) use a more mature pattern, where the elements of the task (arm and trunk rotation, contralateral step forward, hips, trunk, and shoulder rotation, forward extension of arm) are performed in an orderly, integrated manner (Roberton, 1977; Wickstrom, 1977).

While a left hemisphere specialization of cerebral functions is most convincingly demonstrated for the processing of speech (Lenneberg, 1967), the left hemisphere has also been demonstrated to be specialized in the putting together of complex sequences of movements (Kimura, 1973). Neuropsychological studies on aphasics (Kimura, 1973) have shown that left hemisphere aphasics had no difficulty reproducing static hand postures but were impaired in the reproduction of complex sequences of movement, both meaningful and meaningless. Attempts to teach aphasics American sign language have failed, due to the high demand for complex sequential movements in this method of communication. Kimura further argued that because aphasics could choose the correct movement when several alternatives were presented, but could not reproduce the movement, the deficit was not on the input side.

Orton (1937) proposed that children with reading and language disorders have difficulty in the "recall of proper sequences." In verbal performance measures they tend to score poorer than their age-equivalent nondisabled peers (Rugel, 1974). In addition, these same children have problems with sequential motor activities (Badian & Wolff, 1977; Lazarus & Kyprie, 1980).

Zurif & Carson (1970) found dyslexics to be significantly inferior in dealing with the temporal aspects of nonverbal auditory and visual information as well as tests of manual dexterity. Similarly, Hurwitz, Bibace, Wolff & Rowbotham (1972) demonstrated that boys with learning-disabilities were inferior to normal boys on items from the Lincoln-Oseretsky Test of Motor Development which depend on rhythmical, temporally-related skills.

On a tapping task that required subjects to keep the rate of an entraining metronome beat and to tap as regularly as possible, boys with a reading disability had greater difficulty than normal boys in maintaining a steady tapping rate when tapping with two hands in alternation, but only with respect to performance of the left hand (Badian & Wolff, 1977). Wyke (1968, 1971) provides evidence for left hemisphere control over the activity of both hands. This finding in conjunction with the left hemisphere's superiority in precise temporal control of motor sequence could account for the inferior performance of the left hand in the reading-disabled group. However, when the rate at which subjects were expected to reproduce intermanual tapping rhythms was reduced (by slowing down an entraining metronome) dyslexics began to perform much closer to normal readers (Wolff, Cohen & Drake, 1984). Increasing speed differentially affected normal and dyslexic readers, the dyslexics performing poor at a lower threshold of speed. Thus, the feature of motor performance which best characterized group differences was the threshold at which movement speed interfered with timing precision.

Bruininks & Bruininks (1977) report the administration of a comprehensive battery of fine and gross motor measures to a sample of learning disabled and nondisabled children. Three subtests (upper limb speed and dexterity, visual-motor control, and upper limb co-ordination) were comprised of several sequential-motor tasks such as finger thumb opposition, rapid placement of dots in circles, pencil tapping, etc. Figure 1 represents standard scores on all eight subtests of this Bruininks-Oseretsky Test of Motor Proficiency for 55 learning disabled and 55 nondisabled children. Learning disabled students performed poorly on all tasks requiring sequencing of motor acts.

In another study published the same year, Williams, Temple & Bateman (1977) assessed the extent to which older "slowly developing" children were similar to chronologically younger but "normally developing" children in basic sensori-perceptual abilities, the ability to learn simple perceptual-motor and higher order cognitive tasks. Both gross and fine perceptual-motor tasks were used to assess learning and in each case the child was asked to perform a series of three independent movement subroutines and to sequence them into a smooth act. The appropriate sequencing of the subroutines was dictated by a low-level analysis of simple visual and auditory information. The learning curves in Figures 2 and 3 clearly show that all groups learned across the five trials. However, the performance of the older (mean age 9 yrs. 2 mon.) slowly developing children on the gross perceptual-motor task was intermediate to that of the 6 and 8 year old normal groups and by the fourth trial of learning was essentially the same as the 6 year olds. On the fine perceptual-motor task, the older slowly developing children functioned consistently throughout learning at a level similar to that of 6 year old normal children.

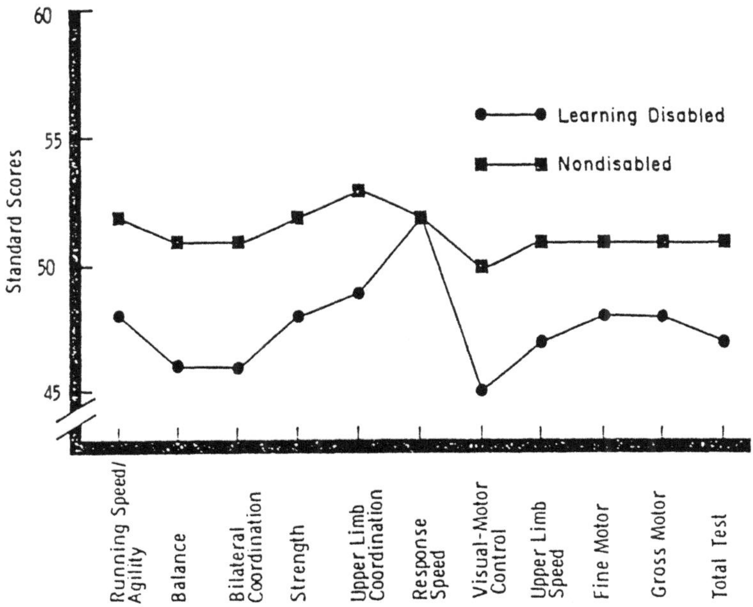

Figure 1. Performance of Learning Disabled and Nondisabled Children. (Reprinted with permission of the authors and publisher from: Bruininks, V.L., & Bruininks, R.H. (1977) MOtor proficiency of learning disabled and nondisabled students. *Perceptual and Motor Skill, 44*, 1131-1137. Fig. 1)

The slowly developing children could perform the individual elements of each gross and fine perceptual-motor task in isolation, but had difficulty when they were required to combine the elements in an orderly series. The authors conclude from this finding that the poor performance of slowly developing children on these tasks was not a function of the movement execution characteristics of the individual acts, but due to differences in efficiency of sensory-analysis processes, the sequential nature of the task and possibly, motor control. It is not clear why motor control would be a critical factor in the sequential condition and not in the individual act condition. Fine control of fingers and hand movements as well as whole body movements requires inhibitory control over associated movements and postural adjustments, which are important both in individual and combinations of acts. Certainly perceptual-motor integration and the sequencing demands of the task play a crucial role in the performance of these slowly developing children. Both inhibitory control and perceptual-motor integration factors will be subsequently discussed.

Figure 2

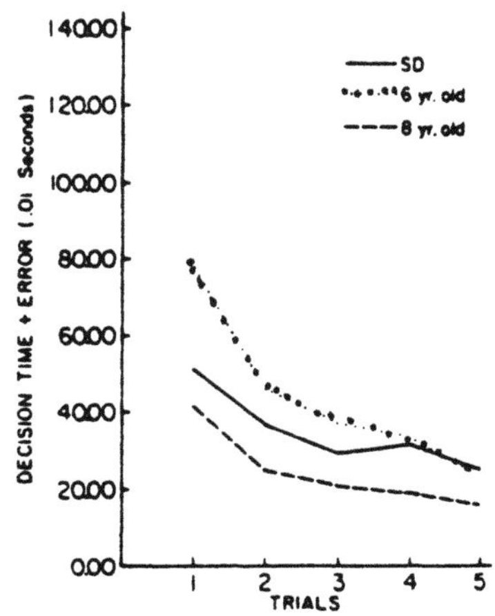

Figure 3

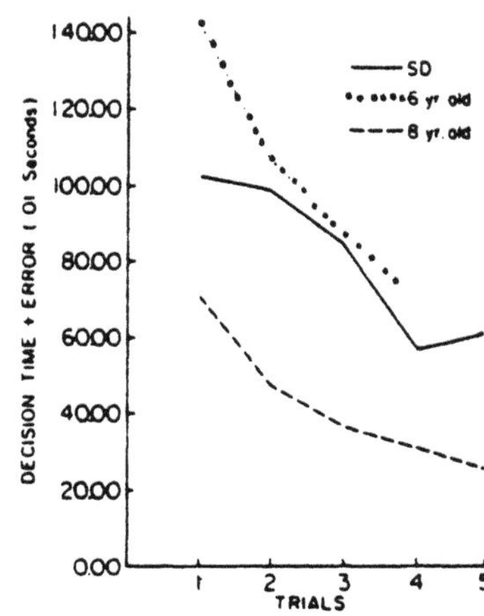

Figure 2. Learning Curves: Gross PM Task. (Reprinted with permission of authors and publisher from: Williams, H.G., Temple, I.G., & Bateman, N.J. (1977) Perceptual motor and cognitive learning in young children. In D.M. Landers, & R.W. Christina (Eds.), *Psychology of Motor Behavior and Sport*, Champaign, Illinois: Human Kinetics Publishers. Fig. 2.)

Figure 3. Learning Curves: Fine PM Task. (Reprinted with permission of authors and publisher from: Williams, H.G., Temple, I.G., & Bateman, N.J. (1977) Perceptual motor and cognitive learning in young children. In D.M. Landers, & R.W. Christina (Eds.), *Psychology of Motor Behavior and Sport*,Champaign, Illinois: Human Kietics Publishers. Fig. 3.)

Halverson and Roberton (1988) found similar serial deficits in a sample of learning disabled boys during a sequential hopping task. Often, associated arm action began at a higher developmental level for the first one to two hops but was forced into a more primitive pattern during subsequent hops. Difficulty in changing direction (turning on extensors and turning off flexors) and hence poor control of force production is a potential cause of this deterioration in performance as the hopping trial progressed.

Multiple discriminant function analysis is a statistical tool often used to determine what test items load heavily on certain variables which discriminate between groups. Using this procedure, Kendrick & Hanten (1980) found finger-thumb opposition and foot-patting to significantly discriminate between a group of normal and learning disabled children. Both of these tasks involve temporal sequencing and were taken from the Devereux Test of Extremity Coordination. The authors conclude that based on the resulting discriminant function prediction equation, 78% of the sample had been correctly classified as learning disabled or nondisabled by previous methods. This data indicates the plausibility of using such sequential-motor tasks as screening tools for early identification of children with learning disabilities.

Several hypotheses could be rendered to explain the inability of learning disabled children to perform well on sequential tasks: a predisposition to use different neuropsychological mechanisms than normal children that are inappropriate for the desired behaviour; a predisposition to use the same neuropsychological mechanisms as normal children but use them ineffectively; a neurophysiological deficit in the transmission of temporally-related events.

Typically, LD children do not exhibit "hard neurological signs" of central nervous system damage. Thus, a neural transmission problem is not likely. Their approach to sequential tasks seems to indicate a predisposition to use different mechanisms than normal children which are not compatible with task demands. A global approach to tasks better subserved by the left hemisphere's sequencing capabilities, results in inferior performance. Communication between the two hemispheres seems to be reduced, with more of a competition between the two hemispheres for processing rights.

Perceptual-Motor Integration

In order to learn and/or perform a gross motor skill, children must be able to process a number of different kinds of task-relevant sensory information, and process it rapidly and accurately in order to be successful in the execution of the act (Whiting, 1972). The most widely researched modalities in terms of their relevance to the performance of motor acts are the visual and kinaesthetic modalities (Hay, 1979, 1981; Whiting & Cockerill, 1972; Whiting, 1972).

The ability to integrate perceptual information which comes through different sensory modalities improves with age (Birch & Belmont, 1965; Birch & Lefford, 1963; Connolly & Jones, 1970; Rudel & Teuber, 1971). In these studies tasks are employed which assess the child's ability to judge the equivalence or nonequivalence of sensory input in the same (intramodal) or different (crossmodal) sensory modalities or to replicate movements presented visually or kinaesthetically in one or the other modality. In general, the integration of information within a modality is more accurate and less variable than the integration of information across modalities (Connolly & Jones, 1970).

Posner (1967) has provided evidence to indicate that visual storage is more efficient than kinaesthetic storage. Given a central processing capacity, he argues that the visual system functions as a "rehearsal" mechanism, whereas the kinaesthetic store is subject to temporal decay. In support of this, Connolly and Jones (1970) found fewer errors in the visual-visual task than in the kinaesthetic-kinaesthetic task. In addition, intra-modal performance was less variable than cross-modal performance. The additional process of translation which a cross-modal match requires, serves to increase variability of performance. There was an increased variability of the visual-kinaesthetic performance over that of the kinaesthetic-visual performance. This result is based on the assumption that translation of information between modalities takes place prior to its being put into short-term memory store. Thus, visual input would be translated into kinaesthetic before being stored in short-term memory, and the susceptibility of the kinaesthetic store to decay increases the variability of performance.

Recent evidence exists to support the premise that with age, communication between the visual and motor systems is refined (Williams, 1973) and that in contrast to younger children, older children make greater use of peripheral feedback (Hay, 1979, 1981).

Traditionally, the learning disabled child has been viewed as having a perceptual deficit resulting from poor sensory integration (Ayres, 1972; Cruickshank, 1967). Support for this view stems largely from their poor performance on tasks designed to measure sensory and perceptual-motor integration (i. e. Developmental Test of Visual Motor Integration, Beery, 1967; Bender-Gestalt Test, Koppitz, 1964; Southern California Sensory Integration Test, Ayres, 1977). However, the emphasis in the conceptualization of the disability has been on the perceptual processing component (i. e. learning disabled children see and hear things "differently" than normal children) rather than on the integration of sensory information with the execution of a motor response.

Early studies on brain-injured children (Birch & Belmont, 1965; Rudel & Teuber, 1971) investigated the claim that cross-modal transfer may be deficient in this population. Although brain-injured children performed more poorly than controls on the intermodal task employed, they performed even worse on those intramodal tasks that involved vision alone (Rudel & Teuber, 1971). The mode of presentation (simultaneous vs. sequential) may have been a more significant factor in their failure to perform as well as normals. When visual information was presented simultaneously, brain-injured children were unable to perform as well as younger controls. Their handicap did not appear to be a specific breakdown of cross-modal transfer or intersensory integration, but rather a difficulty with simultaneous apprehension of sensory information, perhaps from the use of a global approach to processing indiscriminant visual input.

Attempts have been made to target the modality or modalities that are deficient in learning disabled children (Kirk & Kirk, 1971). When a child is administered the Illinois Test of Psycholinguistic Abilities (Kirk & Kirk, 1971) a profile emerges from which clinicians devise their remediation program. Figure 4 is a profile of psycholinguistic ages for a child of age 5 years 11 months diagnosed as having a visual-channel disability. The practitioner would then convert these age scores to standard scaled scores and determine which particular abilities are significantly deficient (i. e. visual association, manual expression, visual closure, visual sequential memory, etc.). A program of training would then be developed to ameliorate this visual channel deficiency. Concurrently, the program would utilize the child's area of strength (in this example, the auditory modality) to teach new material.

One difficulty with this diagnostic and remediation technique is that it assumes that the deficit can be remediated. It also does not explicate the underlying reason for the child's inability to perform in a particular modality. A poor score on visual sequential memory may, in fact, be a function of the sequential component of the task.

Test batteries such as the Bruininks-Oseretsky Test of Motor Proficiency purport to evaluate visual-motor control through subtests such as copying a horizontal diamond with the preferred hand or copying overlapping pencils with the preferred hand. Failure on such tasks may reflect numerous problems, some of which may be perceptual-motor integration problems, but there is no way of identifying these factors.

The concept of perceptual and/or perceptual-motor disorders in learning disabilities remains unclear in the literature. Excluding those children who have obvious structural problems in the visual and auditory domains (i. e. extremely poor visual acuity), the task of integrating sensory information for motor output may be a function of preferential processing of information from one modality over another, the relative salience of sensory cues from different modalities, or the efficiency of feedback utilization in the integration of perceptual and motor components which demands mental attentional energy. Lack of adequate processing of the visual information in the Bruininks-Oseretsky copy the design subtest would result in failure on this task. Individuals whose approach is dominated by rigid structures would have difficulty utilizing perceptual information which varies from situation to situation. Their responses would tend to be governed by the salient information in the environment rather than the appropriate feedback necessary to integrate perception with action.

In terms of remediation, it would be valuable to know the preferential processing modality of children with learning problems. The two clusters of children identified in the introduction (language impairment, visual-spatial difficulties) would likely prefer processing information through the visual and auditory modes, respectively. However, since their deficits are usually much more complex than would be predicted from this unidimensional approach to processing modalities, other variables would have to be taken into account when setting up a treatment program. The characteristics of the task as well as other characteristics of the learner (i. e. field dependency) provide input for evaluating the functional relationship between an individual's processing capacity and task demands. Brown (1982) and Temple & Williams (1977) have discussed the importance of considering such relationships.

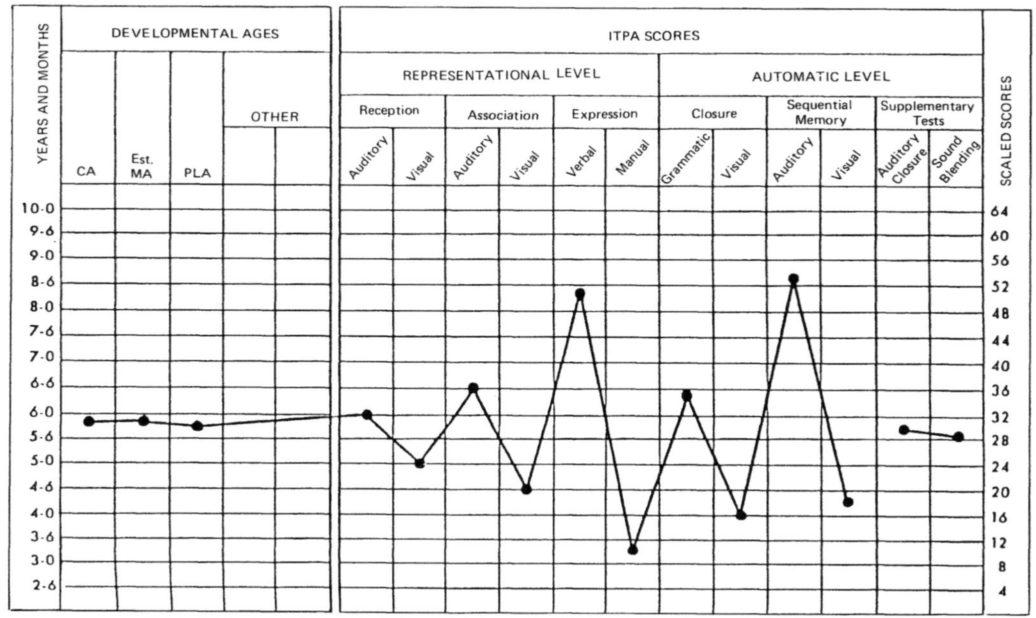

Figure 4. Profile of psycholinguistic ages for a child with visual disability. (Reprinted with permission of publisher from: Kirk, S.A., & Kirk, W.D. (1971) *Psycholinguistic learning disabilities: Diagnosis and remediation*, Chicago: University of Illinois Press. Fig. 6-3.)

Lateralization

The notion of impaired cerebral dominance (lack of establishment of a dominant hemisphere for language) in learning disability was first proposed by Orton in 1937. He hypothesized in his model that the normal course of language development involves bilaterality of language representation, which later becomes lateralized to the left hemisphere. Subsequently it is postulated that lateralization of language is a developmental phenomenon (Lenneberg, 1967). Lenneberg (1967) drew his conclusions from the multitude of evidence that young children are less likely to become aphasic when they have left hemisphere damage. He implied that there was some residual capability in the right hemisphere to compensate for early damage to the left hemisphere, concluding that laterality of language was developmental.

However, there is another way to interpret Lenneberg's observations. The ability of the right hemisphere to compensate for left hemisphere damage does not necessarily mean that there was not some innate propensity for langauge in the left hemisphere. The plasticity of the young brain can account for the right hemisphere's ability to subserve speech.

In the case of the LD child, lateralization is presumed to be incomplete or defective in some way, resulting in inefficient suppression of the activity of the right hemisphere by the left hemisphere and producing competing mirror images within the central nervous system (Orton, 1937). This reasoning has been put forth to explain the many reversal errors observed in the reading, writing, and spelling skills of LD children.

While this explanation is attractive in its simplicity, it is based on faulty assumptions. Many empirical studies on lateralization of language do not support the developmental viewpoint. Rather, the opposite position may be true, as the left hemisphere (for most people) appears to be specialized for language at birth (Entus, 1977; Gardiner & Walter, 1976; Glanville, Best & Levenson, 1977; Molfese, 1977; Trehub & Rabinovitch, 1972). Anatomical evidence of a larger planum temporal (adjacent to Wernicke's area for speech) in the left hemisphere than in the right in neonates as well as adults lends further support for this position (Wada, Clark & Hamm, 1975; Witelson & Pallie, 1973). This evidence supports an attentional model of cerebral dominance, where the fundamental role of each hemisphere is to direct attention to the opposite side of space (Kinsbourne, 1970), rather than a structural-developmental model. Kinsbourne states that perceptual asymmetries can be attributed to unequal activation of the two hemispheres. During verbal tasks, there is a tendency for the left hemisphere to be "primed" or activated to process the material from the right ear or right visual field, attending more to the right side and reciprocally inhibiting the activity on the left side (right hemisphere). As a child becomes older, this process comes under increasing degrees of cortical control.

Perceptual studies of laterality and learning disability have generally used two procedures to measure cerebral asymmetry: visual half-field tachistoscopic presentation (Bryden, 1965) and more commonly, dichotic listening (Kimura, 1961). In the visual modality, stimuli are presented briefly (less than 150 msec.) to the left and right visual fields through a tachistoscope which allows the material to go either to the left or right hemisphere (pathways from the nasal hemiretinas project only to the contralateral hemisphere, while pathways from the temporal hemiretinas project only to the ipsilateral hemisphere). Stimulus material usually consists of words or letters (language) and faces (nonverbal or spatial). In the auditory modality, different stimuli are presented briefly (200-400 msec.) and simultaneously to the right and left ears, and the subject is required to identify one or both stimuli, or to discriminate between them. Stimulus material usually consists of letters, syllables, numbers, or words (language) and music, environmental sounds, or tones (nonverbal).

The results of most lateralized visual and auditory perception studies agree that a right visual field advantage and a right ear advantage exists for language-related material for both learning disabled and normal children, although the performance of the LD group is usually inferior to that of the controls (Kershner, 1977; Marcel, Katz, & Smith, 1974; Marcel & Rajan, 1975; McKeever & Huling, 1970; Olson, 1973). In addition, the control groups often show greater asymmetry than the LD groups (Bryden, 1970; Hynd, Obrzut, Weed & Hynd, 1979; Kershner, 1977; Leong, 1976; Marcel et al., 1974; Marcel & Rajan, 1975; McKeever & Huling, 1970; Obrzut, Hynd, Obrzut & Leitgeb, 1980; Olson, 1973; Witelson, 1977). One particular study found no asymmetry in either group (Zurif & Carson, 1970). However, intersubject variability in this study was high and they tested a fairly small sample of children (n = 14 for each group), rendering the results difficult to interpret.

This fairly consistent finding of a right visual field advantage and a right ear advantage in the population of learning disabled children argues against Orton's hypothesis of incomplete lateralization of language and lends support to the view that impaired cerebral dominance may not be an underlying factor in the poor performance of children with learning disorders.

Several inferences have been made regarding the underlying mechanism involved in the deficient performance of LD children on tasks designed to measure cerebral asymmetry. Witelson (1977) proposed a left hemisphere interference or dysfunction explanation for poor performance in linguistic processing. The dyslexic children in her study were as accurate on tactile and visual spatial tasks as the control children, but showed no difference in accuracy between the left and right visual fields or the left and right hands. The control group showed greater accuracy for stimuli (spatial tasks) presented in the left visual field and in the left hand. She interpreted the results as implicating bilateral processing of spatial functions. It is possible that a functioning, spatial, holistic cognitive mode (that may be represented bilaterally) is being preferentially utilized in cases where linguistic, sequential, analytical processing would produce better performances. In a skill such as reading, heavy reliance on one cognitive mode (especially the holistic mode) is likely to be detrimental to learning. This inference, however, from her data alone, is suspect, as left hemisphere dysfunction would be expected to cause a disproportionately poorer performance by the right ear, not evidenced in her results. It is attractive in that it offers consistency with the cognitive style literature on field dependency cited earlier.

An additional underlying factor proposed by Kinsbourne (1975) can possibly account for the performance differences in Witelson's data. Kinsbourne's (1975) conceptual model of cerebral dominance follows the assumption that the left hemisphere is specialized for language at birth. This view underlies his attentional model of cerebral dominance discussed earlier. Based on this model, Hynd, Obrzut and associates suggest that the performance differences observed between learning disabled and normal children in a series of studies on dichotic listening and time sharing tasks may reflect variability in selective attention on the part of the LD children rather than the degree of lateralization (Hynd et al., 1979; Hynd & Obrzut, 1981 a, b; Hynd, Obrzut & Obrzut, 1981; Obrzut et al., 1980; Obrzut, Obrzut, Hynd & Pirozzolo, 1981). Results of the time sharing task suggest that normal children may use a "verbal strategy" which activates the left hemisphere and positively influences their processing ability, resulting in fewer errors in right ear reports, a strategy not utilized by the learning disabled group. However, the disparity in performance scores between the two groups make statistical comparison of degree of asymmetry scores difficult and inconclusive.

An attentional model of cerebral asymmetry tends to fit the empirical data much more readily than a structural model. If the left hemisphere in 98% of right handers is lateralized for language, then following a structural model, one would expect that the right ear advantage would be much greater than the proposed 80% of the population. Performance differences, in an attentional model, may be due to functional differences in the ability to switch attention between hemispheres during a task; an ability that is known to be deficient in learning disabled children (to be discussed in the following section on Cortical Disinhibition).

Methodological problems can account for some of the confusion in the literature on lateralization. First of all, it is highly unlikely that the group or population labelled learning disabled, reading disabled, or dyslexic in each study is representationally the same. As stated earlier, at least two (and likely other) clusters of children emerge who have quite different profiles when examined on a number of tasks (i. e. short term memory, auditory reception, manual dexterity). In the studies cited, the experimental group is usually taken from either a school setting where the child is identified as learning disabled according to a number of criteria, or from a clinical setting. In some studies the clinic group display a lesser degree of asymmetry than the school group (Witelson, 1977). A high degree of variability usually accompanies the performance scores of LD children, further evidence of a heterogeneous sample. Secondly, stimuli material for the perceptual tasks often involve word recognition, a skill already deficient in the experimental group, placing the control group with more experience in reading skills at an unfair advantage. Thirdly, differing statistical choices used for comparing groups make interpretations across studies vulnerable to error.

Other methodological problems such as various measures of laterality contribute to the overall ambiguity, but more importantly, the literature suffers from conceptual problems. Assumptions relating behaviourial, neurophysiological and neuropsychological information are often unfounded. Associations between anatomical data (larger planum temporal in the left hemisphere) and behaviourial correlates (right ear advantage for language) are merely inferences and not hard facts. Poor performances on behaviourial measures do not necessarily imply a cognitive impairment or dysfunction and deviations from the norm of left lateralization of language (i. e. left-handers and ambidextrals) does not mean that the individual is deficient in some form of cognitive functioning.

The term lateralization emerges in the literature under a number of different headings and methods of investigation. Studies in perceptual asymmetry (Caplan & Kinsbourne, 1981; Kershner, 1977; Leong, 1976) infer lateralization of function for the processing of specific stimuli within a given modality. Other studies infer lateralization of function from such indices as handedness, eyedness, and footedness, behaviourial measures of preference or proficiency (Ingram, 1973; Porac & Coren, 1976). It is usually assumed that if an individual is right-handed, language is represented in the left hemisphere (98% of the time), and that the more consistent the hand usage, the greater the degree of lateralization. This form of measurement of lateralization is not necessarily consistent with that measured from dichotic listening tasks or visual half-field studies, as a person could show a right ear advantage for verbal stimuli but be relatively ambidextrous and/or left-eye dominant. Many studies report measures of lateralization from handedness questionnaires which involve relatively simple overlearned tasks such as writing, hammering a nail, or cutting with scissors. However, it has been demonstrated that the most pronounced hand differences are seen on demanding tasks (Steingruber, 1975; Todor & Doane, 1977). Thus, measures of hand preference which may not reflect relative hand proficiency may be unreliable measures of lateralization, and add to the low correlations found between measures of perceptual asymmetry and behaviourial measures of hand usage.

Orton (1937) emphasized the importance of consistent sidedness in learning, by pointing out the abnormally high incidence of mixed dominance (i. e. right-eyed, left-handed, right-footed) in the LD population. He assumed that the more consistent the hand, foot, and eye usage (at least in terms of preference) the more lateralized the individual. There is, however, no convincing evidence that handedness (or for that matter, footedness, or eyedness) is related to degree of lateralization (Rasmussen & Milner, 1975; Zangwill, 1960). Other than the observation that handedness and footedness tend to be correlated (Annett & Turner, 1974), footedness has no special significance in terms of lateralization of language. Consistency of handedness and footedness does appear to be related to upper and lower limb co-ordination and primary mobility patterns as assessed in the Bruininks-Oseretsky Test of Motor Proficiency (Bruininks, 1978) and a Motor Development Assessment for Pre-Schoolers (Lazarus, 1983). Intuitively it may seem that consistent eyedness and handedness should be related, but again, convincing evidence for a correlation between the two is lacking. Anatomically, each eye projects to both hemispheres, whereas distal portions of the hand are controlled by the contralateral hemisphere (Kolb & Whishaw, 1980). In this regard, there is little neurological data to support the presence of any relationship between ocular and cerebral dominance (Porac & Coren, 1976).

The higher incidence of left-handers and ambidextrals in the learning disability population than in the normal population remains an enigma. A purely statistical explanation for the high incidence of left-handers can be outlined if one assumes a distinction between pathological and natural left-handers. Unilateral brain damage is likely to switch a person from one hand dominance to the other (Kinsbourne & Hiscock, 1978). Given that there are more infants born right-handed (90%) than left-handed (10%), and an equal probability of right and left hemisphere damage, there are going to be more pathological left-handers than pathological right-handers. Thus, there would be an overrepresentation of left-handers in many pathological groups. Kinsbourne (1975) has argued that the left occipitoanterior presentation of the fetal head during childbirth contributes to a higher incidence of left hemisphere damage and thus inflates the incidence of pathological left-handers.

Leisman & Ashkenazi (1980) found structural and neurological differences between dyslexics and normal children through the use of computerized tomography (CT) scans and electroencephalography (EEG). The CT scan of normal subjects indicated that the left parieto-occipital region (language and speech areas) was larger than the right. In contrast, the CT scan of dyslexic subjects indicated the reversal of cerebral asymmetry (right parieto-occipital region larger than left) or more often, equivalent cerebral hemispheres. The EEG data also supported differences between the two groups, the normal group demonstrating greater sharing or communication between the two cerebral hemispheres. However, in a more recent study, it has been demonstrated that most LD children with subtle yet classical neurological signs which lateralize clearly can be expected to have normal CT scans (Denckla, LeMay & Chapman, 1985). These apparent contradictions could be the result of the different samples tested (dyslexic vs. LD) or the degree of resolution of the CT scan and hence the capability of detecting anatomical differences. With the current and projected high resolution of magnetic resonance (MR) scanning as well as the functional capabilities of positron emission tomography (PET), the potential structural and/or functional differences between the learning disabled and nondisabled may become apparent in the near future.

In summary, incomplete cerebral dominance as an underlying mechanism responsible for learning problems has not been experimentally validated. In fact, it appears that learning disabled children possess the same functional lateralization of language as normal children. Their poor performance on tasks of cerebral asymmetry require further investigation to elucidate underlying mechanisms. Attentional processes, and in turn, inhibitory control processes, appear to play a role in the performance of tasks designed to measure cerebral asymmetry.

Cognitive Disinhibition

The nervous system has two kinds of neurons, excitatory and inhibitory. Several anatomical structures such as the corpus callosum and basal ganglia serve a major role in inhibiting stimuli or signals. The inhibitory system serves many purposes in behaviour: curbing impulsiveness, attending to one task for a period of time, interrupting highly overlearned responses, decreasing distractibility, overriding automatic responses such as reflexes, and maintaining an appropriate level of arousal. In one way or another, some or all of these abilities appear to be deficient in learning disabled children, implying a common inhibitory control deficiency and/or a functional deficiency in the ability to allocate appropriate attention to task relevant information. The following categories will be discussed as possible separate manifestations of a common disinhibition problem.

Selective and Sustained Attention: Consider several different tasks. A child is asked to attend to a warning light and then respond to a stimulus light by moving to a target with his/her index finger (typical Reaction Time paradigm). Children become increasingly faster with age in response to a visual cue (Haywood, 1979; Pierson & Montoye, 1958; Surwillo, 1977; Todor, 1975, 1978). Additionally, younger children are more variable in their response (Surwillo, 1977; Todor, 1975, 1978). When a similar task is performed by LD children their performance profile across trials is very irregular i. e. they perform fast on some trials and slow on others, leading one to believe that they lack the ability to maintain appropriate attention all of the time. Neurophysiological evidence supports this contention. Autonomic measures of vigilance, such as heart rate and skin conductance, reveal that in normal children and adults, vigilance is accompanied by increased parasympathetic activity, that is, decreased heart and respiratory rate (Pribram & McGuinness, 1975) and increased skin conductance (Birch & Demb, 1959). An optimal foreperiod (about 2 sec.) for responding reflects encoding time, a process which is relatively automatic in nature given an intact nervous system (Posner, 1978). Learning disabled children perform as well as normals in the optimal foreperiod condition (relatively automatic) but with longer foreperiods (requiring conscious effort or attention) controls are better able to maintain a readiness to respond than LD children (Dykman, Ackerman, Holcomb & Boudreau, 1983). This is reflected in a shorter period of heart rate deceleration in the LD children.

Hynd and Obrzut (1981a) postulated that the poorer performance of LD children on dichotic listening tasks is not necessarily an indication of lack of cerebral asymmetry but more likely a difficulty in selective attention (a notion proposed by Kinsbourne); selective attention being the ability to attend and respond to specific sets of stimuli with preselected features within a multitude of stimuli (Ross, 1976). Learning disabled children tend to be more distractible on school tasks than control children, implying a difficulty in selectively processing task relevant information, perhaps attending to irrelevant features that are detrimental to task performance (Hallahan, Gajar, Cohen & Tarver, 1978; Tarver & Hallahan, 1974; Tarver, Hallahan, Kauffman & Ball, 1976). When stimuli (relevant and irrelevant) are displayed temporally close together, performance by LD children is inferior to that of controls (Pihl & Niauro, 1982; Vrana & Pihl, 1980). No performance differences exist when the stimuli are separate.

Observable group differences (LD vs. controls) in selective attention could be due to several factors: a) LD children use the same processing mode as the controls but use it less effectively; b) LD children use a different (perhaps global as opposed to focal) processing mode; c) controls have developed the ability to actively ignore irrelevant stimuli; d) controls have developed the ability to engage in effortful processing (Hasher & Zacks, 1979); e) LD children perceive as salient, information that is irrelevant to the task.

Impulsivity: Other tasks requiring inhibition that are performed poorly by LD children are measures of cognitive and motor tempo. In problem-solving tasks where there is a high degree of response uncertainty, such as the Matching Familiar Figures Test, children who respond quickly and make many errors are said to be impulsive whereas children who respond slowly and make few errors are said to be reflective (Kagan, 1965). This measure of cognitive inhibition has been found to be correlated with age, IQ, academic performance (Kagan, 1965, 1967) and verbal control of motor behaviour (Meichenbaum & Goodman, 1969).

In the normal population, changes from impulsive to reflective occur with increasing age (Kagan, 1965; Maccoby, Dowley, Hagen & Degerman, 1965). No such developmental trend has been found for the learning disabled (Cullinan, Epstein, Lloyd & Noel, 1980). In fact the learning disabled, as a group, cluster more towards the impulsive end of this continuum (Cullinan et al., 1980; Roberts, 1979), suggesting that they adopt a rather inefficient strategy in approaching problem-solving tasks.

On measures of motor tempo such as walk-slowly, draw-a-line-slowly, and reel-up-slowly, the ability to slow down a movement has been found to be correlated with measures of intellectual ability (Maccoby et al., 1965), age (Constantini & Hoving, 1973), and cognitive tempo (Constantini, Corsini, & Davis, 1973). That is, children who score on the impulsive end of this continuum (as do LD children) have difficulty overriding a highly overlearned response such as walking pace. Recent evidence by Todor, Lazarus & Reichel (1982) found that difference scores during a walk-slow task tended to be smaller for LD children than for the controls. Similar results were found by D'Amato and Herr (1982) on a "move a ball slowly" task. Although the data are statistically weak, replication of these types of studies with a larger sample size warrants investigation, as verification of the trend would support the position of a general inhibition problem in learning disabled children. Difficulties in changing tempo suggests that LD children tend to perform tasks in a very stereotypic manner and experience difficulty when variations in routine behaviours are introduced. Haptic training to modify impulse and attention control deficits of LD children has proven somewhat successful (Locher, 1985).

Associated Movements: The phenomenon of associated movement during voluntary movement represents another form of disinhibition. Associated movements are defined by Fog & Fog (1963) as movements which accompany a motor function, especially an intended one, but which are extraneous and not relevant to the goal. The occurrence of such extraneous movements has been termed motor overflow, mirror movements, imitative movements, associated movements, and synkinesis. Most authors agree that motor overflow (henceforth this term will be used) occurs in young children as a normal, developmental phenomenon, but that persistence of such movements into adulthood may, and usually, reflects a neurological deficit.

Developmental data to date on motor overflow have focused on normal and atypical populations (Abercrombie, Lindon & Tyson, 1964; Cohen, Taft, Mahadeviah & Birch, 1967), the atypical mainly consisting of children with obvious neurological deficits such as cerebral palsy and mental retardation and not specifically children diagnosed as learning disabled. Such studies have relied heavily on subjective evaluations of overflow (i. e. Fog's clip pinching task, Fog's foot-to-hands test, Zasso's finger lifting test, Cohen's repetitive thumb to fingers task). Results generally indicate that inhibition of motor overflow is progressive through age groups and greater in normal than atypical children (Abercrombie et al., 1964; Cohen et al., 1967; Fog & Fog, 1963).

More specifically, the frequency of motor overflow tends to decline rapidly to about the age of nine and then level off (Cohen et al., 1967; Connolly & Stratton, 1968). This trend is present but significantly delayed in the aberrantly functioning (Cohen et al., 1967). In addition, through conscious effort, subjects are capable of voluntarily inhibiting but not extinguishing motor overflow (Cambier & Dehen, 1977; Cohen et al., 1967).

The amount of force or degree of motor effort greatly influences the amount of measured overflow, i. e. the greater the force, the greater the overflow. Failure to control for individual differences in the exertion level of the primary or intended act and trial-to-trial variability in the force exerted has made it difficult to discern the shape of the developmental trend from the current body of literature as well as confounding group and sex differences. Todor and Lazarus (1986a) utilized a technique for quantifying overflow as well as a measurement of each individual's maximum volitional force. The test was administered to a sample of nondisabled right-handed children (M = 8.0 years). The contention that force level effects the amount of overflow was supported. The study not only found greater overflow with greater force, but a lateral asymmetry emerged, indicating more overflow when the left (non-dominant) hand was active (Figure 5). Sex differences were also observed, more overflow evident in males than in females. In a subsequent study testing nondisabled children of various ages, the intensity or magnitude of overflow was found to decrease dramatically between the ages of 6.5 and 8.5 years with no significant age differences beyond 8.5 years (Lazarus & Todor, 1987).

Lazarus (1988) has employed this technique for measuring motor overflow in a sample of learning disabled children. Although the analysis is incomplete at this time, preliminary perusal of the data indicates greater overflow in this population of children over that of normal age-matched controls, again suggesting a lack of inhibitory control over irrelevant motor output.

Theoretical considerations of motor overflow are sparse and inconclusive. Most attempts at explications have relied on available information regarding anatomical pathways, with little research attempting to explain the underlying mechanism involved. Motor overflow is most likely being transmitted through either of the following two pathways: the ipsilateral (uncrossed) pyramidal pathway (Cambier & Dehen, 1977; Haerer & Currier, 1966; Zulch & Muller, 1969); or the lateral descending rubrospinal tract (Green, 1967; Zulch & Muller, 1969). It is assumed that, in the normal population free of neurological damage or dysfunction, the crossed pyramidal fibres exhibit an inhibitory effect on the uncrossed fibres in order to allow bilateral independent usage of the two hands. Thus, in the LD population, the apparent general inhibitory control deficiency seemingly allows activity to travel bilaterally, even when unilateral movement is desired. Further investigation of this phenomenon is needed in order to provide an explanation regarding underlying mechanisms.

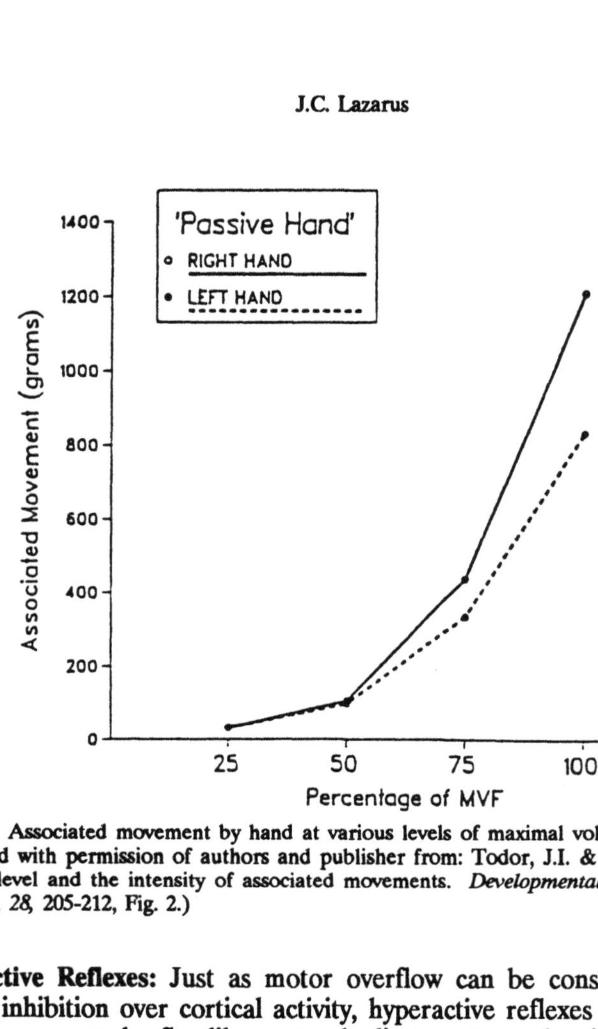

Figure 5. Associated movement by hand at various levels of maximal volitional force (MVF). (Reprinted with permission of authors and publisher from: Todor, J.I. & Lazarus, J.C. (1986) Exertion level and the intensity of associated movements. *Developmental Medicine and Child Neurology, 28*, 205-212, Fig. 2.)

Hyperactive Reflexes: Just as motor overflow can be considered a lack of cortical inhibition over cortical activity, hyperactive reflexes or inappropriate and/or exaggerated reflex-like postural adjustments can be viewed as a lack of cortical inhibition over brainstem and spinal activity. Casual observation of overactive primitive postural reflexes (i. e. Tonic Neck Reflex, Tonic Labrynthine Reflex) in learning disabled children are indicative of another manifestation of a general lack of inhibitory control. At a subcortical level, postural reflexes represent relatively inflexible neural organizations which are elicited usually with a single stimulus. In the normal condition these primitive organizations are evident early in infancy and are eventually replaced by voluntary purposive movement. This is not to say that they disappear from the nervous system. If one considers a hierarchy of motor functions of which reflexes are a basic unit (Easton, 1972), these early and more primitive forms of organization are normally inhibited and succeeded by more mature types of organization.

Through appropriate techniques, reflexes such as the Asymmetrical Tonic Neck Reflex can be elicited in normal children up to about the age of 8 or 9 years (Parr, Routh, Byrd & McMillan, 1974; Zemke, 1980). In pathological conditions such as the physically-handicapped, postural reflexes can be elicited throughout adulthood, indicating either that mature organizations are not present, or that more primitive forms of organization are not under inhibitory control and emerge to interfere with higher levels of skill (Freides, Barbati, VanKampen-Horowitz, Sprehn, Iversen, Silver & Woodward, 1980). Children with less obvious deficits (learning disabled) also display overactive reflexes (Freides et al., 1980; Lazarus & Kyprie, 1980), Asymmetrical Tonic Neck Reflexes being elicited in children up to the age of 14 years (Lazarus & Kyprie, 1980). Many LD children who do not appear awkward in their movement patterns show evidence of reflex activity. This suggests that these primitive forms of organization emerge due to a general lack of inhibition of stereotypic movements rather than the absence of mature neural organizations (more probable in pathological states such as cerebral palsy).

Inherent in all complex skills is the flexibility of their serial organization (Lashley, 1951). Although the movement patterns of learning disabled children may stem from relatively mature neural organizations, they may differ in their characteristics, evidencing relative inflexibility of their serial organization. Wolff (1982) indicated that a structural perspective that assumes a developmental arrest or regression in the timing for motor control would suggest therapeutic approaches to differentiate the timing of existing motor stereotypes rather than suppress them by negative reinforcement.

Although conventional neurological examinations do not typically reveal "hard signs" of central nervous system damage in the learning disabled population, irregular cutaneous reflex responses have recently been recorded in some of these children (Rowlandson & Stephens, 1985) In this study, eight of fifteen LD children tested showed an abnormal cutaneous reflex response, usually a difference between right and left sides. The authors suggest that this provides evidence of the failure of long-loop reflex pathways to develop normally, that is, there is an impairment of (inhibitory) cortical control of spinal mechanisms (and perhaps brainstem mechanisms).

Poor Vestibular Integration: An immature neurological system that displays overactive reflexes is also likely to evidence immaturity in other areas of neurological development such as vestibular integration. There is growing evidence that direct stimulation of the vestibular apparatus enhances the motor development of both normal and developmentally delayed infants (Clark, Kreutzberg & Chee, 1977; Kantner, Clark, Allen & Chase, 1976). Maclean and Baumeister (1982) found that brief periods of vestibular stimulation have demonstratable effects on muscular tonicity, gross motor skills, fine motor skills, and reflexive behaviour in their small sample of developmentally delayed infants. It has been argued that semicircular canal stimulation enhances the maturation of synaptic connectivity within the inhibitory centres of the cerebellum (Kreutzberg, cited in MacLean & Baumeister, 1982), which may be a necessary prerequisite for maturation of reflexive behaviour in favour of coordinated voluntary movement. Thus the integrity of the vestibular system could be another indicator of a general deficit in inhibitory control. Normative data on the postrotary nystagmus response indicates a lack of age differences in normal children aged 3 through 10 years (Ayres, 1976; Kimball, 1981; Punwar, 1982). Although several authors have identified the existence of hyporeactive and/or hyperreactive vestibular responses in samples of learning disabled children (Ayres, 1978; DeQuiros, 1976; DeQuiros & Schrager, 1978), recent research on the vestibular ocular response and optokinetic nystagmus have found no differences in vestibular function between normal and learning disabled children (Polatajko, 1985, 1987). As suggested by Polatajko, these discrepancies may be a function of the tests used to measure vestibular functioning. In one study, no differences between groups were found in static postural sway on a force platform in normal and dyslexic children (Brown, Haegerstrom-Portnoy, Herron, Galin, Yingling & Marcus, 1985). However, Horak, Shumway-Cook, Crowe & Black (1988) looked at learning disabled children with abnormal co-ordination, and found (a) normal vestibular responses as measured by the vestibular ocular response (as did Polatajko); (b) deficits in sensory organization for postural orientation as measured by postural sway on a force platform (unlike Brown et al.), suggesting difficulty in integrating multimodal sensory information. This would be consistent with the types of sensory integration problems reported by others in this particular subgroup of children (Ayres, 1972; DeQuiros, 1976; DeQuiros & Schrager, 1978).

In summary, the notion of a general inhibitory control deficit in learning disabled children can account for many observable behaviours that typify this population. Selective and sustained attention, impulsivity, excessive motor overflow or associated movements, hyperactive primitive postural reflexes, and poor vestibular integration are all phenomenon that have been identified as characteristic of learning disabled children as a group.

Summary and Future Directions

The notion of a learning disability seems to defy definition, population, and etiology. The often heard declaration "These children can't learn!" is a misinterpretation of their capabilities. They do, in fact, learn but not in a manner compatible with the expectations of the educational system as it exists today. If one is measuring biogenetic intelligence, then given the same mental capacity as age-equivalent peers, the LD child potentially possesses the equivalent structural intellect as any nondisabled child. This would be comparable to Cattell's fluid intelligence. If one is measuring performance on standardized IQ tests, in spite of the classic verbal-performance discrepancy often cited in LD children, they emerge overall within the normal range of intelligence (80-120). However, if one is measuring competence at any given moment (i. e. intellectual phenotype), one is referring to the child's repertoire of psychological schemes available for use and comparable to Cattell's crystallized intelligence. It is this type of measurement that differentiates nondisabled and learning disabled children.

The second cluster of children outlined in the introduction whose major deficits lie in the visual-spatial-motor domain comprise the minority of children classified as learning disabled. Their problems tend to be multiple and more obvious to the inexperienced onlooker. Most would show evidence of cortical inhibition problems possibly stemming from structural deficits (i. e. severe visual acuity problems, mild cerebral palsy). Given the complexity of their deficits, I would venture to suggest that these children are the true learning disabled group. Early clinicians (i. e. Kephart, Strauss) likely dealt with these type of children with their more obvious perceptual-motor problems.

The major cluster of children referred to as learning disabled, reading disabled, or dyslexic also exhibit inefficiency of movement as evidenced throughout this review. I propose that these children be viewed as not that unlike poor performers within a nondisabled population of children. Considerable evidence suggests that the LD category is primarily one of underachievement (Algozzine & Sutherland, 1977; Wepman, Cruickshank, Deutsch, Morency & Strothers, 1975; Ysseldyke, Algozzine, Shinn & McGue, 1982). A study comparing school-identified LD children with a group of low-achieving students not identified as LD on a large battery of tests commonly used with LD children indicated considerable similarities between the groups; in fact, an average of 96% of the scores were within a common range, and the performance of LD and low-achieving children on many subtests were identical (Ysseldyke et al., 1982). The authors interpreted the findings in terms of misclassifications (either failing to identify LD children or labelling non-LD students as LD) but I contend that the two groups may only differ in the degree of compatibility between their available psychological structures and task demands.

The characteristics of LD children discussed in this paper suggest the development of a psychological structure which is incompatible with the current mode of instruction in our educational system (i. e. emphasis on problem-solving, divergent thinking, analytical, logical reasoning). These children appear to develop rigid, inflexible structures, which make learning, especially novel material, an arduous task. They appear to overlearn tasks in context and have great difficulty using feedback to flexibly monitor their performance when the organization of the movement demands alteration. Much of the behaviour of learning disabled children can be viewed as responses to salient features or clusters of features in their environment. They fail to sample fully from the available cue set producing stereotypic behaviour on a variety of tasks which would be performed more effectively through effortful processing. Attempts to re-educate early motor milestones may be extremely difficult to achieve, unless the focus is placed on the interruption of monotonous patterns of behaviour and the development of logical, cognitive structures or programs which are transferrable to various situations.

This review points to several future directions in research on learning-disabilities. Most studies cited in this paper have been product-oriented. It is the belief of this author that a process-oriented approach encompassed in an organismic theory will produce the type of research that may be able to answer some of the baffling questions that arise concerning the learning disabled population. The following represents several feasible avenues of research:

1) Measures of cognitive style potentially give insight into learning approaches adopted by learning disabled children and perhaps should be incorporated not only into research paradigms, but also into assessment procedures designed for children suspected of being learning disabled.

2) Sequencing difficulties, both language and motor, appear to be markers for children with learning problems. Since motor tasks can be designed to be relatively free of the influence of prior experience, they may prove a fruitful avenue of investigation for their potential use in the early screening of children suspected of having learning problems.

3) To date, little study has been given to the role that active primitive postural reflexes play in the performance of other tasks (i. e. crossing the midline). A potential avenue of research would be to investigate this relationship in a sample of learning disabled children over a period of time and include several measures of tasks suspected to be related to degree of reflex integration and/or known to be performed poorly by LD children. Refined and quantifiable measures of the Asymmetrical Tonic Next Reflex and other postural reflexes would be needed.

4) The crucial role of attention and inhibition mechanisms in the development of normal motor competence has been discussed elsewhere (Todor & Lazarus, 1986b). Deficiencies in inhibitory control processes seem to contribute a great deal to poor performance on a number of motor control measures. Future research in learning-disabilities should involve the investigation of the hypothesis that these children as a group suffer from a form of functional cerebral disinhibition.

5) With recent additions to brain imaging capabilities (positron emission tomography [PET] magnetic resonance imaging [MRI], computerized tomography [CT]), the potential structural and/or functional differences between LD and nondisabled may become apparent as well as the relationship of such differences to inefficient motor performance.

Author Notes

1. Send request for reprints to Jo-Anne C. Lazarus, Department of Physical Education and Dance, University of Wisconsin - Madison, 2000 Observatory Drive, Madison, Wisconsin, USA, 53706.

References

Abercrombie, M. L. F., Lindon, R. L., & Tyson, M. C. (1964). Associated movements in normal and physically handicapped children. *Developmental Medicine and Child Neurology, 6*, 573-580.

Algozzine, B., & Sutherland, J. (1977). Non-psychoeducational foundations of learning disabilities. *The Journal of Special Education, 11*, 91-98.

Annett, M., & Turner, A. (1974). Laterality and the growth of intellectual abilities. *British Journal of Educational Psychology, 44*, 37-46.

Ayres, A. J. (1972). *Sensory integration and learning disorders.* Los Angeles, CA: Western Psychological Services.

Ayres, A. J. (1976). *Southern California postrotary nystagmus tests.* Los Angeles, CA: Western Psychological Services.

Ayres, A. J. (1977). *Southern California sensory integration tests.* Los Angeles, CA: Western Psychological Services.

Ayres, A. J. (1978). Learning disabilities and the vestibular system. *Journal of Learning Disabilities, 11*, 18-29.

Badian, N. A., & Wolff, P. H. (1977). Manual asymmetries of motor sequencing in boys with reading disabilities. *Cortex, 13*, 343-349.

Beery, K. E. (1967). *Developmental test of visual motor integration: Administration and scoring manual.* Chicago, IL: Follet.

Bender, L. (1958). Problems in conceptualization and communication in children with developmental alexia. In P. H. Hock & J. Zubin (Eds.), *Psychopathology of communication* (pp. 155-176). New York, NY: Grune & Stratton.

Birch, H. G., & Belmont, L. (1965). Auditory-visual integration, intelligence and reading ability in school children. *Perceptual and Motor Skills, 20*, 295-305.

Birch, H. G., & Demb, H. (1959). The formation and extinction of conditioned reflexes in "brain damaged" and mongoloid children. *Journal of Nervous and Mental Diseases, 129*, 162-170.

Birch, H. G., & Lefford, A. (1963). Intersensory development in children. *Monographs of the Society for Research in Child Development, 28*, 1-48.

Boder, E. (1973). Developmental dyslexia: A diagnostic approach based on three atypical reading-spelling patterns. *Developmental Medicine and Child Neurology, 15*, 663-687.

Brown, A. L. (1982). Learning and development: The problems of compatibility, access and induction. *Human Development, 25*, 89-115.

Brown, B., Haegerstrom-Portnoy, G., Herron, J., Galin, D., Yingling, C. D., & Marcus, M. (1985). Static postural stability is normal in dyslexic children. *Journal of Learning Disabilities, 18*, 31-34.

Bruininks, R. H. (1978). *Bruininks-Oseretsky test of motor proficiency.* Circle Pines, MN: American Guidance Service, Inc.

Bruininks, V. L., & Bruininks, R. H. (1977). Motor proficiency of learning disabled and nondisabled students. *Perceptual and Motor Skills, 44*, 1131-1137.

Bryden, M. P. (1965). Tachistoscopic recognition, handedness, and cerebral dominance. *Neuropsychologia, 3*, 1-8.

Bryden, M. P. (1970). Laterality effects in dichotic listening: Relations with handedness and reading ability in children. *Neuropsychologia, 8*, 443-450.

Cambier, J., & Dehen, H. (1977). Imitation synkinesia and sensory control of movement. *Neurology, 27*, 646-649.

Caplan, B., & Kinsbourne, M. (1981). Cerebral lateralization, preferred cognitive mode, and reading ability in normal children. *Brain and Language, 14*, 349-370.

Case, R. & Globerson, T. (1974). Field independence and central computing space. *Child Development, 45*, 772-778.

Clark, D. L., Kreutzberg, J. R., & Chee, F. K. W. (1977). Vestibular stimulation influence on motor development in infants. *Science, 196*, 1228-1229.

Cohen, H. J., Taft, L. R., Mahadeviah, M. S., & Birch, H. G. (1967). Developmental changes in overflow in normal and aberrantly functioning children. *The Journal of Pediatrics, 71*, 39-47.

Connolly, K., & Jones, B. (1970). A developmental study of afferent-reafferent integration. *British Journal of Psychology, 61*, 259-266.

Connolly, K., & Stratton, P. (1968). Developmental changes in associated movements. *Developmental Medicine and Child Neurology, 10*, 49-56.

Constantini, A. F., Corsini, D. A., & Davis, J. E. (1973). Conceptual tempo, inhibition of movement and acceleration of movement in 4-, 7-, and 9-year old children. *Perceptual and Motor Skills, 37*, 779-784.

Constantini, A. F., & Hoving, K. L. (1973). The relationship of cognitive and motor response inhibition to age and IQ. *Journal of Genetic Psychology, 123*, 309-319.

Cruickshank, W. M. (1967). *The brain-injured child in home, school, and community.* New York, NY: Syracuse University Press.

Cullinan, D., Epstein, M. G., Lloyd, J., & Noel, M. (1980). Development of cognitive tempo in learning disabled and normal children. *Learning Disability Quarterly, 3*, 46-53.

D'Amato, G., & Herr, P. M. (1982). Inhibition of motor movement in children with learning disabilities. *Perceptual and Motor Skills, 54*, 1077-1078.

DeAvila, E. A., Havassy, B., & Pascual-Leone, J. (1976). *Mexican-American schoolchildren: A neo-Piagetian analysis.* Washington, DC: Georgetown University Press.

Delacato, C. H. (1959). *The treatment and prevention of reading problems.* Springfield, IL: Charles C. Thomas.

Denckla, M. B. (1972). Clinical syndromes in learning disabilities: The case for "splitting" vs. "lumping". *Journal of Learning Disabilities, 5*, 401-406.

Denckla, M. B., LeMay, M., & Chapman, C. A. (1985). Few CT scan abnormalities found even in neurologically impaired learning disabled children. *Journal of Learning Disabilities, 18*, 132-135.

DeQuiros, J. B. (1976). Diagnosis of vestibular disorders in the learning disabled. *Journal of Learning Disabilities, 9,* 39-47.

DeQuiros, J. B., & Schrager, O. L. (1978). *Neuropsychological fundamentals in learning disabilities.* San Rafael, CA: Academic Therapy Publications.

Dykman, R. A., Ackerman, P. R., Holcomb, P. J., & Boudreau, A. Y. (1983). Physiological manifestations of learning disability. *Journal of Learning Disabilities, 16,* 46-53.

Easton, T. A. (1972). On the normal use of reflexes. *American Scientist, 60,* 591-599.

Entus, A. K. (1977). Hemispheric asymmetry in processing of dichotically presented speech and nonspeech stimuli by infants. In S. Segalowitz and F. A. Gruber (Eds.), *Language development and neurological theory* (pp. 63-73). New York, NY: Academic Press.

Farnham-Diggory, S. (1978). *Learning disabilities: A psychological perspective.* Cambridge, MA: Harvard University Press.

Farnham-Diggory, S. (1980). Learning disabilities: A view from cognitive science. *American Academy of Child Psychiatry, 12,* 570-578.

Fog, E., & Fog, M. (1963). Cerebral inhibition examined by associated movements. In R. MacKeith & M. Bax (Eds.), *Minimal cerebral dysfunction* (pp.52-57). London: National Spastics Society.

Freides, D., Barbati, J., VanKampen-Horowitz, L. J., Sprehn G., Iversen, C., Silver, J. R., & Woodward, R. (1980). Blind evaluation of body reflexes and motor skills in learning disability. *Journal of Autism and Developmental Disorders, 10,* 159-171.

Friedman, M. P., Guyer, B. L., & Tymchuk, A. (1976). Cognitive style and specialized hemispheric processing in learning disability. In R. Knights & K. Bakker (Eds.), *The neuropsychology of learning disorders: Theoretical approaches* (pp. 275-263). Baltimore, MD: University Park Press.

Frostig, M. (1964). *The Marianne Frostig developmental test of visual perception.* Palo Alto, CA: Consulting Psychologists.

Gardiner, M. F., & Walter, D. O. (1976). Evidence of hemispheric specialization from infant EEG. In S. Harnad, R. W. Doty & L. Goldstein (Eds.), *Lateralization in the nervous system* (pp.481-500). New York, NY: Academic Press.

Glanville, B. B., Best, C. T., & Levenson, R. (1977). A cardiac measure of cerebral asymmetries in infant auditory perception. *Developmental Psychology, 13*, 55-59.

Goodenough, D. R. (1976). The role of individual differences in field dependence as a factor in learning and memory. *Psychological Bulletin, 4*, 675-694.

Green, J. B. (1967). An electromyographic study of mirror movements. *Neurology, 17*, 91-94.

Guyer, B. L. & Friedman, M. P. (1975). Hemispheric processing and cognitive styles in learning disabled and normal children. *Child Development, 46*, 658-668.

Haerer, A. F., & Currier, R. D. (1966). Mirror movements. *Neurology, 16*, 757-760.

Hallahan, D. P., Gajar, A. H., Cohen, S. B., & Tarver, S. G. (1978). Selective attention and locus of control in learning disabled and normal children. *Journal of Learning Disabilities, 11*, 231-236.

Halverson, L. E., & Roberton M. A. (1988) Comparison of the developmental levels of learning disabled and nondisabled boys in hopping. *Psychology of Motor Behavior and Sport Abstracts.*

Hasher, L., & Zacks, R. T. (1979). Automatic and effortful processes in memory. *Journal of Experimental Psychology: General, 108*, 356-388.

Haubenstricker, J. L. (1982) Motor development in children with learning disabilities. *Journal of Physical Education, Recreation, and Dance, 53*(5), 1-43.

Hay, L. (1979). Spatial-temporal analysis of movements in children: Motor programs versus feedback in the development of reaching. *Journal of Motor Behaviour, 11*, 189-200.

Hay, L. (1981). The effect of amplitude and accuracy requirements on movement time in children. *Journal of Motor Behaviour, 13*, 177-186.

Haywood, K. (1979). Age differences in movement times and distances. *Perceptual and Motor Skills, 48*, 309-310.

Horak, F. B., Shumway-Cook, A., Crowe, T. K., & Black, F. O. (1988). Vestibular function and motor proficiency of children with impaired hearing, or with learning disability and motor impairments. *Developmental Medicine and Child Neurology, 30,* 64-79.

Hurwitz, I., Bibace, R. M. A., Wolff, P. H., & Rowbotham, B. M. (1972). Neuropsychological function of normal boys, delinquent boys, and boys with learning problems. *Perceptual and Motor Skills, 35,* 387-394.

Hynd, G. W., & Obrzut, J. E. (1981a). Development of reciprocal hemispheric inhibition in normal and learning disabled children. *The Journal of General Psychology, 104,* 203-212.

Hynd, G. W., & Obrzut, J. E. (1981b). Reconceptualizing cerebral dominance: Implications for reading and learning disabled children. *The Journal of Special Education, 15,* 447-457.

Hynd, G. W., Obrzut, J. E., & Obrzut, A. (1981). Are lateral and perceptual asymmetries related to WISC-R and achievement test performance in normal and learning disabled children? *Journal of Consulting and Clinical Psychology, 49,* 977-979.

Hynd, G. W., Obrzut, J. E., Weed. W., & Hynd, C. R. (1979). Development of cerebral dominance: Dichotic listening asymmetry in normal and learning disabled children. *Journal of Experimental Child Psychology, 28,* 445-454.

Ingram, D. (1973). Motor asymmetries in young children. *Neuropsychologia, 13,* 95-101.

Kagan, J. (1965). Reflection-impulsivity and reading ability in primary grade children. *Child Development, 36,* 609-628.

Kagan, J. (1967). Biological aspects of inhibition systems. *American Journal of Diseases in Children, 114,* 507-512.

Kantner, R. M., Clark, D. L., Allen, L. C., & Chase, M. F. (1976). Effects of vestibular stimulation on nystagmus response and motor performance in the developmentally delayed infant. *Physical Therapy, 56,* 414-421.

Kendrick, K. A., & Hanten, W. P. (1980). Differentiation of learning disabled children from normal children using four co-ordination tasks. *Physical Therapy, 60,* 784-788.

Keogh, B. K., & Donlon, G. (1972). Field dependence impulsivity and learning disabilities. *Journal of Learning Disabilities, 5,* 331-336.

Kershner, J. R. (1977). Cerebral dominance in disabled readers, good readers and gifted readers: Search for a valid model. *Child Development, 48,* 61-67.

Kimball, J. G. (1981). Normative comparison of the Southern California postrotary nystagmus test: Los Angeles vs. Syracuse data. *American Journal of Occupational Therapy, 35,* 21-25.

Kimura, D. (1961). Cerebral dominance and the perception of verbal stimuli. *Canadian Journal of Psychology, 15,* 166-171.

Kimura, D. (1973). The asymmetry of the human brain. *Scientific American, 228,* 70-80.

Kinsbourne, M. (1970). The cerebral basis of lateral asymmetries in attention. *Acta Psychologica, 33,* 193-201.

Kinsbourne, M. (1975). The ontogeny of cerebral dominance. *Annals of the New York Academy of Sciences, 263,* 244-250.

Kinsbourne, M., & Hisock, M. (1978). The ontogeny of cerebral dominance. *Annals of the New York Academy of Sciences, 263,* 244-250.

Kirk, S. A., & Kirk, W. D. (1971). *Psycholinguistic learning disabilities: Diagnosis and remediation.* Chicago, IL: University of Illinois Press.

Kolb, B., & Whishaw, I. Q. (1980). *Fundamentals of human neuropsychology.* San Francisco, CA: W. H. Freeman and Company.

Koppitz, E. M. (1964). *The Bender-Gestalt test for young children* (2nd ed.). New York, NY: Grune & Stratton.

Lashley, K. S. (1951). The problem of serial order in behaviour. In L. A. Jeffress (Ed.), *Cerebral mechanisms in behaviour* (pp. 112-136). New York, NY: John Wiley & Sons.

Lazarus, J. C. (1983). *Motor development assessment for pre-schoolers.* Unpublished manuscript, University of Michigan.

Lazarus, J. C. (1989). *The relationship between cognitive and motor inhibition in learning disabled children.* Unpublished manuscript, University of Wisconsin-Madison.

Lazarus, J. C., & Kyprie, P. M. (1980, Nov). *Perceptual-motor development in learning disabled children.* Paper presented at the 24th Annual Convention of the Council for Exceptional Children, Windsor, Ontario, Canada.

Lazarus, J. C., & Todor, J. I. (1987). Age differences in the magnitude of associated movement. *Developmental Medicine and Child Neurology, 29,* 726-733.

Leisman, G., & Ashkenazi, M. (1980). Etiological factors in dyslexia: IV. Cerebral hemispheres are functionally equivalent. *Neuroscience, 11,* 157-164.

Lenneberg, E. (1967). *Biological foundations of language.* New York, NY: John Wiley & Sons.

Leong, C. K. (1976). Lateralization in severely disabled readers in relation to functional cerebral development and synthesis of information. In R. M. Knights & D. J. Bakker (Eds.), *The neuropsychology of learning disorders: Theoretical approaches* (pp. 221-231). Baltimore MD: University Park Press.

Locher, P. J. (1985) Use of haptic training to modify impulse and attention control deficits of learning disabled children. *Journal of Learning Disabilities, 18,* 89-93.

Maccoby, E. E., Dowley, E. M., Hagen, J. W., & Degerman, R. (1965). Activity level and intellectual functioning in normal preschool children. *Child Development, 36,* 761-770.

MacLean, W. E. Jr., & Baumeister, A. A. (1982). Effects of vestibular stimulation on motor development and stereotyped behaviour of developmentally delayed children. *Journal of Abnormal Child Psychology, 10,* 229-245.

Marcel, T., Katz, L., & Smith, M. (1974). Laterality and reading proficiency. *Neuropsychologia, 12,* 131-139.

Marcel, T., & Rajan, P. (1975). Lateral specialization for recognition of words and faces in good and poor readers. *Neuropsychologia, 13,* 489-497.

Mattis, S. (1978). Dyslexia syndromes: A working hypothesis that works. In A.L. Benton & D. Pearls (Eds.), *Dyslexia: An appraisal of current knowledge* (pp. 43-58). London: Oxford University Press.

McKeever, W. F., & Huling, M. D. (1970). Lateral dominance in tachistoscopic word recognitions of children at two levels of ability. *Quarterly Journal of Experimental Psychology, 22,* 600-604.

Meichenbaum, D., & Goodman, J. (1969). Reflection-impulsivity and verbal control of motor behaviour. *Child Development, 40,* 785-798.

Molfese, D. L. (1977). Infant cerebral asymmetry. In S. J. Segalowitz & F. A. Gruber (Eds.), *Language development and neurological theory* (pp.21-35). New York, NY: Academic Press.

Obrzut, J. E., Hynd, H. W., Obrzut, A., & Leitgeb, J. L. (1980). Time sharing and dichotic listening asymmetry in normal and learning disabled children. *Brain and Language, 11,* 181-194.

Obrzut, J. E., Obrzut, A., Hynd, G. W., & Pirozzolo, F. J. (1981). Effect of directed attention on cerebral asymmetries in normal and learning disabled children. *Developmental Psychology, 17,* 118-125.

Olson, M. E. (1973). Laterality differences in tachistoscopic word recognition in normal and delayed readers in elementary school. *Neuropsychologia, 11,* 343-350.

Orton, S. T. (1937). Reading, writing, and speech problems in children. New York, NY: Norton.

Overton, W. F., & Reese, H. W. (1973). Models of development: Methodological implications. In J. R. Nesselroade & H. W. Reese (Eds.), *Life-span developmental psychology: Methodological issues* (pp. 65-86). New York, NY: Academic Press.

Parr, C., Routh, D. K., Byrd, M. T., & McMillan, J. (1974). A developmental study of the asymmetrical tonic neck reflex. *Developmental Medicine and Child Neurology, 16,* 329-335.

Pascual-Leone, J. (1975). *A neo-Piagetian structural model of Witkin's psychological differentiation.* Unpublished manuscript, York University.

Pascual-Leone, J., & Goodman, D. (1979). Intelligence and experience: A neo-Piagetian approach. *Instructional Science, 8,* 301-367.

Petrauskas, R., & Rourke, B. (1979). Identification of subgroups of retarded readers: A neuropsychological multivariate approach. *Journal of Clinical Neuropsychology, 1,* 17-37.

Pierson, W. R., & Montoye, H. J. (1958). Movement time, reaction time, and age. *Journal of Gerontology, 13,* 418-421.

Pihl, R. O., & Niauro, R. (1982). Learning disability: An inability to sustain attention. *Journal of Clinical Psychology, 38,* 632-634.

Polatajko, H. J. (1985). A critical look at vestibular dysfunction in learning disabled children. *Developmental Medicine and Child Neurology, 27,* 283-292.

Polatajko, H. J. (1987). Visual-ocular control of normal and learning disabled children. *Developmental Medicine and Child Neurology, 29,* 477-485.

Porac, C., & Coren, S. (1976). The dominant eye. *Psychological Bulletin, 83,* 880-897.

Posner, M. I. (1967). Characteristics of visual and kinaesthetic memory codes. *Journal of Experimental Psychology, 75,* 103-107.

Posner, M. I. (1978). *Chronometric explorations of mind: The Third Paul M. Fitts Lectures.* Hillsdale, NJ: Lawrence Erlbaum.

Pribram, K. H., & McGuinness, D. (1975). Arousal, activation, and effort in the control of attention. *Psychological Review, 82,* 116-149.

Punwar, A. (1982). Expanded normative data: Southern California postrotary nystagmus test. *The American Journal of Occupational Therapy, 36,* 183-187.

Rasmussen, T., & Milner, B. (1975). Clinical and surgical studies of the cerebral speech areas in man. In K. J. Zulch, O. Creutzfeldt, & G. Galbraith (Eds.), *Otfrid Foerster symposium on cerebral localization* (pp.238-255). Heidelberg: Springer-Verlag.

Roberton, M. A. (1977). Stability of stage categorizations across trials: Implications for the 'stage theory' of overarm throw development. *Journal of Human Movement Sciences, 3,* 49-59.

Roberts, T. (1979). Reflection-impulsivity and reading ability in seven-year old children. *British Journal of Educational Psychology, 49,* 311-315.

Ross, A. (1976). *Psychological aspects of learning disabilities and reading disorders.* New York, NY: McGraw-Hill.

Rowlandson, P. H., & Stephens, J. A. (1985) Cutaneous reflex responses recorded in children with various neurological disorders. *Developmental Medicine and Child Neurology, 27,* 434-447.

Rudel, R. G., & Teuber, H. L. (1971). Pattern recognition within and across sensory modalities in normal and brain-injured children. *Neuropsychologia, 9,* 389-399.

Rugel, R. P. (1974). WISC subtest scores of disabled readers: A review with respect to Bannatyne's recategorization. *Journal of Learning Disabilities, 7,* 48-55.

Satz, P., & Van Nostrand, G. K. (1973). Developmental dyslexia: An a evaluation of a theory. In P. Satz, & J. Ross (Eds.), *The disabled learner: Early detection and intervention* (pp. 212-248). Rotterdam, The Netherlands: Rotterdam University Press.

Senf, G. M. (1972). An information-integration theory and its application to normal reading acquisition and reading disability. In N. D. Bryant, & C. E. Kass (Eds.), *Leadership training institute in learning disabilities: Final report, Vol 2.*, (pp. 303-392). Tucson, Arizona: University of Arizona.

Shiffrin, R. M., & Schneider, W. (1977). Controlled and automatic human information processing: II. Perceptual learning, automatic attending, and a general theory. *Psychological Review, 84,* 127-190.

Steingruber, H. J. (1975). Handedness as a function of test complexity. *Perceptual and Motor Skills, 40,* 263-266.

Strang, J. (1979). *Nonverbal learning disabilities.* Unpublished manuscript, University of Windsor.

Surwillo, W. W. (1977). Developmental changes in the speed of information processing. *Journal of Psychology, 96,* 97-102.

Tarver, S. G., & Hallahan, D. P. (1974). Attention deficits in children with learning disabilities: A review. *Journal of Learning Disabilities, 7,* 560-569.

Tarver, S. G., Hallahan, D. P., Kauffman, J., & Ball, D. (1976). Verbal rehearsal and selective attention in children with learning disabilities: A developmental lag. *Journal of Experimental Child Psychology, 22,* 375-385.

Temple, I. G., & Williams, H. G. (1977). Rate and level of learning as functions of information-processing characteristics of the learner and the task. *Journal of Motor Behavior, 9,* 179-192.

Thomas, J. R., & Bender, P. R. (1977). A developmental explanation for children's motor behaviour: A neo-Piagetian interpretation. *Journal of Motor Behaviour, 9,* 81-93.

Todor, J. I. (1975). Age differences in integration of components of a motor task. *Perceptual and Motor Skills, 41,* 211-215.

Todor, J. I. (1978). Cognitive considerations in the development of motor ability: A neo-Piagetian view. In L. L. Gedvilas, & M. E. Kneer (Eds.), *Proceedings of the NAPECW/NCPEAM national conference* (pp. 40-45). Chicago, IL: Office of Publication Services.

Todor, J. I., & Doane, T. (1977). Handedness classification: Preference versus proficiency. *Perceptual and Motor Skills, 45*, 1041-1042.

Todor, J. I., & Lazarus, J. C. (1982). Cognitive style and the rate and mode of learning. *Psychology of Motor Behavior and Sport Abstracts* (pp. 145). University Park, Maryland.

Todor, J. I., & Lazarus, J. C. (1986a). Exertion level and the intensity of associated movements. *Developmental Medicine and Child Neurology, 28*, 205-212.

Todor, J. I., & Lazarus, J. C. (1986b). Inhibitory influences on the emergence of motor competence in childhood. In L. D. Zaichowsky, & C. Z. Fuchs (Eds.), *Psychology of motor behavior: Development, control, learning and performance* (pp. 239-255). Ithaca, NY: Movement Publications.

Todor, J. I., Lazarus, J. C., & Reichel, M. (1982). Unpublished data, University of Michigan.

Torgeson, J. (1977). The role of nonspecific factors in the task performance of learning disabled children. *Journal of Learning Disabilities, 10*, 33-39.

Trehub, S. E., & Rabinovitch, M. S. (1972). Auditory-linguistic sensitivity in early infancy. *Developmental Psychology, 6*, 74-77.

Vellutino, F. R. (1978). Toward an understanding of dyslexia: Psychological factors in specific reading disability. In A. L. Benton, & D. Pearls (Eds.), *Dyslexia: An appraisal of current knowledge* (pp. 61-111). New York and London: Oxford University Press.

Vrana, F., & Pihl, R. O. (1980). Selective attention deficit in learning disabled children. *Journal of Learning Disabilities, 13*, 42-46.

Wada, J. A., Clark, R., & Hamm, A. (1975). Cerebral hemispheric asymmetry in humans. *Archives of Neurology, 32*, 239-246.

Wepman, J. M. (1960). Auditory discrimination, speech and reading. *Elementary School Journal, 60*, 325-333.

Wepman, J. M., Cruickshank, W. M., Deutsch, C. P., Morency, A., & Strothers, C. R. (1975). Learning disabilities. In N. Hobbs (Ed.), *Issues in the classification of children* (Vol. 1, pp. 300-317). San Francisco. CA: Jossey-Bass.

Whiting, H. T. A. (1972). Overview of the skill learning process. *Research Quarterly, 43,* 266-294.

Whiting, H. T. A., & Cockerill, I. M. (1972). The development of a simple ballistic skill with and without visual control. *Journal of Motor Behaviour, 4,* 155-162.

Wickstrom, R. L. (1977). *Fundamental motor patterns.* Philadelphia, PA: Lea & Febiger.

Williams, H. G. (1973). Perceptual-motor development as a function of information processing. In M. G. Wade, & R. Martens (Eds.), *Psychology of motor behavior and sport* (pp. 344-356). Champaign, IL: Human Kinetics Publishers.

Williams, H. G., Temple, I. G., & Bateman, N. J. (1977). Perceptual-motor and cognitive learning in young children. In D. M. Landers, & R. W. Christina (Eds.), *Psychology of motor behavior and sport* (pp. 471-493). Champaign, IL: Human Kinetics Publishers.

Witelson, S. F. (1977). Developmental dyslexia: Two right hemispheres and none left. *Science, 195,* 309-311.

Witelson, S. F., & Pallie, W. (1973). Left hemisphere specialization for language in the newborn. *Brain, 96,* 641-646.

Witkin, H. A., Dyk, R. B., Faterson, H. F., Goodenough, D. R., & Karp, S. A. (1962). *Psychological differentiation.* New York, NY: John Wiley & Sons.

Witkin, H. A., Goodenough, D., & Karp, S. (1967). Stability of cognitive style from childhood to young adulthood. *Journal of Personality and Social Psychology, 7,* 291-300.

Witkin, H. A., Oltman, P. K., Raskin, E., & Karp, S. A. (1971). *Manual for embedded figures test, children's embedded figures test, and group embedded figures test.* Palo Alto, CA: Consulting Psychologists Press, Inc..

Wolff, P. H. (1982). Theoretical issues in the development of motor skills. In M. Lewis, & L. R. Taft (Eds.), *Developmental disabilities: Theory, assessment, and intervention* (pp. 117-134). New York, NY: Spectrum Publications, Inc.

Wolff, P. H., Cohen, C., & Drake, C. (1984) Impaired motor timing control in specific reading retardation. *Neuropsychologia, 22,* 587-600.

Wolff, P. H., & Hurwitz, I. (1976). Sex differences in finger tapping: A developmental study. *Neuropsychologia, 14,* 35-41.

Wong, B. (1979a). The role of theory in learning disabilities research. Part I. An analysis of problems. *Journal of Learning Disabilities, 12,* 585-595.

Wong, B. (1979b). The role of theory in learning disabilities research. Part II. A selective review of current theories of learning and reading disabilities. *Journal of Learning Disabilities, 12,* 649-658.

Wyke, M. (1968). Influence of direction on the rapidity of bilateral arm movements. *Neuropsychologia, 7,* 189-194.

Wyke, M. (1971). The effect of brain lesions on the performance of bilateral arm movements. *Neuropsychologia, 9,* 33-42.

Ysseldyke, J. E., Algozzine, B., Shinn, M. R., & McGue, M. (1982). Similarities and differences between low achievers and students classified learning disabled. *The Journal of Special Education, 16,* 73-85.

Zangwill, O. L. (1960). *Cerebral dominance and its relation to psychological function.* London: Oliver and Boyd.

Zemke, R. (1980). Incidence of ATNR response in normal preschool children. *Physical and Occupational Therapy in Pediatrics, 1,* 31-37.

Zulch, K. J., & Muller, N. (1969). Associated movements in man. In P. J. Vinken, & G. W. Bruyn (Eds.), *Disturbances of nervous function: Handbook of clinical neurology* (Vol. 1, pp. 404-426). Amsterdam: North Holland Publishing Company.

Zurif, E. B., & Carson, H. (1970). Dyslexia in relation to cerebral dominance and temporal analysis. *Neuropsychologia, 8,* 351-361.

Problems in Movement Control
G. Reid (editor)

THE SYNDROME OF PHYSICAL AWKWARDNESS

A.E. Wall
Greg Reid
Department of Physical Education
McGill University

and

John Paton
Department of Physical Education and Sport Sciences
University of Alberta

Children who are particularly agile on the playing field, nimble at dance, or dextrous with a musical instrument are a source of wonderment to professionals and pride for parents. Their movement skills are increasingly being viewed as a unique form of "intelligence" (Gardner, 1983) and the scientific investigation of such expertise (eg Allard & Burnett, 1985; French & Thomas, 1987 ;Wall, 1986) holds promise in understanding the motor skill acquisition process. At the other end of the continuum are youngsters who are awkward in movement and feel the anguish of peer ridicule and professional disinterest. Not only is it important to develop remedial strategies for their psycho-educational well being, but increased knowledge of their condition may lead also to advances in understanding motor skill acquisition for everyone (Reid, 1989).
Awkward children, apart from those with more obvious movement disorders such as cerebral palsy, were probably first recognized by Collier in the early 1900's when he described such children as "congenitally maladroit" (Ford, 1966). R. Tait McKenzie (1926), well known physician, sculptor and physical educator, recognized the increasing task demands which children face with age and the problems with which less-skilled children must cope if their movement patterns do not develop in accordance with their age.

One of the earliest descriptions of children with movement difficulties was offered by Orton (1937, p. 121):

> Such children are often somewhat delayed in learning even the simpler movements such as walking and running, and have great

> difficulty in learning to use their hands and to copy motions shown to them. They are slow in learning to dress themselves and are clumsy in their attempts to button their clothes, tie their shoes, handle a spoon, and in other simple tasks.

He also placed the problem of awkwardness in a socio-cultural context when he noted that feelings of inferiority result from exposing the youngsters' limitations in unavoidable physical competition.

Annell (1949) reported on a group of 78 Swedish children between ages 6 and 17 years who displayed motor dysfunction but whom had normal or above average intelligence. The clinical description of one eight year old is remarkably similar to that proposed by Orton (1937). The boy:

> ...learnt to dress himself late and still dresses slowly, finding it difficult to do up buttons, and cannot tie his shoe-laces without their coming undone. He has not wanted to learn to ride a bicycle or to skate ... His gait is slightly side-stepped like that of a small child.

Walton, Ellis and Court (1962) provided case descriptions of five children who they referred to as "clumsy" and proposed the existence of a clumsiness syndrome. The issue of recognizing awkwardness as a specific entity was also addressed in an editorial published in the British Medical Association Journal (1962). The authors stressed the need to acknowledge the common occurrence of clumsy children who were characterized as being awkward in movement and highlighted the importance of their early identification because:

> Failure to recognize that the symptoms are genuine and not due to naughtiness may lead to aggravation of the symptoms and so to a variety of behaviour problems, and it means in addition that the children cannot be given the specialized help and support which they need. (p. 1666)

Physically awkward children may have been recognized for many years by a select group of scholars, but they have not been the focus of widespread research or remedial efforts. More commonly, such disorders of movement control are considered tangential to more central concerns (eg. perceptual difficulties, learning problems). The purpose of this chapter is to review the available literature regarding definition, incidence, identification, etiology and clinical manifestations of physical awkwardness. Also we will describe findings from three broad research strategies; neurological, information processing and knowledge-based. We will conclude with sketching some remedial suggestions and point to future research directions. In this manner we hope to achieve a broader objective, that of describing physically awkward children as a viable subgroup of youngsters worthy of our research efforts. In fact, knowledge and understanding in this area is likely to contribute to advances in our understanding of developmental skill acquisition.

Definition

A commonly accepted working definition of physical awkwardness has eluded the professional literature. In fact, as noted in Table 1 there have been a number of terms used over a 60 year period to label the condition. Yet, as Table 1 shows, there has been considerable agreement that physical awkwardness or clumsiness refers to individuals who are cognitively competent, and who have no known neuromuscular involvement. In those cases where authors have included children with neuromuscular problems they have differentiated these children from those with no organic impairment. While there is considerable agreement that these children have no known neuromuscular problems, it is not uncommon for authors to postulate that some awkwardness may be a mild form of cerebral palsy (Dare & Gordon, 1970; Denckla, 1984, Gubbay, 1975a, p. 33).

It has generally been accepted that awkwardness is directly related to the culturally-normative demands of a child's social milieu (Table 1). Awkwardness is thus culturally dependent and one can hypothesize that an environment which placed minimal motor demands upon children would not recognize the condition. This notion is supported by the observation that awkwardness in adults of Western societies is not generally highlighted because there are few cultural demands which place significance on movement competence. Children however are constantly being confronted with the need to solve movement problems; in dressing themselves, in gym class, on the playground, with musical instruments or construction hobbies. It is only in recent years that ecologically-valid test items, reflecting the notion of culturally-normative demands, have been included in quantitative and qualitative measures of physical proficiency. Consequently the degree of physical proficiency in such culturally-normative tasks has been empirically measured during the last decade only.

One common problem that emerges from an analysis of the literature on physical awkwardness is the difficulty of finding a cause or causes for the phenomenon. As noted in the column labelled "unclear etiology" (Table 1) nearly every author during the past 60 years has mentioned this problem. Clearly more work needs to be done in this area.

Finally, three terms seem to have been commonly used to describe these childrens' movement difficulties: developmental apraxia, clumsiness, and physical awkwardness. Developmental apraxia (or dyspraxia) appears to be the favoured term in neurological and medical circles. Apraxia refers to the inability to carry out voluntary movements and has been used so extensively in

Table 1: Physical Awkwardness - 60 Years of Definitions

AUTHOR(S)	Neuromuscular Involvement	Cognitive Competence	Culturally Normative Demands	Degree of Proficiency	Unclear Aetiology	Term
McKenzie (1926)			1			
Orton (1937)		Average	1	1		Dev. Apraxia
Orton (1946)	None			1	1	Dev. Apraxia
Annell (1949)		Avg. to Below	1	1	1	Motor Infantilism
Brit Med Jnl (1962)	Some C.P.	Average		1	1	Clumsy
Walton et al (1962)	None	Average	1	1	1	Dev Apraxia/Clumsy
Gubbay et al (1965)	None	Average	1	1	1	Clumsy, Apraxia
Brenner et al (1967)	Some	Average	1	1	2	Clumsy
Reuben & Bakwin (1968)	None		1	1	1	Apraxia
Illingworth (1968)	Min C.P.	Average		1	1	Delayed Motor Dev't
Bakwin (1968)	None	Average	1	1		Dev Clumsiness
Gordon (1969)	Minimal	Average	1	1	1	Clumsy
Dare & Gordon (1970)	Minimal	Average	1	1	2	Clumsy
Gubbay (1975)	None	Average	1	2	2	Aprax/Dev Clumsiness
Henderson & Stott (1977)						Clumsy
Gubbay (1978)	Mixed	Average	1	2	2	Dev Aprax/Clumsy
McKinlay (1978)	None	Average	1	1	1	Clumsy
Keogh et al (1979)	None	Average		2		Clumsy
Hulme et al (1982)	None	Average		2		Clumsy
Henderson & Hall (1982)	Mixed	Below to above Avg	2	2		Dev Clumsiness
Taylor (1982)	None	Average	2	2		Physically Awkward
Wall (1982)	None	Average	1	1	1	Physically Awkward
Knuckey & Gubbay (1983)	Mixed	Average	2	2	2	Clumsy
Denckla (1984)	Mixed	Average				Dev Dyspraxia/Clumsy
Clifford (1985)	None	Average	2	2		Physically Awkward
Wall et al (1985)	None	Average	1	1	1	Physically Awkward
Cermak (1985)	Mixed	Average	1	1	1	Dev Dyspraxia
Hulme & Lord (1986)	None	Average	1	1	1	Clumsy Children
van Dellen & Geuze (1988)		Average	1	1	1	Clumsy Children
Henderson et al (1989)		Average	1	1	1	Children with movement difficulties

Note: 1 = Mentioned in article; 2 = Supported by empirical evidence in article

adult neurology that it has come to infer the loss of the ability to execute movements that were previously possible (Gubbay, 1975, p. 41). Therefore authors who are concerned with children who have always been ineffective and inefficient with voluntary movements have used the term developmental apraxia or developmental dyspraxia (eg. Cermak, 1985; Denckla, 1984; Gubbay, 1975a). Educators have preferred the terms clumsy or physical awkwardness, the latter being less pejorative. Furthermore, as Henderson and Hall (1982) point out, the term clumsy is sometimes used to describe children who bump into things frequently because they are distractible or hyperactive. The term physically awkward seems more restrictive to children whose primary problem stems from movement difficulties rather than other behaviours.

For the purposes of this chapter we will adopt Wall's definition (1982) of physical awkwardness as it captures the essence of Table 1. Physical awkwardness refers to "children without known neuromuscular problems who fail to perform culturally-normative motor skills with acceptable proficiency" (p. 254). Culturally-normative skills are those that are commonly used by a majority of children at certain ages within a given socio-cultural setting.

Identification, Incidence and Etiology

Determining the incidence of physical awkwardness is intrinsically tied to identification procedures and definition. A widely accepted conceptual definition which is tied to identification procedures has not emerged. Authors have used various defining criteria. Coupled with some agreement that the criteria of awkwardness may change with age and culture (Henderson & Hall, 1982; Wall, 1982), it is not surprising, perhaps, that the wide range of identification procedures has produced considerable variance in estimates of incidence, from 4 to 15% of school aged children (Table 2).

Empirical studies on identification are rare. Keogh, Sudgen, Reynard and Calkins (1979) recognized the elusive nature of identification when they questioned if three different assessment methods would identify the same 71 month old children as awkward. The procedures used were (a) a teacher checklist for the classroom teacher who rated movement skills such as handwriting, knowledge of body parts, jumping and catching (b) observation sessions by trained physical educators who concentrated on locomotor and ball activities during gym classes, and (c) a traditional motor performance test including balance, standing long jump, footwork, tire-run and ball throwing and catching items. There was only minimal agreement among the three procedures since a somewhat different group of boys was identified as physically awkward by each assessment method. In fact, Keogh et al. (1979) noted that only about 20-30% of boys already receiving attention for their movement problems were identified as awkward. They recommended a multiple measures process to identify individual children for remediation.

Table 2: Incidence of Physical Awkwardness

Author(s)	Year	Incidence
Annell	1949	8%
Keogh	1966	7% severe 13% moderate
Keogh	1968	7%
Rutter	1970	5% severe 15% moderate
Gubbay	1975	6%
Booth	1976	4% severe 10% moderate
Keogh et al	1979	9%
Taylor	1982	27% of reading disabled group 13% of control group

Gubbay (1975a) also asked classroom teachers to fill in a questionnaire about children's sporting ability, handwriting and clumsiness. While the teachers identified significantly poorer performance among the awkward youngsters than the control subjects they were less than 50% accurate in judging awkward children as having difficulties in sport, handwriting, etc.

Henderson and Hall (1982) compared four methods of identifying physically awkward children: (a) classroom teachers who were well-informed regarding the nature of awkwardness and normal motor development, (b) a test of motor performance, which later was modified and published as the Test of Motor Impairment - Henderson Revision (Stott, Moyes & Henderson, 1984), (c) neurodevelopment scores, and (d) the subjective judgement of a pediatrician. Contrary to Keogh et al. (1979) the assessment methods used by Henderson and Hall identified a similar group of youngsters as physically awkward. Of particular interest was the agreement between the teachers and the other measures. Recently Todd (1988) also noted the close agreement between a skilled clinician/teacher who worked with awkward children and the Test of Motor Impairment in identifying physically awkward children. It appears that teachers may accurately identify such children if knowledgeable about awkwardness and if they restrict their attention to movement competence rather than factors such as impulsivity.

More research is required however to determine the boundaries of teacher competence in assessing awkwardness. Henderson and Hall (1982) worked closely with teachers who in turn were dealing with children under 8 years of age. Gubbay (1975a) however appears not to have discussed awkwardness with teachers but they were also dealing with older students. As Henderson and Hall (1982) pointed out, the nature of awkwardness might change with age making it more difficult for teachers to identify older children. Future research should address the process of identification and include factors such as age of children, training of teachers and the detail and time requirements of testing methods.

One test that has been specifically developed to identify physically awkward children is the Test of Motor Impairment - Henderson Revision (Stott, Moyes & Henderson, 1984). The authors selected items and scoring procedures which were designed to differentiate among the lower end of the performance continuum, in fact those who scored at the fifth and 15th percentile ranks. The test items measure manual dexterity, static and dynamic balance, and ball skills. There is also an observational checklist which describes some of the qualitative dimensions of movement. Another test designed for physically awkward children is described by Gubbay (1975a). The items include whistling through pouted lips, skipping, rolling a tennis ball with the feet, throwing and catching a tennis ball, tying shoe laces, threading beans, piercing pinholes and placing shapes into the appropriate slots. The evolution of the test, scoring criteria and percentiles are included in his pioneering book *The Clumsy Child* (1975a).

Motor performance is the end product of numerous interacting physiological, psychological and sociological systems. It is not surprising that the etiology of physical awkwardness would be quite diverse and complicated. For example, considering only physiological systems, it is acknowledged that any number of central nervous system abnormalities might result in clumsiness despite an intact motor system (Gubbay, 1975a, p. 2). While most authors recognize that the causes are obtensibly unknown (Table 1) clinical investigation has shed some light on potential neurological factors. These will be dealt with in a subsequent section.

The etiology of physically awkwardness has been viewed at different levels of analysis. As mentioned, some investigators (eg. Gubbay, 1975a) have adopted a neurological analysis and therefore have explored EEG's and specific regions of the brain which might show damage. At this level of analysis are hypothesized factors such as metabolic problems, drug toxicity, blood incompatibility, maternal drug ingestion and vitamin deficiencies. These of course are commonly identified as potential causes for other developmental disorders such as mental retardation or learning disabilities.

At a psychological level information processing scholars have looked for a specific deficit within a series of cognitive operations. Proponents of a knowledge based approach emphasize the types of knowledge that the physical awkward child lacks. Finally, a sociological perspective would particularly highlight the environmental factors of education, parental support and community resources to understand the condition. All levels of analysis have a viable place in research efforts and only thorough investigations at each level will a complete portrait of the problem be produced.

Characteristics of Children who are Physically Awkward

Physical Characteristics

Table 3 outlines the major developmental indicators of physical awkwardness. One of the most common indicators has been a general delay in motor development. Late walking and general coordination difficulties have often been included. They are described as children who drop things, bump into others and often fall. Two other common developmental characteristics are problems with handwriting and self care. Included with the latter are slow dressing, difficulties with shoelaces and brushing teeth. Handwriting ineptitude is often listed with poor spatial organization, problems with construction play (eg. blocks) and use of scissors. Balance difficulties, a lack of skill in throwing and catching, and problems with gait have also been mentioned. It is clear from Table 3 however that most of the physical developmental indicators have not emerged from empirical investigations, rather from case reports or clinical summaries. There is an obvious need for more data-based descriptions of the motor development of physically awkward children from theoretical viewpoints such as the component approach to motor development (Roberton, 1982).

In addition to more accurate developmental descriptions of motor skills there is a need to further delineate the quality of movements associated with physical awkwardness. This could occur in a skill-specific or general manner. Gait is a specific skill in which difficulties have been mentioned yet the pattern of abnormality has not been clarified. It remains simply (and vaguely) a problem of gait! A more detailed description of the intricacies of gait and concomitant problems in children with movement difficulties would represent a skill specific description. In contrast, Haubenstricker (1982) and Denckla (1984) have identified a number of general movement characteristics commonly exhibited by children with movement problems. These include inconsistency or larger trial-to-trial variation in performance, perseveration, mirroring a leader's movements rather than separating their directions from him/her, asymmetry in movements usually requiring bilateral responses, falling after performance, extraneous movements, rhythmical difficulties, an inability to control force and inappropriate motor planning.

Table 3: The Developmental Indicators of Physical Awkwardness

AUTHOR(S)	Delayed Motor Development	Slow to Dress	Writing Problems	Balance	Ball Skills	Gait Problems
McKenzie (1926)						
Orton (1937)			1	1		1
Orton (1946)						
Annell (1949)		1	1			1
Brit Med Jnl (1962)	1		1	1		1
Walton et al (1962)	1	1	1			
Gubbay et al (1965)			2			
Ford (1966)	1	1				
Brenner et al (1967)	2		2			1
Reuben & Bakwin (1968)	1	1	1		1	1
Illingworth (1968)	1	1	1			
Bakwin (1968)	1					
Gordon (1969)	1		1			
Dare & Gordon (1970)	1	1	1	1		
Gubbay (1975)	2	2	2			1
Henderson & Stott (1977)						
Gubbay (1978)			2			1
McKinlay (1978)	1		1	1		
Keogh et al (1979)						
Adler (1982)	2	2			2	
Hulme et al (1982)						
Henderson & Hall (1982)				2	2	
Taylor (1982)	1			2	2	
Wall (1982)	1			1	1	
Knuckey & Gubbay (1983)						
Denckla (1984)	1		1	1		1
Clifford (1985)				2	2	
Wall et al (1985)	1			1	1	
Cermak (1985)	1	1	1	1	1	
Paton (1986)				2	2	
Hulme et al (1986)		1	1			
van Dellen & Geuze (1988)						
Henderson et al (1989)						

Note: 1 = Mentioned in article; 2 = Supported by empirical evidence in article

The height and weight of physically awkward children do not differ from their peers, as assessed in studies from Australia (Gubbay, 1975, p. 133) and Canada (Paton, 1986). While their physical fitness has not been studied extensively (Table 4) the empirical evidence that does exist suggests a low level of fitness performance. Paton (1986) described the physical fitness of 23 boys and 18 girls, ranging in age from 6 to 11. A striking result was the low percentile score for the boys and girls on the push-up, 5 and 4 respectively. While some degree of co-ordination is required to perform this item it is a culturally-normative activity which taps muscular endurance. The majority of youngsters could not do one push-up! On other tests measuring abdominal endurance, leg power, flexibility and cardiovascular endurance the physically awkward children were usually below the 30th percentile. These findings were interpreted as consistent with Wall's (1982) contention that movement problems lead to physical activity avoidance which in turn results in low physical fitness. However, Paton's subjects did not carry excess fat as indicated by average skinfold measures. Skinfold thickness is used as an estimation of body fat. These data are in contrast with earlier suggestions that physically awkward children may be obese (Gordon, 1969; Illingworth, 1968).

Only one study has addressed the long range effects of awkwardness. Knuckey and Gubbay (1983) completed a follow-up investigation of awkward children eight years after their original assessment. Gubbay had reported that the awkward children in his original study (1979) were "...significantly inferior to their controls in handwriting, sporting ability, popularity and academic performance..." The young adults, 16-20 years, were reassessed on five of the original tests. The awkward children were divided into three groups according to the degree of their awkwardness: mild, moderate and severe. The results indicated that whereas the control group was significantly better than the others on all five tests when originally assessed, they were better on only two tests when reassessed. The authors contend that with time the groups merged together since the mild and moderate groups had improved to the levels of the controls. However, the severely awkward children were significantly less proficient than the controls on four of the five tests. The data may support a developmental or maturation lag hypothesis for other than the most severely affected but may also reflect the inability of the tests to differentiate among older persons. Further longitudinal research should address this issue.

Social-Affective Characteristics

Physical awkwardness is also related to social-emotional difficulties (Table 4). The prevailing thought is that the movement problems lead to the affective problems rather than vice-versa. However, as noted by Wall, McClements, Bouffard, Findlay and Taylor (1985), lack of confidence and negative affect toward physical activity are likely to result in less participation which prevents an increase in skill, thus reinforcing the tendency to dislike situations requiring

Table 4: Correlates of Physical Awkwardness

AUTHOR(S)	Social Difficulties	Behavioural Difficulties	Low Self Esteem	Avoids Physical Activity	Fitness Level
McKenzie (1926)					
Orton (1937)	1		1		
Orton (1946)					
Annell (1949)	1	1			
Brit Med Jnl (1962)		1			
Walton et al (1962)	1				
Gubbay et al (1965)		1	1		
Ford (1966)			1	1	obese
Brenner et al (1967)	2	2	2		
Reuben & Bakwin (1968)	1	1			
Illingworth (1968)		1			obese
Bakwin (1968)		1			
Gordon (1969)	1				obese
Dare & Gordon (1970)	1	1	1		
Gubbay (1975)	2	2	1	1	
Henderson & Stott (1977)	1		1		
Gubbay (1978)					
McKinlay (1978)	1	1	1		
Keogh et al (1979)	1	1			
Adler (1981)	2		2	2	
Hulme et al (1982)					
Henderson & Hall (1982)	2				
Shaw et al (1982)	1		2		
Taylor (1982)	1	1	1	1	1
Wall (1982)	1	1	1	1	1
Knuckey & Gubbay (1983)					
Denckla (1984)	1	1			
Cermak (1985)	1	1	1	1	
Clifford (1985)	2	1	2	2	
Wall et al (1985)	1	1	1	1	1
Paton (1986)					2
Hume & Lord (1986)					
van Dellen & Geuze (1988)					
Henderson et al (1989)	1		2		

Note: 1 = Mentioned in article; 2 = Supported by empirical evidence in article

motor competence. Therefore the relationship between movement problems and affect is likely reciprocal rather than unidirectional.

Findings which link motor impairments to lower self-esteem, fewer playmates and emotional difficulties appear to be widespread among industrial nations which place considerable importance upon physical activity prowess and sport. Such findings have emerged from Australia (Gubbay, 1975), Canada (Causgrove, 1987; Clifford, 1985), England (Henderson, May & Umney, 1989), the United States (Cratty, Ikeda, Martin, Jennett & Morris, 1970; Shaw, Levine & Belfer, 1982) and Sweden (Adler, 1982).

Cratty et al. (1970) used the Piers-Harris Self-Concept scale with physically awkward children who acknowledged that peers made fun of them. The awkward subjects demonstrated lower self-concepts than their more skilled counterparts. These results were corroborated by Henderson et al. (1989) using a modified version of the same instrument. Shaw et al. (1982) compared a group of children who were delayed by at least one year in math, reading or writing with a group of children who were equally delayed academically but also motorically. The children with motor delays scored lower on self-esteem, rated themselves as lower in social relationships with peers of the same gender, and were found to be less happy. The children with motor difficulties were also perceived by their mothers as being less popular. Thus, motor difficulties appear to add additional challenges and problems to children with other learning problems. The low peer status of children with motor impairments has also been demonstrated by Adler (1981).

The apparently immense impact of physical awkwardness on ones social-emotional well-being is best understood in the context of cultures which place enormous value on physical prowess (perusal of sports coverage in general, salaries in professional sport and linkage of political prestige with international sport championships attest to this statement) and in the nature of physical activity itself. Orton (1937) astutely observed many years ago that "a considerable measure of feeling of inferiority seems to be unavoidable...especially as these children grow to the age when they enter active physical competition where their limitations must be rather piteously exposed" (p. 193). Movements which are physically awkward are open for public scrutiny (Wall, 1982); and they often generate immediate negative feedback (Griffin, 1985).

Not surprisingly children who have movement difficulties do not enjoy physical education or competition (Adler, 1982), may be truant from school on gym days (Gubbay, 1975a), have a history of quitting community sponsored physical activity programs (Clifford, 1985) and prefer individual rather than group activities and younger playmates (Clifford, 1985). Among the strategies that they might employ to avoid embarrassment in physical activities are acting silly or foolish to cover up their ineptitude, gravitating to intellectually challenging but sedentary activities, becoming overly aggressive during physical activity or simply avoiding activities with a myriad of excuses (Cratty, 1975; Gubbay, 1975a).

Recently Henderson et al. (1989) have made a significant step to understand the affective responses of children with movement difficulties. Not only is their study empirical rather than clinical, but they have selected dimensions of behaviour which are relatively robust theoretically; goal setting, locus of control and self-esteem (previously discussed). Henderson et al. showed that children with motor difficulties set goals without regard for the feedback they received. That is, whether they were told they had improved or not was unrelated to their goal on the next attempt. The authors postulated that long term failure on similar motor tasks rendered them unable to set realistic levels of aspiration. In fact it was common for the youngsters to set particularly *high* and unrealistic goals. This was explained logically by the observation that goals outside the realm of possibility are never realistic and therefore the impact of failure is minimized since there was no initial standard established or expectation. Finally, the children with movement difficulties were significantly less likely to assume responsibility for any outcome compared to a control group. Rather they attributed success and failure to persons other than themselves. An external locus of causality has been linked with learning difficulties but recent reviews suggest that persons who meet with failure in learning situations tend to accept responsibility for failure but not success (Dudley-Marling, Snider & Tarver, 1982). Clearly, more research which builds on these notions is required.

Related Educational Characteristics

Physical awkwardness is often associated with other learning problems. In fact, movement difficulties were first recognized as a characteristic of children who came to professional attention due to other school related problems. Only in recent years have authors focused primarily on their movement attributes, relegating other learning problems to secondary status.

Difficulties with speech, math, reading and handwriting as well as hyperactive behaviour have been associated with awkwardness (Cermak, 1985; Gubbay, 1975a; Henderson & Hall, 1982). Usually these children perform more successfully on the verbal than the performance portion of IQ tests (Gubbay, 1975a).

Taylor (1982) examined the incidence of physical awkwardness in both reading disabled and average elementary school children. She found 27.7 percent of the reading disabled group to be physically awkward whereas only 13 percent of the average readers fell into this category. Exploring the problem in a similar way Henderson and Hall (1982) postulated that a subcategory of awkward children likely exist who have associated reading or learning problems but that the motor impairment is the only problem with another subcategory. For optimal research purposes we are likely to benefit most from learning about the "pure" physically awkward child who does not come "contaminated" with other learning difficulties and their social -affective influences. In remedial programs and attempts to define physical awkwardness, it will be necessary to acknowledge the associated learning problems which occasionally accompany the motor difficulties.

Neurological Perspectives

Early investigations sought a better understanding of physical awkwardness by extensive study of developmental history and neurology. A reading of case histories (eg. Reuben & Bakwin, 1968; Gubbay et al., 1965; Gubbay, 1975a; Walton et al., 1962) suggests a number of general abnormalities in children who are physically awkward. However, larger empirical studies either refute earlier tentative conclusions or point out that neurological pathology and developmental histories are so heterogeneous that specific conclusions are unwarranted.

Walton et al. (1962) reported findings of five youngsters, two of whom were born prematurely, one who had a difficult delivery and another who had whooping cough at three months. This suggested birth injury or neonatal trauma might be logical etiological candidates of awkwardness. Cermak's (1985) review also concluded that a relationship between awkwardness and neonatal problems seemed plausible. The data however are equivocal. Gubbay (1975a) summarized from his comparative study of physically awkward and nonawkward children that "Prematurity, postmaturity, abnormal delivery and neonatal illness were not commoner in the clumsy group..." and that "(1) a history of past neurological illness and (2) all abnormal perinatal factors failed to disclose significant differences between the two groups" (p. 141).

The neurological evidence is equally mixed. Despite physical awkwardness there do not appear to be any defects in the pyramidal, extrapyramidal or cerebellar pathways which control voluntary movements (Walton et al., 1962). While no lesions have been recorded, some authors have favoured an explanation of cerebral disorganization based upon, in part, some evidence of mixed dominance (Gubbay et al., 1965; Walton et al., 1962). Thus confusion in cerebral dominance remains a working hypothesis as a correlate to awkardness.

Gubbay (1975a,b) has provided the most complete and cautious description of electroencephalography in physical awkwardness. There is evidence that children who are physically awkward show more EEG abnormalities than control groups but diffuse rather than focal abnormalities predominate. Also there is no common pattern among the youngsters.

Denckla (1984) reported a study by Nichols and Chen (1981) investigating children with "neurologically soft" signs such as uncoordinated or involuntary movements. Approximately half of the youngsters were rated as neurologically normal and about 44 percent as neurologically suspicious. Obvious neurological deficits were largely absent. These data, coupled with earlier work (eg. Gubbay, 1975a; Walton et al., 1962) point to the difficulties researchers have had describing the neurological correlates of awkwardness. Only mild chorea appears with any regularity (Gubbay, 1975a). It is possible that the testing procedures are not sensitive to such mild pathology or that awkwardness is associated with a heterogeneous neurological background ranging from subtle anatomical difficulties to physiological malfunctions. As yet no obvious neurological problems exist and consequently definitions of awkwardness, as noted previously, assume a neurologically intact system.

An immature central nervous system might be associated with awkwardness. The longitudinal data of Knuckey and Gubbay (1983) are consistent with this notion since their awkward children were closer to average motor proficiency as young adults. Conversely, however, Walton et al. (1962) concluded that "there is no evidence that in our children the defect is a simple abnormality of maturation which is corrected with the passage of time" (p. 610). Future research must explore the neurological underpinnings of awkwardness with the recognition that diversity is likely to characterize the condition.

Information Processing Perspectives

The cognitive orientation of information processing has attracted a number of authors in their attempt to unravel the complexities of awkwardness. According to this perspective awkwardness is the product which follows a series of discrete steps (structural features) and operations (control processes) upon incoming environmental stimuli and items retrieved from memory. Thus, a breakdown at any stage could theoretically result in awkwardness. A conceptual advantage would occur if a specific structural feature or control process could be implicated. Remedial strategies would benefit as well (Dare & Gordon, 1970). Thus an information processing analysis has been pursued in a number of studies with physically awkward children.

Perceptual processing is posited to occur in the early portion of information processing models (eg. Whiting, 1969; Marteniuk, 1976). Hulme, Biggerstaff, Moran and McKinlay (1982) compared visual, kinesthetic and cross-modal processing by physically awkward and control youngsters. The experimental task was estimating the length of straight lines. In the visual condition a standard line was presented by the experimenter and then removed. The subject was then requested to tell the experimenter to extend another line until it was the same length as the standard. The kinesthetic condition had the child move a handle along a linear-positioning apparatus to a stop and then reproduce the movement when the stop was removed. In the cross-modal condition the stimuli were presented in either visual or kinesthetic modes and reproduced in the contrasting mode. The awkward children were found to be less accurate than the control group on visual, kinesthetic and cross model judgements. A follow up study (Hulme, Smart & Moran, 1982) ruled out the possibility that the results were due to memory deficits or eye-movement problems. There were no significant correlations between kinesthetic judgements and motor skill with the awkward children in the study by Hulme, Biggerstaff et al. (1982). As cogently noted by Hulme and Lord (1986), however, this might be due to the limited assessment of kinesthetic sensitivity.

In a more extensive evaluation of kinesthetic perception, Lazlo and Bairstow (1983) reported that eight out of 14 awkward children could be labelled kinesthetically blind because of their marked inability to process kinesthetic information. Smyth and Glencross (1986) used a reaction time paradigm and produced results consistent with Hulme and colleagues as well as Lazlo and Bairstow (1983). Awkward children were slower than nonawkward children in reacting to kinesthetic stimulation. A more detailed discussion of perceptual difficulties of awkward children can be found in a review by Hulme and Lord (1986).

While Hulme, Biggerstaff et al. (1982) demonstrated that awkward children were less accurate than nonawkward controls on a task of visual judgement, Smyth and Glencross (1986) have shown that awkward children do not show deficits on the speed of visual information processing. Such findings are not necessarily incongruent since one could be quite fast but less accurate in perception. Nonetheless more research is required for a more substantive conclusion to be drawn regarding the visual processing of awkward children.

In summary, there is some evidence supporting kinesthetic impairments among awkward children but there is a paucity of evidence linking such problems to their motor deficits. Thus, from an information processing perspective the perceptual processing of awkward youngsters may be impaired but its effect on the execution of motor skills is unclear. It is possible that only a select group of awkward children have perceptual difficulties and including "other" awkward children in experimental designs may mask the real relationship between awkwardness and perceptual impairment. It is also conceivable that there is no single factor related to awkwardness and thus one factor such as perception is not likely to have a major influence on the outcome, that is, motor output.

Most models of information processing include a stage of perceptual processing (described above), decision making and response processing. The central decision making stage includes response selection which is the process of choosing an appropriate response in light of the environmental stimuli (Stelmach, 1982). Response processing refers to organizing the motor commands which in turn execute the response. Manipulating stimulus-response compatibility is argued to influence response selection while precuing subjects in advance about movement characteristics of upcoming responses is believed to effect response programming (Rosenbaum, 1980).

van Dellen and Geuze (1988) have shown that awkward children have particular difficulties with response selection. On a choice reaction time task the awkward children were significantly slower than the nonawkward youngsters and were markedly affected by the incompatible stimulus-response condition. This suggests that their ability to select appropriate responses to environmental stimuli may be impaired. However the data from Smyth and Glencross (1986) did not support a deficit in response selection. Further research which explores the methodological differences will be required to resolve these contradictory findings. Only van Dellen and Geuze (1988) have systematically explored response programming but their data were not clear cut enough to warrant firm conclusions.

Summarizing the information processing literature of awkward children is tenuous because of a limited data base. Yet there seems to be some evidence of slow kinesthetic (Smyth & Glencross, 1986) and inaccurate kinesthetic and visual-spatial (Lazlo & Bairstow, 1983; Hulme, Biggerstaff, et al., 1982) information processing. However, the precise link to motor performance deficits is cloudy. The data are equivocal regarding specific weaknesses in response selection (Smyth & Glencross, 1986; van Dellen & Geuze, 1988) and inconsistent regarding response programming.

The information processing paradigm should remain an attractive one as researchers unravel the problems associated with physical awkwardness. Not only might a greater theoretical understanding emerge but it is conceivable that remedial strategies will be identified as these youngsters processing strengths and weaknesses are clarified.

A Knowledge-Based Approach

In 1985, a new approach to the problem of physical awkwardness was taken by Wall, McClements, Bouffard, Findlay and Taylor. Argueing that physical awkwardness was a developmental problem that might best be viewed from a knowledge-based perspective, they suggested that children who exhibit motor skill difficulties probably have a relatively impoverished knowledge-base in the physical activity domain.

They outlined an heuristic approach to motor development that divides knowledge about action into two key categories: structural capacity and acquired knowledge. The first refers to the anatomical and physiological potential that a person inherits. The second refers to knowledge that is gained through experience which increases with development.

Wall and his colleagues label acquired knowledge in the physical domain: knowledge about action. They divide such knowledge into five main categories: procedural, declarative, affective, and metacognitive knowledge and metacognitive skill.

Procedural Knowledge

Procedural knowledge refers to the storage of action schemas that control the execution of skilled movement (Wall et al., 1985). Such knowledge is stored in schema form and is controlled by a hetararchial control system that depends on countless feedforward and feedback loops. At the specific skill level, procedural knowledge represents the entire action sequence, including the stimulus identification, perceptual decision-making phases, as well as the selection and execution of responses.

An action sequence includes both the internal processing and the resulting overt behavioural response. Thus, the execution of a given motor skill depends on the use of procedural knowledge that has been acquired through learning and experience. Hence, the motor skill repetoire that children develop depends on the quality and quantity of practice that they have experienced.

Viewed from a developmental perspective, procedural knowledge represents the breadth and depth of skills that a person has acquired in a variety of domain-specific activities. Thus, the soccer player has an extensive procedural knowledge base related to various kicks, defensive moves, and heading skills as the swimmer acquires proficiency and an extensive procedural base in front crawl, backstroke, breaststroke, and other aquatic skills.

Wall and his colleagues suggest that one might assess the developmental level of a person's procedural knowledge base by evaluating the number of automatized skills that a person has acquired. Skillful individuals are those with a large repetoire of automatized skills that can handdle a broad array of task demands. In contrast, physically awkward children have relatively impoverished skill repetoires.

Children's skill proficiency should increase proportionally with age and reflect the increasing complexity of their physical activity, sport, and social environments. Unfortunately, a cycle of behaviours centered on their inadequate motor performance negatively affects the development of procedural knowledge in physically awkward children. Let us briefly examine this cycle of behaviours that has been called the physically awkward syndrome (Wall, 1982; Wall et al., 1985).

Due to their lack of physical proficiency, physically awkward chidren often withdraw from physical activity and sport settings. They realize that they do not have sufficient skill to enjoy participating in game situations and they use a variety of techniques to avoid the failure experiences associated with such involvement. Physical activity during the school years is largely based on ball and team game activities which demand quick, skilled responses in fast changing environments. Furthermore, such activities are performed in a public environment where peers can evaluate performance. The negative feedback and ridicule experienced by less-skilled children has been previously noted (Griffith, 1985).

Thus, it is not surprising that physically awkward chidren withdraw from physical activity which results in a lack of physical practice opportunities. Such reduced practice time further inhibits the development of culturally-normative skill which, in turn, heightens the performance differences that already exist between them and their peers. By definition then, physically awkward children will have less procedural knowledge than their age-matched peers. Furthermore, the proficiency with which they can perform the skills that they have developed will also be less than adequate.

Declarative Knowledge

Declarative knowledge about action refers to the conceptual knowledge that people develop and store within the action domain. Wall et al. (1985) purport that factual knowledge about morphological, biomechanical and environmental constraints increases with development. A number of studies (French & Thomas, 1987) show that declarative knowledge about the self and others in action situations increases with age and appropriate experience. The use of words, phrases and sentences to communicate about action increases dramatically throughout the preschool years (Bruner, 1983; Huttenbocher, Smiley & Charney, 1983; Olson, 1975).

Individuals involved in sport activities can readily document the vocabulary that develops within that domain. In fact, phrase books on baseball and hockey have been published that provide definitions of such esoteric phrases as "he's got the right stuff, today" and that was a "good penalty". Experts in a variety of domains develop extensive declarative knowledge bases (French & Thomas, 1987). Furthermore, they use such knowledge to augment the procedural knowledge that they have acquired. A person's declarative knowledge base is particularly important in the early stages of learning when verbal-cognitive processing is required to develop the "image of an action" (Fitts & Posner, 1967; Whiting & den Brinker, 1982).

Wall et al. (1985) suggest that physically awkward children possess a rather limited movement vocabulary in contrast to those who are more physically skilled due to their lack of proficiency and involvement in physical activity. Todd (1988) has shown however that with basic skills such as catching, their declarative knowledge base may be equal to their skilled peers and the difficulties remain primarily in the procedural area.

Affective Knowledge

Affective knowledge about action refers to the subjective feelings that people develop in the action domain. As children learn and perform physical skills, they develop feelings about their actions and the situations in which they perform them. Youngsters who are able to handle the demands of play and sport situations learn to enjoy the time they spend in such activities. Successful experiences generate feelings of competence that results in the development of a positive self-concept (Harter, 1978, 1981, 1982). Unfortunately, children who do not have the culturally-normative skills to meet the demands of play and sport environments, often exhibit feelings of learned helplessness which is characterized by a lack of motivation, minimal persistence in the face of difficulties, and a general withdrawal from challenging situations (Gibson, 1980; Griffin, 1985; Griffin & Keogh, 1982).

Smith (1978) reports that people who consistently experience success are usually those with high achievement needs. In contrast, people who often experience failure are usually placed in the low achievement needs group. Clearly, physically awkward children would be placed in the latter category within the physical activity domain. Of prime importance to our discussion is the fact that individuals in the high achievement needs group attribute their success to personal effort and ability, whereas, individuals with low achievement needs generally have unclear reasons for their success when they do succeed, yet they always attribute their failures to a lack of ability. Unfortunately, such an attribution pattern is a relatively stable one that leads to less personal effort on the part of low achievers. This pattern is congruent with the earlier observation that physically awkward children withdraw from physical activity much more readily and often than their more-skilled peers.

In sum, negative feelings of competence and confidence in physically awkward children can adversely affect their motivational state which, in turn reduces the opportunity to acquire the very culturally-normative skills that are important for success and enjoyment in physical activity settings.

Metacognitive Knowledge

Metacognitive knowledge refers to an awareness of what one knows. As children develop, they begin to realize what they can do and cannot do. For example in relation to procedural knowledge about action, they know that they can perform certain skills better than others. The preschool child on a slide knows whether she needs help to get down a steep slide or not. The young swimmer knows whether she can do the front crawl better than the breaststroke.
In the same way, from a declarative knowledge perspective, children know whether they understand the rules of a game, appreciate offensive and defensive strategies, and know what the key cues are when learning a new skill. From an affective perspective, they know how they feel about performing certain skills. The preschool child knows whether she likes to be deep water or not and certainly knows whether she wants to try skiing down a steep hill.

Wellman (1984) contends that as children grow older they develop an organized set of concepts about the operation of their minds. They become aware of the variables that affect their cognitive processing; for example, they become aware of the fact that they can mentally plan and rehearse future actions.

In short, children develop metacognitive knowledge about their procedural, declarative,and affective knowledge about action. The extent and validity of such metacognitive knowledge will depend on the quality and quantity of the knowledge children have acquired within a given domain. Clearly, those with relatively few physical skills, minimal declarative knowledge, and negative feelings toward participation in physical activity will have a less developed metacognitive knowledge base. Physically awkward children exhibit exactly these characteristics in clinical settings.

Metacognitive Skill

Metacognitive skills are responsible for the executive control of cognitive activity. Such high-level procedural knowledge is the final major category of knowledge about action. Metacognitive skills include both the conscious control of action as well as automatized executive control procedures related to the planning, monitoring, and evaluating of learning and performance.

Recent studies of planning suggest that it is a heterachial process that involves both top-down and bottom-up processing (Bouffard, 1986; Pea, 1982). It is an tentative process that depends on the knowledge base of the person, the demands of the task at hand, and the person's repetoire of planning strategies. Expert-novice studies have shown that skilled athletes use both conscious and unconscious strategies within game and learning situations. Furthermore, they realize that conscious planning processes are more effective if they are used prior to or after a performance rather than during the execution of skilled action.

The monitoring of performance whether in a game or practice situation is an important metacognitive skill that distinguishes those with expertise from those who are novices. The ability to change strategies during the course of fast-paced sports like cricket and tennis in response to subtle changes in the environment is the mark of the skilled athlete.

The evaluation of performance is another crucial metacognitive skill. Understanding the key variables that underlie task demands, being able to remember key plays, being able to analyse why a strategy or action was successful, are the characteristics of expert performance. Again, recent expert-novice studies support these observations (Glaser & Bassok, 1989), as well as a recent study of physically awkward children mentionned in an earlier section (Henderson et al., 1989)

In addition to the planning , monitoring and evaluating aspects of metacognitive skills, expert athletes demonstrate superior memory and visual imagery skills. The work of Allard and Burnett (1985) demonstrates the use of chunking, by skilled athletes in basketball and Starkes' (1987) study of field hockey show that such techniques are needed in decision making tasks related to play selection. Furthermore, recent studies on the use of mental imagery show that this powerful technique is used more effectively by those who are skilled in the physical domain (Feltz & Landers, 1983).

The above brief outline of metacognitive skills adumbrates some of the executive control strategies that skilled individuals use in both learning and performance situations. When we consider that physically awkward children have only a few physical skills in their procedural repetoire and their declarative knowledge base may be limited, one can readily predict that their metacognitive skills will also be underdeveloped. Clinical experience shows that this is the case. Often physically awkward children do not know how to approach a movement problem, they have no idea how to analyze the demands of a task; quite simply, they do not have the planning skills that are required to learn on their own. In the same way, they have great difficulty changing strategies in response to environmental demands and are unable to accurately evaluate their performance in an effective manner.

A knowledge-based approach to the problem of physical awkwardness stresses the developmental nature of the problem. It emphasizes the direct effect of a lack of practice on skill acquisition and highlights the interactive effect that such a lack of procedural knowledge has on the development of declarative, affective, and metacognitive knowledge. Even more importantly, it stresses the negative effects that accrue over time when a person does not have sufficiently developed metacognitive skills to control their own learning and performance.

Educational Management

In addition to treatment or management suggestions in a number of papers (eg. Cermak, 1985; Dare & Gordon, 1970; Denckla, 1984; Gubbay, 1978; Haubenstricker, 1982; McKinlay, 1978; Shaw et al., 1982; Sudgen, 1984) there have been at least three books (Arnheim & Sinclair, 1979; Cratty, 1975; Gordon & McKinlay, 1980) devoted to the practical problems of teaching and programming for physically awkward children (Table 5). Hence this particular section will be brief. We will highlight some recurring themes and issues as well as outline some newer notions.

At least since the editorial by the British Medical Journal on awkward children in 1962, authors have stressed that the condition of movement difficulties should be recognized as a serious problem necessitating assistance and that it is not the result of laziness, disinterest or naughtiness. Recognizing the problem may itself reduce the social pressure on the child (Gubbay, 1978). Dare and Gordon (1970) suggested that honest and frank discussion of the problem occur with the parents, teachers and child. This should dispel myths associated with awkwardness and strike a common front for management. Adults must realize the psychosocial ramifications of awkwardness and appreciate the long term nature of remedial efforts. As Haubenstricker (1982) noted, it is unreasonable to assume that a program of several weeks would alleviate a problem which may have existed for many years.

The early identification of the problem is also important. Early childhood is a period of rapid gains in movement skills, it is likely to be a time when children are willing to practice and, the psychosocial correlates may have less influence (Haubenstricker, 1982). Also, despite the recent data regarding young adults by Knuckey and Gubbay (1983) it is unlikely that maturation from childhood to adolescent reduces the severity of the problem (Walton et al., 1962). Hence, early attention is called for.

Awkward children require extensive instruction, possibly on a one-to-one basis, with clearly defined objectives in mind. Denckla (1984 p. 254) reminds us once again that "there is no evidence that you get anything other than what you teach". Thus the content of programs should reflect fitness activities and movement skills which have a high probability of being required in the child's environment. After all, it is essentially their problem on age appropriate and culturally normative physical skills which define their condition of awkwardness (Wall, 1982).

Table 5: Recommendations of Remedial Strategies for Physically Awkward Children

AUTHOR(S)	Call For Remediation	Need For Progression	Prescription of 1 or 2 Skills	Need For Parental Information	Need For Counselling
McKenzie (1926)					
Orton (1937)	1	1	1	1	
Orton (1946)		1	1		
Annell (1949)					
Brit Med Jnl (1962)	1				
Walton et al (1962)	1	1			
Gubbay et al (1965)	1			1	
Ford (1966)			1		
Brenner et al (1967)					
Reuben & Bakwin (1968)					
Illingworth (1968)					
Bakwin (1968)	1			1	
Gordon (1969)	1	1	1	1	1
Dare & Gordon (1970)	1		1	1	1
Gubbay (1975)					
Henderson & Stott (1977)	1			1	
Gubbay (1978)	1	1	1		1
McKinlay (1978)	1	1		1	
Keogh et al (1979)					
Hulme et al (1982)					
Henderson & Hall (1982)	1				
Shaw et al (1982)	1			1	1
Taylor (1982)	1	1	1	1	1
Wall (1982)	1	1	1	1	1
Knuckey & Gubbay (1983)					
Denckla (1984)	1			1	1
Cermak (1985)	1	1			
Clifford (1985)	1	1	1	1	1
Wall et al (1985)	1	1	1	1	1
Hume & Lord (1986)					
van Dellen & Geuze (1988)					
Henderson et al (1989)					

Note: 1 = Mentioned in article; 2 = Supported by empirical evidence in article

Wall et al.(1985) have argued that knowledge of action is a fundamental developmental phenomenon. Thus the children should be assisted in performing new skills but also in knowing about the skill. For example, Sugden (1984) pointed out a number of important factors in catching which included; recognizing that a ball was about to be thrown, picking up cues from the thrower regarding speed and direction of the ball even before release, attention to the ball's trajectory and organizing their own response to the ball. Children should therefore be assisted in learning to perform physical skill as well as knowing about performing.

Physically awkward children have a deficient movement repetoire and require much practice to acquire new skills and refine others (Machiori et al., 1987). Sufficient practice opportunities must be built into the ongoing program. Also it is likely wise to concentrate on activities in which the child's motivation is relatively high in order to maximize the chances of enough practice occurring. Finally, instructors should always be sensitive to the functionality of what they are teaching. Always throwing a ball directly to a child may be necessary early in learning, but as some skill is developed the child should be challenged to make minor hand and arm as well as body adjustments in order to catch the ball. After all, on the functional playground, a ball is seldom thrown directly to you!

In the current volume, Vallerand and Reid discuss motivational issues surrounding such children as the physically awkward. They point out that some children experience sufficient failure which leads to a helplessness attitude toward many movement tasks. Attribution retraining (Dweck, 1975) was designed to alleviate this feeling and involves teaching the children to take credit for their successes as a reflection of new abilities. A comprehensive management program with physically awkward children should incorporate attribution retraining.

Despite excellent instruction and enthusiasm by the children, it is possible that certain activities will remain quite difficult for them. By early adolescence, awkward youngsters should receive leisure counselling which will not only explore the values of leisure but also point to activities which match their needs and strengths (Taylor, 1987). Fast moving ballgames may remain a mystery to the awkward youngster but he/she may cope or even excel in swimming, wrestling, skating or skiing (Shaw et al., 1982). There are also a host of outdoor activities such as canoeing, which do not emphasize competition. The instructors role therefore becomes not only one of a teacher but also a facilitator of activity.

Future Directions

As a reading of this chapter shows, the syndrome of physical awkwardness has been approached from a number of perspectives. A process to establish a definition of physical awkwardness seems to be an essential next step in the development of this field. An examination of past and current research on this topic indicates that physical awkwardness is a developmental problem that should be viewed from a relatively broad perspective. Theorists should closely examine the relationship between the knowledge-based and the information processing perspectives as both approaches identify important parameters for the identification, evaluation, instruction, and counselling of physically awkward individuals. More theoretical contributions need to be made with suitable feedback and criticesms of them. A central objective of such work must be the development of an appropriate definition of the syndrome and the key characteristics and parameters that underly it.

Agreement on a definition would allow for the development and refinement of checklists and ratings scales to facilitate the identification of those children who are at risk. Approximately 10-15% of school-age children have have been categorized as physically awkward; hence, there is considerable urgency to complete this task. Preschool, kindergarten, and early primary grade identification programs need to be refined and implemented.

In addition to the identification process, it is important that more research be done on the evaluation of the physical skills repertoire of such children. The evaluation of physical proficiency in body management, simple, reactive, and complex skills need to be improved. Given the evidence generated from a knowledge-based approach to motor development, it would seem important to develop evaluation procedures to assess the conceptual, affective, and metacognitive aspects as well. Such evaluation procedures should reflect the cultuarlly normative expectations of children and youth of both genders and at different ages.

The development and use of data-based computer systems might facilitate this process, especially if they include self-evaluation and family evaluation procedures that are user friendly. The McGill Physical Activity Selection System makes use of such computer technology at the present time.

The prescription of skills for instruction is an extremely important process that requires more attention and research. Given the fact that the acquisition of a physical skill or set of skills requires considerable time and practice, it is especially important that prescription procedures be developed to carefully match the skills that a given shild will be encouraged to learn. Clearly, such a process must include an appreciation of the physical activity, sport, and play demands of each child based on age, gender, family history, and community situation. An evaluation of the skills, knowledge base about action, fitness level, interests and participation history must be completed. The availability of suitable instruction, progressive learning opportunities, and the time and place to practice and use a given skill must be considered. Entry skills such as running, biking, swimming and skating should be given high priority as they can facilitate involvement in many related activities.

A conceptual model of skill instruction need to be developed that takes a holistic view of the knowledge base of the person, appreciates the demands of the skills-to-be-learned, recognizes the learning environment factors that facilitate skill acquisition, and stresses the use of flexible instructional strategies to meet the needs of physically awkward individuals.

As indicated above, the careful prescription of skills-to-be-learned should be an essential first step in the learning process. The use of individual skill profiles that reflect a person's developmental level on simple, reactive, and complex skills would facilitate this process.

As outlined in this chapter, physically awkward individuals, by definition, develop a rather limited physical skill repertoire; evidence is also accumulating that indicates that they also have relatively meagre declarative and metacognitive knowledge about action. Furthermore, the picture of the syndrome of physical awkwardness that seems to be emerging suggests that they often have relatively weak physical self-concepts and, at best, variable motivation.

Research needs to be done on the relationship among the development of procedural, declarative and metacognitive knowledge, the importance that domain-specific knowledge has in the skill acquisition process, and means to increase the use of such metacognitive or learning-how-to-learn skills as predicting planning, evaluating, monitoring, and self-checking. Such research is currently underway in the cognitive domain.
Physically awkward children require plenty of progressive practice if they are to acquire proficiency in culturally-normative motor skills. The design, structure and use of the learning environment requires much more research. Means must be found to allow for personal choice and adjustment of task difficulty, enhance information feedback, encourage self monitoring and evaluation, and facilitate progressive practice through the innovative design and use of equipment and apparatus at home, on the playground, and in the gymnasium.

An important objective in the instructional progress must be the designing of strategies to encourage physically awkward individuals to practice effectively on their own, or with supportive others, not only during scheduled instruction but during their free time as well. They need to be taught how to use the equipment, apparatus, and physical layout of their environment, indoors and outdoors, to facilitate their own skill learning. Much more attention needs to be paid to the fundamental role of the learning environment in the skill acquisition process; especially to adopting it to individual needs.

Author Notes

1. Send request for reprints to Greg Reid, Department of Physical Education, McGill University, 475 Pine Avenue West, Montreal, Quebec, H2W 1S4.

References

Adler, H. (1981). Children with problems in physical education in school I. Social factors, school performance, and attitudes towards physical education and sport. *Acta paedopsychiatra, 47,* 313-326

Adler, H. (1982). Children with problems in physical education in school II. Physical factors and psychosocial problems. *Acat paedopsychiatra, 48,* 33-46.

Allard, F. & Burnett, N. (1985). Skill in sport. *Canadian Journal of Psychology, 39*, 294-312.

Annell, A. L. (1949). School problems in children of average or superior intelligence: A preliminary report. *Journal of Mental Science, 95,* 901-909.

Arnheim, D. D., & Sinclair, W. A. (1979). *The clumsy child: A program of motor therapy* (2nd ed). St. Louis, MO: C. V. Mosby.

Bouffard, M. (1986). Knowledge, anticipation and the solution of movement problems by mentally retarded adolescents. Unpublished doctoral dissertion. University of Alberta, Edmonton, Alberta.

Causgrove, J. (1987). *A study of the motor learning of physically awkward children under three instructional conditions.* Unpublished master's thesis, University of Alberta, Edmonton.

Cermak, S. (1985). Developmental dyspraxia. In E. A. Roy (Ed). *Neuropsychological studies in apraxia and related disorder* (pp. 225-248). North-Holland: Elsevier Science Publishers B. V.

Chi, M. T. H. (1978). Knowledge structures and memory development. In R. S. Siegler (Ed.), *Children's thinking: What develops?* (pp. 73-96). Hillsdale, NJ: Lawrence Erlbaum.

Clifford, L. D. (1985). *A profile of the leisure pursuits of seven physically awkward children.* Unpublished master's thesis, University of Alberta, Edmonton.

Clumsy Children (1962). British Medical Journal, 2, 1665.

Cratty, B. J. (1975). *Remedial motor activity for children.* Philadelphia, PA: Lea and Febiger.

Cratty, B. J., Ikeda, N., Martin, M. M., Jennett, C., & Morris, M. (1970). *Movement activities, motor ability and the education of children.* Springfield, IL: Charles C. Thomas.

Dare, M. T., & Gordon, N. (1970). Clumsy children: A disorder of perception and motor organisation. *Developmental Medicine and Child Neurology, 12,* 178-185.

Denckla, M. B. (1984). Developmental dyspraxia: The clumsy child. In M. D. Levine & P. Satz (Eds.), *Middle childhood: Development and dysfunction* (pp. 245-260). Baltimore, MD: University Park Press.

Dudley-Marling, C. C., Snider, V., & Tarver, S. G. (1982). Locus of control and learning disabilities: A review and discussion. *Perceptual and Motor Skills, 54,* 503-514.

Dweck, C. S. (1975). The role of expectations and attributions in the allevation of learned helplessness. *Journal of Personality and Social Psychology, 31,* 674-685.

Feltz, D.L. & Landers, D.H. (1983). The effects of mental practice on motor skill learning and performance: A meta-analysis. *Journal of Sport Psychology, 5,* 25-57.

Fitts, P.M. & Posner, M.I. (1967). *Human Performance.* Belmont, CA: Brooks/Cole.

French, K.E. & Thomas, J.R. (1987). The relation of knowledge development in children's basketball performance. *Journal of Sport Psychology, 9,* 15-32.

Ford, F. R. (1966). *Diseases of the nervous system* (5th ed). Springfield, IL: Charles C. Thomas.

Gardner, H. (1983). *Frames of Mind.* New York: Basic Books.

Gibson, B. J. (1980). *An attributional analysis of performance outcomes and the alleviation of learned helplessness on motor performance tasks: A comparative study of educable mentally retarded and non-retarded boys.* Unpublished doctoral dissertation, University of Alberta, Edmonton.

Glaser, R. & Bassok, M. (1989). Learning theory and the study of instruction. *Annual Review of Psychology, 40*, 631-666.

Gordon, N. (1969). Helping the clumsy child in school. *Special Education, 58*, 19-20.

Gordon, N., & McKinlay, I. (1980). *Helping clumsy children.* Edinburgh: Churchill Livingstone.

Griffin, P.S. (1985). Boys participation styles in a middle school physical education team sport unit. *Journal of Teaching in Physical Education, 3*, 100-110.

Griffin, N. S., & Keogh, J. F. (1982). A model for movement confidence. In J. A. S. Kelso & J. E. Clark (Eds.), *The development of movement control and co-ordination* (pp. 213-236). New York, NY: John Wiley & Sons.

Gubbay, S. S. (1975a). *The clumsy child.* Toronto: W. B. Saunders.

Gubbay, S. S. (1975b). Clumsy children in normal schools. *The Medical Journal of Australia, 1,* 233-236.

Gubbay, S. S. (1978). The management of developmental apraxia. *Developmental Medicine and Child Neurology, 20,* 643-646.

Gubbay, S. S. (1979). The clumsy child. In F. C. Rose (Ed.), *Pediatric neurology* (pp. 145-160). Oxford: Blackwell.

Gubbay, S. S., Ellis, E., Walton, J. N., & Court, S. D. M. (1965). Clumsy children: A study of apraxic and agnosic defects in 21 children. *Brain, 85*, 295-312.

Harter, S. (1978), Effectance motivation reconsidered: Toward a developmental model. *Human Development, 21,* 34-64.

Harter, S. (1981). The development of competence motivation in the mastery of cognitive and physical skills: Is there still a place for joy? In G. C. Roberts & D. M. Landers (Eds.), *Psychology of motor behavior and sport - 1980* (pp. 3-29). Champaign IL: Human Kinetics.

Harter, S. (1982). The perceived competence scale for children. *Child Development, 53,* 87-97.

Haubenstricker, J. L. (1982, May). Motor development in children with learning disabilities. *Journal of Physical Education, Recreation and Dance,* 41-43.

Henderson, S. E., & Hall, D. (1982). Concomitants of clumsiness in young schoolchildren. *Developmental Medical and Child Neurology, 24,* 448-461.

Henderson, S. E., May D. S., & Umney, M. (1989). An exploratory study of goal-setting behaviour, self-concept and locus of control in children with movement difficulties. *European Journal of Special Needs Education, 4* (1), 1-15.

Hulme, C., Biggerstaff, A., Moran, G., & McKinlay, I. (1982). Visual, kinaethetic and cross-modal judgements of length by normal and clumsy children. *Developmental Medicine and Child Neurology, 24,* 461-471.

Hulme, C., & Lord, R. (1986). Clumsy children - A review of recent research. *Child: Care, Health and Development, 12,* 257-269

Hulme, C., Smart, A., & Moran, G. (1982). Visual perceptual deficits in clumsy children. *Neuropsychologia, 20*(4), 475-481.

Illingworth, R. S. (1968). The clumsy child. In M. Bax & R. McKeith (Eds.), *Minimal cerebral dysfunction* (pp. 26-27). London: Heinemann Medical Books.

Keogh, J. F., Sugden, D. A., Reynard, C. L., & Calkins, J. A. (1979). Identification of clumsy children: Comparisons and comments. *Journal of Human Movement Studies, 5,* 32-41.

Knuckey, N. W., & Gubbay, S. S. (1983). The clumsy child: A prognostic study. *Australian Pediatrics Journal, 19,* 9-13.

Lazlo, J. I., & Bairstow, P. J. (1983). Kinaesthesis: Its measurement, training and relationship to motor control. *Quarterly Journal of Experimental Psychology, 35A,* 411-421.

McKenzie, R. T. (1926). The functions and limits of sport in education. *The Canadian Medical Association Journal, 16,* 630-632.

McKinlay, I. (1978). Strategies for clumsy children. *Developmental Medicine and Child Neurology, 20,* 494-495.

Machiori, G. E., Wall, A. E., & Bedingfield, E. W. (1987). Kinematic analysis of skill acquisition in physically awkward boys. *Adapted Physical Activity Quarterly, 4,* 305-315.

Marteniuk, R. G. (1976). *Information processing in motor skills.* New York, NY: Holt.

Nichols, P. L., & Chen, T. (1981). *Minimal brain dysfunction: A prospective study.* Hillsdale, NJ: Lawrence Erlbaum.

Orton, S. T. (1937). *Reading, writing and speech problems in children.* New York, NY: Norton.

Paton, J. F. (1986). *The fitness performance of physically awkward children.* Unpublished master's thesis, University of Alberta, Edmonton.

Pea, R. D. (1982). What is planning development the development of? In D. Forbes & M. T. Greenberg (Eds.), *Children's planning strategies* (No. 18, pp. 5-27). San Francisco, CA: Jossey-Bass.

Reid, G. (1989). Ideas about motor behavior research with special populations. *Adapted Physical Activity Quarterly, 6*(1), 1-10.

Reuben, R. N., Bakwin, H. (1968). Developmental clumsiness. *Pediatric Clinics of North America, 15,* 601-610.

Roberton, M.A. (1982). Describing "steps" within and across motor tasks. In J.A.S. Kelso & J.E. Clark (Eds.), *The development of movement control and co-ordination* (pp. 293-308). New York: John Wiley & Sons.

Rosenbaum, D. A. (1980). Human movement initiation: Specification of arm, direction, and extent. *Journal of Experimental Psychology: General, 109,* 444-474.

Shaw, L., Levine, M. D., & Belfer, M. (1982). Developmental double jeopardy: A study of clumsiness and self-esteem in children with learning problems. *Journal of Developmental and Behavioral Pediatrics 3,* 191-196.

Smith, M.F.R. (1978). Attribution, achievement motivation, and task difficulty in physical education. Paper presented at the B.C. Conference on the Teaching of Physical Education. Victoria, B.C.

Smyth, T. R., & Glencross, D. J. (1986). Information processing deficits in clumsy children. *Australian Journal of Psychology, 38,* 13-22.

Starkes, J.L. (1987). Skill in field hockey: Nature of cognitive advantage. *Journal of Sport Psychology, 9*, 146-160.

Stelmach, G. E. (1982). Information processing framework for understanding human motor behavior. In J. A. S. Kelso (Ed.), *Human motor behavior: An introduction* (pp. 63-91). Hillsdale, NJ: Lawrence Erlbaum.

Stott, D. H., Moyes, F. A., & Henderson, E. E. (1984). *A test of motor impairment/Henderson revision.* San Antonio: Psychological Corporation.

Sugden, D. A. (1984). Issues in teaching children with movement problems. *British Journal of Physical Education, 15*, 68-70.

Taylor, M.J. (1988). *Physical awkwardness and reading disability. A descriptive study*. Unpublished master's thesis. University of Alberta, Edmonton, Alberta.

Todd, T. (1988). *A comparison of metacognitive and procedural knowledge of ball catching by physically awkward and non-awkward children.* Unpublished master's thesis, McGill University, Montreal, Quebec.

van Dellen, T., & Geuze, R. H. (1988). Motor response processing in clumsy children. *Journal of Child Psychology and Psychiatry, 29*, 489-500.

Wall, A. E. (1982). Physically awkward children: A motor development perspective. In J. P. Das, R. F. Mulcahy, & A. E. Wall (Eds.), *Theory and research in learning disabilities* (pp. 253-268). New York, NY: Plenum Press.

Wall, A.E. (1986). A knowledge-based approach to motor skill acquisition. In M.G. Wade & H.T.A. Whiting (Eds.). *Motor development in children: Aspects of co-ordination and control* (pp. 33-47). Dordrecht: Martinus Nyhoff Publishers.

Wall, A. E., McClements, J., Bouffard, M., Findlay, H., & Taylor, M. J. (1985). A knowledge-based approach to motor development: Implications for the physically awkward. *Adapted Physical Activity Quarterly, 2*, 21-42.

Walton, J. N., Ellis, E., & Court, S. D. M. (1962). Clumsy children: Developmental apraxia and agnosia. *Brain, 85*, 603-612.

Wellman, H.M. (1984). The development of concepts of the mental world. *Behavioral and Brain Sciences, 7*, 651-652.

Whiting, H. T. A. & den Brinker, B.V. (1982). Image of the act. In J.P. Das, R.F. Mulcahy & A.E. Wall (Eds.). *Theory and Research in Learning Disabilities*, (pp. 217-235). New York: Plenum Press.

SECTION IV:

ATHLETES WITH DISABILITIES

Problems in Movement Control
G. Reid (editor)

SPORT, SOCIETY, AND INDIVIDUALS WITH DISABIITIES

Karen P. DePauw
Department of Physical Education, Sport & Leisure Studies
Washington State University

"Sports are cultural practices embedded in a whole range of social processes in which humans interact with one another" (Sage, 1987, p. 273). In the broadest sense, sport is a cultural phenomenon and a reflection of society. Hollands (1984) contends that play, games, leisure and sport are elements of a contemporary popular culture and have far more impact and importance than readily acknowledged.

Professional issues within physical education and sport science must be seen in the context of a general concern and critical awareness of events which are occurring in society as a whole. Gruneau (1978) insists that sport can be studied in relation to the general features of social organization in order to gain a more coherent and comprehensive understanding of institutional arrangements and cultural values in the whole society and the place of sport activities within them (p 82). Historically, sport has been viewed as the domain of the elite and not the masses. Sport has been dominated by men and masculinity. Sport has played a significant role in the preservation of patriarchal social order (Hall, 1985). Further, Theberge (1985) has argued that sport as a gendered cultural form bears significant relation to gender segregation and inequality in other realms of social life (p. 193).

Sport has been an exclusive club; a club for the "majority". Therefore not only have women experienced exclusion but so have the other minorities, persons of ethnic backgrounds and individuals with disabilities. But this is changing. The inclusion of "minorities" (women, ethnic minorities, disabled individuals) in sport is but a reflection of some level of acceptance of these same "minorities" in society in general (DePauw, 1986).

The social world is constituted and reproduced through and in human action (Giddens, 1977, p. 166). Inasmuch as sport is a product of society, society can be seen as an agent for change in sport and sport as an agent for the transformation of social relations in society.

Sport sociologists have investigated the personal characteristics and backgrounds of sport participants and coaches including personal-social attitudes and values, birth order, motivation, social stratification and sport involvement, and sport socialization. Specifically, social class, ethnicity, race, and gender as factors in sport participation have been investigated. Disability as a similar factor has yet to be systematically studied.

The study of social organization and behaviour requires a concern with meanings and values within cultural settings that are part of a historical process (Zeitlin, 1973). The core of social reality is viewed as the human being trying to make sense out of social situations. When extended to research, emphasis must be placed upon understanding culture and social norms in historical and comparative contexts. Historical sensitivity is critical to understanding society, as a whole, and its component parts.

Inasmuch as society has influenced, will continue to influence, and to be influenced by sport for individuals with disabilities, an examination of the interrelation among sport, society, and individuals with disabilities is important. To accomplish such an end, this review has been divided in four sections: (a) societal treatment of individuals with disabilities throughout history, (b) the evolution of sport for individuals with disabilities, (c) research efforts on sport and disabled athletes, and (d) identification of future trends and issues.

Societal Treatment of Individuals with Disabilities: Historical Perspectives

Societal acceptance of individuals with disabilities has changed over the past three thousand years. The attitudes and actions of society toward individuals with disabilities have spiralled around a continuum from exclusion to inclusion (DePauw, 1986). Historical trends have occurred repeatedly along this continuum due to changes in the social and economic conditions, religious beliefs, laws and knowledge of facts (Hewett & Forness, 1974).

"Social myths are constantly in the making--compelling in their simplicity, and alluring because we want to believe them" (Smith, 1985, p. 9). Throughout history, many perceptions or beliefs have been accepted as facts and evolved into social myths. An example is the concept the portions of the human race are inherently inferior, and that status is not modifiable. Portions of the human race considered inferior at one time or another, include certain racial and ethnic groups, women, individuals with disabilities, those in lower social classes, and so on.

Historically, those who were different in appearance and/or behaviour were treated in variety of ways ranging from cruel to humane. Those who were different have been destroyed, tortured, exorcised, sterilized, ignored, exiled, exploited, and even considered divine (Hewett & Forness, 1974, p. 9). They have also been pitied, cared for, categorized, and educated. The general trend has been toward "progressive inclusion and acceptance" of individuals with disabilities in society (DePauw, 1986).

Four determiners have been identified by Hewett and Forness (1974) which depict the historical treatment of individuals with disabilities. These four determiners are: (a) *threat to survival* due to harsh treatment by the physical and social environment, (b) *superstition* in relation to appearance and behaviour of those with differences, (c) *science* or the natural, lawful, and objective approach to explaining differences, and (d) *service* including the care, humane treatment, education, and societal acceptance of those with differences (p. 10).

Primitive and Ancient Period (3000 B.C. to 500 B.C.)

During the Primitive and Ancient period, survival and superstition were the two main determiners of the treatment of individuals with disabilities. These manifested themselves through the natural elements, demonology, and religious beliefs.

Most commonly, babies with obvious abnormalities were killed. Due to the harsh natural environment, those individuals who were weak typically did not survive very long. Individuals who behaved differently might either be feared or considered possessed. Those possessed with "good spirits" were revered; those with "bad spirits" were indulged to prevent revenge. Mental illness of ancient time was treated by a crude skull operation called trephining and/or exorcism.

Greek and Roman Period (500 B.C. to A.D. 400)

During the Greek and Roman period, the treatment of individuals with disabilities was based upon survival and superstition with a brief moment of humanitarian reform. The factors affecting survival included the harsh physical environment, infanticide, eugenics, harsh treatment, and even exile. It was allowable for parents of physically deformed and female children to let them die. The survival of the fitness doctrine was in effect; not only in terms of the environment but also in terms of severe punishment and discipline. In addition, abandonment of children, or exile, was widespread.

Initially during this period, mental illness was thought to be caused by the gods taking away one's mind. Thus, purification, exorcism and demonology were the primary practices of the times.

Later during this period, an attempt was made to scientifically understand individuals with disabilities and to treat them accordingly. Hippocrates considered mental illness a disease of natural causes and not the anger of the gods. Not only was care for mentally ill individuals advocated by Plato but also other humane treatment such as hydrotherapy, massage, sunshine, exercise, and abstinence from meat (Hewett & Forness, 1974). Unfortunately, this moment of humanitarism was all too brief.

Middle Ages (A.D. 400 to 1500)

Although survival and superstition continued as determiners during the Middle Ages, religion and religious conviction became the major factors influencing the treatment of individuals with disabilities. Infanticide was no longer an accepted practice and individuals with differences were allowed to live. Even so, their life was still hard due to the harshness of both the physical and social environments.

The behaviour of physically impaired and "feebleminded" individuals was believed to be influenced by Satan (Hewett & Forness, 1974). With the onset of Christianity, mentally retarded individuals were viewed as "children of God" while mentally ill individuals were thought to be possessed of the "devil" (Lilly, 1983). The treatment of individuals with disabilities varied with the believed etiology. Mentally retarded individuals were considered "blessed" and gained prestige by becoming court jesters. Mild forms of exorcism, torture, witchburning, and demonology remained the practice for mentally ill individuals.

Although there were isolated attempts at acceptance, understanding and humanitarian treatment of individuals with differences, behaviour based upon deep religious conviction would ultimately have the effect of setting the stage for persecution on the grounds of any difference (physical, mental, religious, etc.).

Sixteenth and Seventeenth Centuries

Early in this time period, severe persecution of those with differences was commonplace. All individuals considered to be heretics were investigated. Along with others, mentally ill persons were tortured and burned at the stake. Witchburning and torture were the results of the demonology of the time. Science and medicine were unable to separate themselves from demonological tradition.

Those with hearing impairments and mental retardation were received different treatment during this period. "Special" education for deaf individuals appeared. Both oral and finger spelling techniques were utilized to teach reading, writing, arithmetic, astronomy, Greek, and so on to deaf children from noble families.

An attempt was made to define mental retardation from a psychological and educational point of view. Mentally retarded individuals were considered idiots, sots, simpletons. These were persons who could not read, write, count to 20, etc. Many mentally retarded individuals became segregated from society in workhouses for the poor and unemployed. In such places, they suffered from loss of contact with normal life and a growing lack of understanding of their problems by the community who banished them (Hewett & Forness, 1974).

Although the period was one of deeply ingrained irrational beliefs and neglect, as well as practices such as witch burning and demonology, a trend toward scientific explanation, humanitarianism, care and education of individuals with disabilities emerged.

Eighteenth Century

More acceptance of individuals with disabilities was noted during the eighteenth century. Demonology gave way to concern for the "rights of man". But the realities of a harsh physical environment remained. Many children died. The carelessness of midwives, and/or general lack of prenatal care, caused a large number of physical deformities in children who were, as a result, not destined to survive infancy nor childhood.

The French Revolution awakened the sense of one's social responsibility as well as the community's responsibility toward its members, including children (Hewett & Forness, 1974). This gave rise to care and education for individuals with disabilities. Mental illness was considered a disease or sickness and classified as mania, melancholia, and dementia. The humane treatment of those with mental illness was established through hospitals and institutions.

The role of the humanitarian teacher was established. Throughout Europe, education and training programmes for both blind and deaf individuals were developed. Schools were established, each equipped with unique methods for teaching one's particular students.

While schools for deaf and blind children appeared, little was done for the child with a physical impairment (Pritchard, 1963). One exception was the introduction of the scientific study of physical deformity in Russia by Peter the Great. This is considered part of the early development of special education in the Soviet Union.

It was also during the Eighteenth century that the role of sensory experience in learning was brought to the forefront. Locke and Rousseau believed that the natural curiosity of the child should be utilized in learning and that children should be allowed to develop in a natural, unrestricted environment.

This period can be characterized by the establishment of the dignity of the individual, and social responsibility. In addition, fear, superstition and hostility toward those with differences were replaced by rational understanding, care, and education.

Nineteenth Century

Science and service were the primary determiners of the treatment of individuals with disabilities during this period. Essentially the threat to survival was minimized and superstition and religious fanaticism all but eliminated. Therefore, attention was focused upon the care and education of individuals with disabilities.

Reform in the treatment of mentally ill persons was given impetus during this period. Mental illness was still considered a result of a disease of the brain, and therefore mental hospitals, or institutions, were established for the treatment and rehabilitation of mentally ill persons.

In addition to the already established institutions for blind, deaf, and mentally ill persons, institutions for mentally retarded individuals were developed. These residential institutions appeared throughout Europe and America during this period.

In the later 19th century in the United States, it was generally accepted that the state had responsibility for the care of retarded individuals. Institutional segregation, either temporary or permanent, was viewed as most effective (Hewett & Forness, 1974).

The beginnings of current educational theory were developed during this period. Because of such persons as Itard, Sequin, Montessori, and others, developmental concepts and concern with the child's total personality emerged. The importance of individualization of instruction was recognized. Effective techniques and approaches were developed to enhance the teaching of deaf (sign language, oral communication) and blind (braille, special writing tablets) individuals. Education, or training, was found to be effective even for severely retarded individuals. In addition, less severely retarded individuals were thought capable of some level of gainful employment.

Although the events of the nineteenth century established care, treatment, and education for individuals with disabilities as the mandates for the twentieth century, they were not able to eliminate all of the inhumane treatment. Yet the fragments of knowledge and understanding accumulated over thousands of years had finally begun to dismantle the cruelty , superstition and neglect of individuals with disabilities. The threat to survival and superstition as determiners of treatment and societal acceptance of those with differences were giving way to scientific investigation and more appropriate treatment and service delivery.

Twentieth Century

Three major events of the 20th century are considered as particularly significant in the treatment of individuals with disabilities and fostered the emergence of special education in the United States (Lilly, 1983). The first event was the development and use of the intelligence (IQ) test. Because the IQ test was based upon the school curriculum of the time, a situation was created in which it was erroneously thought that the IQ scores could predict school achievement. In general, children who had not been exposed to the school curriculum scored low on the test and as a result, were thought to be mentally retarded, and were labelled as such.

Second, in the early 1900s child labour and compulsory school attendance laws were passed. The result was "education for all" not just the elite. The elimination of children from the work force created an influx of children into the schools. As a result, these "industrial children" were to experience difficulties with education. They were administered the IQ test and it was concluded that they did not do well because they were retarded. Special classes were soon developed which included a watered down curriculum for these "morons". These children who had difficulty with school were those who had not previously been exposed to formal education.

The third significant event was the decision rendered in the case of Brown vs. Board of Education of Topeka, Kansas in 1954. The court stated that schools would be integrated because separate but equal for black children was illegal. Many black children experienced difficulty in "integrated" education and as a result, many of them were placed in special education classes. This social movement of integration in society created new problems in the schools and a new category of retardation; the educable mentally retarded.

From these three major events emerged special education. Their influence firmly established the early belief that the problem of those requiring special education (and labelled "handicapped") was "in the child"; no examination of the school curriculum was made (Lilly, 1983). Many of these individuals placed in special education were not necessarily "handicapped in society" but they were "handicapped in school".

With the passage of the Education of All Handicapped Children's Act (PL 94-142), such concepts as individualized education, mainstreaming, integration, and least restrictive environment became commonplace. Special education was required and it became the responsibility to the public educational agency.

In the United States, the legal mandates of the 1970s (Education of All Handicapped Children's Act, Rehabilitation Act, Amateur Sports Act of 1978) provided for equal opportunity, non discrimination on the basis of "handicap", accessibility, education, and sport for individuals with disabilities. These laws, as well as laws enacted throughout the world, reflected a change in society's response to individuals with disabilities and their place in society; a legislated step toward "progressive inclusion and acceptance". Individuals with disabilities were gradually gaining more acceptance. Increased awareness fostered more inclusion, and less isolation and exclusion of disabled individuals within the activities of society.

Trends

The treatment of individuals with disabilities has changed over the course of time. At least four major trends can be identified. (a) For all disabled individuals, steady progress has been made from exclusion to inclusion. (b) For those with obvious and/or severe impairments, treatment which began as remediation and isolation has now become that of compensation. (c) For individuals with mild and less obvious impairments (mild mental retardation, learning disabilities), the neglect of their problems early in history and isolation gave way to protection and finally challenge. (d) For individuals with disabilities who were first neglected, then identified and over-identified, attention is now more focused upon the individual rather than the label.

Although differences can be seen across nations, the attitudes and behaviour of societies in general have changed so that individuals with disabilities have more opportunities and can experience more inclusion within society. Acceptance of those with disabilities is replacing rejection. Attitudes toward those with disabilities are now progressing from mere acceptance to expectation of full participation in society.

History of Sport for Individuals with Disabilities

Sport opportunities for individuals with disabilities have been created as a result of changes in societal attitudes and behaviours toward individuals with disabilities. Prior to World War I, athletes with disabilities had virtually no opportunities for sports competition with the exception of deaf individuals.

International Perspectives

Deaf individuals were the first to participate in organized sport. This phenomenon can be explained by the facts that (a) deaf individuals, born of noble families, were the first to receive tutoring/special education (in the 1600s), (b) the first public school for disabled individuals was established for deaf individuals, (c) the first residential (educational) institutions were established for deaf individuals, and (d) the French revolution awakened a sense of social responsibility for individuals with disabilities. As a result, the International Sports Committee for the Deaf (CISS) was founded in Paris, in 1924, and thus became the first organization to sanction sport competition for any disability group (Ammons, 1986; Stein, 1986).

In the ensuing 60 plus years, this European organization expanded from the original 6 affiliated nations into the present 45 and was the first of the disabled sport organizations to be recognized by the International Olympic Committee (IOC). This recognition came in 1955 after 30 years of sponsoring sport events for deaf individuals.

Since their inception, the World Summer Games and World Winter Games for the Deaf have seen international competitions held every four years in an Olympic format. Events include but are not limited to, alpine skiing, nordic skiing, speed skating, volleyball, tennis, wrestling, basketball, swimming, track and field events, badminton, and soccer.

Although individuals with physical impairments existed long before the 20th century, it was not until after the World Wars that significant progress was made in sport opportunities for them (DePauw, 1985a; Huber, 1984). As a consequence of these wars, men (and a few woment) who were once able bodied and accepted by society were still considered "normal" even though many had become physically impaired. This "acceptance" fostered the need for rehabilitation of the war veterans. This attitude was ultimately extended to those with other physical impairments and physically disabled children.

In 1960, the International Stoke Mandeville Games Federation (ISMGF) was formed under the leadership of Guttman to sanction all international competition for individuals with spinal cord injuries (Huber, 1984). In that same year, the United States entered its first international competition for wheelchair athletes (Lipton, 1970).

During the 1960s, international sport competition were expanded to include other disability groups not eligible for the World Games for the Deaf or the international wheelchair competitions. In 1963, the International Sports Organization for the Disabled (ISOD) was created to provide international sport opportunities for blind, amputee, and other locomotor disabled individuals (Lindstrom, 1984). In such a role, the founders of the ISOD intended for it to become "the" international organization for disabled sport; a structure parallel with the IOC (International Olympic Committee).

In 1968, the International Cerebral Palsy Society (ICPS) sponsored the first international games for individuals with cerebral palsy in France. ICPS continued to sponsor this international competition every two years until 1978 when Cerebral Palsy-International Sports and Recreation Association (CP-ISRSA) became recognized by ISOD as the official sanctioning body for cerebral palsy sports (Huber, 1984).

As an outgrowth of expanded opportunities and interest in competition for blind athletes, the International Blind Sports Association (IBSA) was formed in 1981 (Stein, 1986). This organization was the last "disability" sport group to seek and attain recognition by ISOD. Thus, each disability group to compete in international (Para-olympic) competition (blind, cerebral palsy, amputee, spinal cord injured) was then represented by separate organizations.

Recently, the International Sports Federation for Persons with Mental Handicap (INAS-FMH) was formed in the Netherlands. The purposes of this association included (a) promoting sporting activities for persons with mental handicaps, (b) training of coaches, trainers, officials, etc., (c) promoting technical and medical research, (d) disseminating information, and so on. The INAS-FMH is considered by many to be the international governing body for sport for mentally retarded/handicapped individuals and Special Olympics as a United States organization.

The most recent addition to the disabled sport scene is the International Coordinating Committee (ICC). It was joint interest in international sport for individuals with disabilities which brought the CP-ISRA, IBSA, ISMGF, and ISOD together in 1982 to form the ICC to coordinate disabled sport worldwide and to negotiate with the International Olympic Committee (IOC) on behalf of athletes with disabilities. In addition to the four founding member organizations, CISS and Federation for Sports for Persons with Mental Handicaps (INAS-FMH) have recently joined.

Although based in the United States, Special Olympics International has chapters throughout the world. Many mentally retarded individuals around the world participate in year-round programs of Special Olympics while some chapters are organized primarily for sending a team to the United States to compete at International Special Olympics. At present there is limited communication between the two "international" organizations serving mentally retarded individuals (International Sports Federation for Persons with Mental Handicaps and Special Olympics, International). Whereas INAS-FMH is recognized by the ICC, Special Olympics has entered into a protocol agreement with the International Olympic Committee for recognition and use of the term "Olympics" as long as it is used with Special. Thus, sole leadership in the international sport arena for mentally retarded individuals has yet to be established.

Essentially the international organizations serving sport for individuals with disabilities tended to pattern themselves after the "able bodied" world, the international Olympic model. In doing so, these groups have created parallel sport structures by disability.

Through alignment with the IOC, recognition, and acceptance of athletes with disabilities and inclusion of disabled athletes in the Olympic movement was sought. Some progress has been made. Disabled athletes have participated in Demonstration Events at the Winter Olympics in Sarajevo (1984) and Calgary (1988) and the Summer Olympics in Los Angeles (1984) and Seoul (1988). Although not yet considered as equals in elite athleticism, some disabled athletes were able to wear the official uniform of their country and march with their country in the opening and closing ceremonies.

United States Perspectives

Organized in 1945, the American Athletic Association for the Deaf (AAAD) became the United States affiliate to the CISS (Ammons, 1986). Originally, the AAAD provided competitive sports opportunities for individuals with hearing impairments through state, regional, and national basketball, softball, and volleyball tournaments. The AAAD currently promotes competition also in sports such as athletics, soccer, badminton, tennis, team handball, water polo, and wrestling. It also promotes participation by U.S. deaf athletes in the World Games for the Deaf (summer and winter).

In 1949, the first national wheelchair basketball tournament was held at the University of Illinois and as a result, the National Wheelchair Basketball Association (NWBA) evolved as the governing body for wheelchair basketball in the United States (Lipton, 1970). The emphasis of this group was placed upon sport, physical activity and competition rather than strictly rehabilitation.

In the early 1950s, while Guttman was organizing the first international competition for wheelchair athletes, Ben Lipton was contemplating the development of organized wheelchair sports, in addition to wheelchair basketball, on the national U.S. level (Huber, 1984). In 1956, Lipton founded the National Wheelchair Athletic Association (NWAA) in recognition of the value of recreational and competitive sports in the rehabilitation and daily lives of physically disabled individuals. Currently, the NWAA sponsors various competitive sports on a state, regional, and national level (Lipton, 1970). Over the years the NWAA has organized and conducted competitions in a variety of Olympic sports including: athletics (track and field), archery, air guns, swimming, weightlifting, and table tennis. With a focus upon sport and participation by athletes with disabilities, the NWAA moved to Colorado Springs to be more closely affiliated with the United States Olympic Committee and within the past year, the NWAA has reorganized itself into a federation of wheelchair sport governing bodies.

In response to a void in winter sport opportunities for physically disabled individuals, the National Handicapped Sports and Recreation Association (NHSRA) was formed in 1977 by a small group of Vietnam veterans with amputations (DePauw, 1985a). Although NHSRA was initially involved primarily with winter sport activities, chapters now promote year-round recreational activities and various levels of competitive sports including water skiing, swimming, scuba diving, sailing, canoeing, river rafting, horseback riding, and skiing. These activities and recreational sports as well as competitive sports are available for individuals with physical (amputee, spinal cord injury, cerebral palsy, and so on) or visual impairments. At the national level, NHSRA sponsors the Handicapped Ski Championships and Winter Festival and sends competitive Alpine and Nordic ski teams to international competitions.

In the 1960s, Presidents Eisenhower and Kennedy initiated a public concern for the fitness and well being of mentally retarded individuals. As a specific response to such concern, Eunice Kennedy Shriver founded International Special Olympics and Special Olympics, Inc. in 1968 and hosted the first International Special Olympics Games in Soldier's Field, Chicago. Special Olympics is the national governing sports body for mentally handicapped individuals in the United States (Songster, 1986). Today, over a million mentally handicapped individuals participate in year-round activities in 16 sports including swimming, gymnastics, bowling, basketball, soccer, track and field events, and equestrian events.
The period encompassing the 1960s can be characterized in terms of the civil rights movement for minority individuals and women. The legislation of the 1970s for disabled individuals came as a result of the civil rights awakening of the 1960s and laid the foundation for increasing opportunities and inclusion of individuals with disabilities. Education for disabled children and non-discrimination on the basis of handicap were mandated.

The passage of the Amateur Sports Act of 1978 was also affected by the civil rights movement and the legislation of the 1970s in that specific reference was made to opportunities for minority athletes, women, and disabled individuals. As a result, several additional sport organizations serving disabled individuals were formed.

The National Association of Sports for Cerebral Palsy was founded in 1978 as the United States governing sport organizing body for individuals with cerebral palsy and similar neurological conditions. In 1986, the NASCP was reorganized as the United States Cerebral Palsy Athletic Association (USCPAA) (Jones, 1988) and continues to sponsor competitions in a variety of events including archery, horseback riding, powerlifting, table tennis, soccer, bowling, swimming,and track and field events.

During this same time, the United States Association for Blind Athletes (USABA) became the national governing sport organizing body for blind and visually impaired individuals (DePauw, 1985a). The USABA organizes competitions for summer and winter events such as alpine and nordic skiing, gymnastics, powerlifting, swimming, track and field, and wrestling.

A small group of amputee athletes founded the United States Amputee Athletic Association (USAAA) in 1981 (DePauw, 1985a). The USAAA sponsors competitions specifically for amputee athletes in summer sports such as archery, stand-up basketball, sit-down and stand-up volleyball, swimming, weightlifting, and track and field events.

The most significant event in the recent history of the disabled sport movement was the passage of PL95-606, The Amateur Sports Act of 1978 (DePauw, 1985b). As a result, the following was included among the purposes listed in the Constitution of the United States Olympic Committee (USOC):

> To encourage and provide assistance to amateur athletic programs and competition for handicapped individuals, including, where feasible, the expansion of opportunities for meaningful participation by handicapped individuals in programs of athletic competition for able-bodied individuals.

To achieve this objective, Group E membership in the USOC and a Committee on Sports for the Disabled were established (DePauw & Clarke, 1986). Group E membership is available to national amateur sports organizations serving the disabled population which sponsor national athletic competitions in two or more sports which are included on the program of the Olympic or Pan American Games. The Committee on Sports for the Disabled (COSD) is a standing committee of the USOC composed of two representatives from each of the Group E members (AAAD, USAAA, USABA, USCPAA, NHSRA, NWAA, and Special Olympics). In addition to representatives of Group E members, the USOC currently appoints five at-large members to serve on the COSD. (Inasmuch as current changes are taking place within the United States Olympic Committee that which is described here is accurate through 1988.)

The COSD essentially serves in a coordinating capacity for amateur athletic activity for individuals with disabilities in the United States. The recognition of athletes with disabilities by the USOC via the COSD represents an important step in the advancement of disabled sport. Some progress has been noted. For example, in 1985, disabled athletes participated in the annual National Sport

Festival sponsored by the USOC. Since that time, disabled athletes have been included in all Sport Festivals.

European and Canadian Perspectives

The history of sport for individuals with disabilities in Europe has followed a somewhat different course than that followed in the United States. Due in part to the size of the countries, and the nature of their governments, sport for individuals with disabilities in western European countries, tends to be organized more by sport than by disability. This is influenced by the system of democratic sport clubs prevalent in Europe. European countries tend to have one officially recognized organization for sport for disabled individuals (e.g. German Sport Federation for the Disabled, Belgian Sport Organization for the Disabled) which are quite commonly affiliated with the nation's able bodied sport organization as well. Most often these sport for disabled organizations include only those with physical and visual impairments (spinal cord injured, cerebral palsy, blind, amputee, etc.). In addition, one can also find separate sport organizations for deaf and mentally retarded individuals. Although Special Olympics programs can be found in European countries, these are organizations primarily outside of the main structure of sport in a given country.

Historically, at least the initial sport for disabled organizations were established in the 1940s and 1950s. Most of these original organizations have broadened in the scope of sports provided and disabled individuals served.

The Canadian system of sport for disabled individuals is philosophical affiliated with the European system but has been influenced by the United States as well. Although activities and organizations exist at the provincial level, there is a national organization entitled Canadian Federation of Sport Organizations for the Disabled. This organization has existed since 1976 although not formally constituted until 1981. The association consists of member organizations and individuals members.

The purpose of the CFSOD is to coordinate those activities common to member organizations for disabled individuals on matters pertaining to promotion, rule integration, coaching integration, and participation in national and international competition an administration involving more than one disability group (Steadward, n.d.). Currently there are five member organizations: Canadian Wheelchair Sports Association (CWSA), Canadian Amputee Sports Association (CASA), Canadian Association of Disabled Skiing (CADS), the Canadian Blind Sports Association (CBSA) and the Canadian Deaf Sports Association (CDSA). The Canadian Cerebral Palsy Sport and Recreation Association holds "associate" membership in CFSOD. Special Olympics in Canada exists as a separate organization.

Concluding Comments

Throughout the world, the sport for the disabled movement has gathered a great deal of momentum over the past few years (Sherrill, 1986). As a result, new national sport groups have been formed and additional sport opportunities for individuals with disabilities have been provided throughout the world. Recent additions include sport for disabled organizations in Australia, New Zealand, Hong Kong, China, Korea, and so on. The creation of such organizations reflects changes in attitudes toward the inclusion of individuals with disabilities in the sport arena not only internationally but nationally as well.

Research Efforts

Although sport for individuals with disabilities has existed for the past 40 years, little research was undertaken until the 1970s. The initial research was conducted primarily in two areas: investigation of disabled athlete's level of conditioning and response to exercise, and wheelchair propulsion. Not only have the research efforts continued in these two areas, but a substantial increase in research activity occurred during the 1980s. Since those initial research efforts, the research has become (a) sport specific, (b) disability specific, (c) performance enhancing, and (d) discipline-oriented (exercise physiology, sociology, etc.) (DePauw, 1988).

Based upon the findings of research, it has been determined that both similarities and differences exist between athletes with disabilities and able bodied athletes (see DePauw, 1987, for summary of selected research findings). (For further information on research in the psychological/sociological area, see the chapter by Sherrill in the current volume). Similarities include response to exercise, application of biomechanical principles to performance, psychological profile, measures of anxiety, sport related injuries, attitudes toward physical activity and sport participation, and enhancement of athletic performance after training.

As expected, some differences found were specifically related to one's disability; functional muscle mass, observable performance, number of injuries related specifically to impairment, and type and extent of training regimens. Socialization into sport appears to be different for individuals with disabilities; whereas friends and community agencies were reported by athletes with disabilities to be the prime stimulators for sport participation, the prime stimulators for able bodied athletes are the family and school (Sherrill, Rainbolt, & Ervin, 1984; Sherrill, Rainbolt, Montelione, & Pope, 1986).

Actually, sport research on individuals with disabilities is in its "growing years". Many research questions are currently being investigated and many more have yet to be asked. Five areas of research were identified by DePauw (1988). There are as follows:

1. Movement efficiency -- research on the mechanics and physiology of movement including wheelchair design, and adapted sport equipment, applied technology

2. Sport Performance -- research on the effectiveness of training regimens and coaching techniques, application of sound principles of sport physiology, biomechanics, psychology, and nutrition for enhancing performance and injury prevention, classification

3. Sport Initiation -- research on the reasons for and the extent of participation in sport, effect upon participation in youth sport programs, recreation, and leisure activities

4. Effects of Sport -- research on the values of and specific sociological, psychological, and physical benefits of participation and competition upon functional capacity for sport and activities of daily living

5. Influences upon Sport -- research on the historical, philosophical, legal, and societal factors influencing sport and athletes with disabilities.

Future Directions

The future of sport for individuals with disabilities will be shaped not only by the findings of a concerted research effort but by political and social factors as well. The following are predictions for the future of sport for individuals with disabilities:

1. Although more multi-disability national sport organizations will emerge,disability specific sport organizations will continue to exist throughout the world.

2. National and international standards for competition will increase.

3. Specialization within sport participation will increase.

4. Classification and competition will become sport specific rather than disability specific.

5. The number of individuals with disabilities participating in sport will significantly increase except at the elite level of competition.

6. The number of individuals with disabilities included within able bodied sport and Olympic sport will increase.

7. Public awareness and acceptance of individuals with disabilities will increase due in part to sport participation.

The future directions of sport for individuals with disabilities as of yet is not fully charted. Significant controversies currently exist which must be addressed and resolved. Among the issues to be faced are the following: (a) sport by ability or disability, (b) sport for participation or competition, and (c) integrated or separate competition. Although it should be argued that these issues can be expressed along a continuum, controversy arises when these are discussed relative to the future direction of national and international sport for individuals with disabilities.

Within the next ten years, these issues and others will not only be addressed but resolved. Inasmuch as sports are cultural practices reflecting societal attitudes and behaviours, the future of sport for individuals with disabilities will be a reflection of society's progressive inclusion and acceptance of individuals with disabilities. How much acceptance and how much inclusion remains to be seen.

Author Notes

1. Send request for reprints to Karen P. DePauw, Department of Physical Education, Sport and Leisure Studies, Washington State University, Pulman, Washington, USA.

References

Ammons, D. (1986). World games for the deaf. In C. Sherrill (Ed.), *Sport and disabled athletes* (pp. 65-72). Champaign, IL: Human Kinetics.

Clarke, K. S. (1986). Perspectives for the future of the disabled in sport. *Adapted Physical Activity Quarterly, 3,* 152-155.

DePauw, K. P. (1985a). History of sports for individuals with disabilities. *Able Bodies, 4,* 1, 3.

DePauw, K. P. (1985b). USOC's commitment to sports for individuals with disabilities. *Palaestra, 1,* 6.

DePauw, K. P. (1986). Toward progressive inclusion and acceptance: Implications for physical education. *Adapted Physical Activity Quarterly, 3,* 1-5.

DePauw, K. P. (1987). Research on sport for individuals with disabilities: State of the art. *Proceedings of the Civitan-I'M SPECIAL International Physical Education and Sport for the Disabled Conference* (pp. 33-61). Tampa, FL: University of South Florida.

DePauw, K. P. (1988). Sport for individuals with disabilities: Research opportunities. *Adapted Physical Activity Quarterly, 5*(2), 80-89.

DePauw, K. P., & Clarke, K. C. (1986). Sport for disabled U.S. citizens: Influence of Amateur Sports Act. In C. Sherrill (Ed.), *Sport and disabled athletes* (pp. 41-50). Champaign, IL: Human Kinetics

Giddens, A. (1977). *Studies in social and political theory.* New York, NY: Basic Books.

Gruneau, R. (1978). Conflicting standards and problems of personal action in the sociology of sport. *Quest, 30,* 80-90.

Guttman, L. (1976). *Textbook of sport for the disabled.* Oxford: H. M. & M. Publishers.

Hall, M. A. (1985). Knowledge and gender: Epistemological questions in the social analysis of sport. *Sociology of Sport Journal, 2,* 25-42.

Hewett, F. M., & Forness, S. R. (1974). *Historical origins.* Boston, MA: Allyn & Bacon.

Hollands, R. G. (1984). The role of cultural studies and social criticism in sociological study of sports. *Quest, 36,* 66-79.

Huber, C. A. (1984). An overview and perspective on international disabled sports: Past, present, future. *Rehabilitation World, 8,* 8-11.

Jones, J. A. (1988). *Training guide to cerebral palsy sports.* Champaign, IL: Human Kinetics.

Lilly, M. S. (1983). *Divestiture in special education: An alternative model for resource and support services.* Unpublished manuscript.

Lindstrom, H. (1984). Sport for disabled: Alive and well. *Rehabilitation World, 8,* 12-16.

Pritchard, D. G. (1963). *Education and the handicapped: 1760-1960.* London: Routledge and Kegan.

Sage, G. H. (1987). Pursuit of knowledge in sociology of sport: Issues and prospects. *Quest, 39,* 255-281.

Sherrill, C. (Ed.). (1986). *Sport and disabled athletes.* Champaign, IL: Human Kinetics.

Sherrill, C., Rainbolt, W., & Ervin, S. (1984). Attitudes of blind persons towards physical education and recreation. *Adapted Physical Activity Quarterly, 1,* 3-11.

Sherrill, C., Rainbolt, W., Montelione, T., & Pope, C. (1986). In C. Sherrill (Ed.), *Sport and disabled athletes* (pp. 189-195). Champaign, IL: Human Kinetics.

Smith, J. D. (1985). *Minds made feeble.* Rockville, MD: Aspen Publications.

Songster, T. B. (1986). The Special Olympics sport programs: An international sport program for mentally retarded athletes. In C. Sherrill (Ed.), *Sport and disabled athletes* (pp. 73-80). Champaign, IL: Human Kinetics.

Steadward, R. D. (1980). Analysis of wheelchair sport events. In H. Natvig (Ed.), *Proceedings of the First International Medical Congress on Sports for the Disabled* (pp. 184-192). Oslo, Norway: Royal Ministry of Church and Education, State Office for Youth and Sports.

Steadward, R. D. (n.d.). *Sports for the physically disabled and birth of the CFSOD.* Unpublished manuscript.

Stein, J. U. (1986). International perspectives: Physical education and sport for participants with handicapping conditions. In C. Sherrill (Ed.), *Sport and disabled athletes* (pp. 51-64). Champaign, IL: Human Kinetics.

Therberge, N. (1985). Toward a feminist alternative to sport as a male perspective. *Quest, 37,* 193-202.

Zeitlin, I. M. (1973). *Rethinking sociology: A critique of contemporary theory.* Englewood Cliffs, NJ: Prentice-Hall.

Problems in Movement Control
G. Reid (editor)
©Elsevier Science Publishers B.V. (North-Holland), 1990

PSYCHOSOCIAL STATUS OF DISABLED ATHLETES

Claudine Sherrill
Department of Kinesiology
Texas Woman's University

Over 100 countries now provide their disabled citizens with opportunities for international level sport competition (Price, 1986). Children, both able-bodied (AB) and disabled, are exposed to a growing number of role models from the sport for disabled movement (Dickinson & Perkins, 1985; Sherrill, 1986a). There is widespread agreement that sport is a means of highlighting ability and affirming competence. Local, regional, and national sport programs for individuals with disabilities are emerging. With this growth, interest in the relationship between motor behaviour and psychosocial status is increasing. Recently several writers have emphasized the importance of extending sport psychology to disabled athletes (Asken & Goodling, 1986; Goodling & Asken, 1987; Ogilvie, 1985).

The purpose of this chapter is to review research on the psychosocial status of disabled athletes. This will be accomplished by identifying and discussing the most frequently used data collection instruments, organizing findings whenever possible in relation to established or emerging theories, and speculating about future directions. Several reviews of psychosocial research on adult disabled athletes (Asken, 1987; DePauw, 1988; Goodling & Asken, 1987; Sherrill, 1986b) and on young handicapped performers (Reid, 1987) already exist, and the contents of these will not be duplicated. This review focuses on theory-related research completed since 1984.

Most existing research is relatively atheoretical and adult-oriented. A major reason for the atheoretical nature of disabled athlete research is its recent origin. The first psychosocial studies of disabled athletes appear to be those of Szyman (1980) and Kennedy (1980). Too few years have elapsed to resolve problems of sampling design, instrument selection, and data collection to have allowed for major theoretical advances.

The creation of a knowledge base underlying the practices of a profession typically requires three stages of inquiry: (a) exploratory, in which researchable ideas evolve and methods of studying these ideas are pilot tested, (b) descriptive, in which a phenomenon is fully and carefully described and findings are generalized from one sample to another, and (c) explanatory, in which the goal is to develop theory that offers insight into the generalizations that evolve from the descriptive stage. Explanation is often conceptualized as a continuous cycle of theory development, theory testing, and theory expansion and/or reformulation. Research on the psychosocial status of disabled athletes is clearly in the exploratory stage.

Contemporary psychosocial research in relation to disabled athletes resembles that conducted in the early stages of sport psychology, 1950-1965. According to Landers (1983), this stage was characterized by empiricism and dominated by personality testing. Most research was descriptive-comparative, and the major thrust was identifying similarities and differences between groups (i.e., males vs. females, athletes vs. nonathletes, beginners vs. advanced performers) on various psychological instruments. Theory was seldom mentioned although the inventories typically used were associated with trait theory (i.e., the study of highly enduring, even lifelong, characteristics, temperament, or disposition). In the 1970s interest expanded to include states (e.g., moods and emotions) that were situation-specific, and researchers began to debate the merits of various approaches: (a) trait or general personality theory, (b) situational theory, largely concerned with states, and (c) interactional theory, which focused on the interactions between the two.

Today sport psychology (Gill, 1986; Kane, 1980; Morgan, 1980) and psychology in general (Endler & Hunt, 1984; Hall & Lindzey, 1978) appear divided in regard to personality theory approaches. Central to the ongoing controversy are the definition of personality, the state-trait distinction (Fridhandler, 1986), concern about person vs. situation variance in predicting athletic performance, and problems regarding generalization. Also, interest in personality theory is diffusing into cognitive psychology.

Rehabilitation psychology and counselling research (Cook, 1987; Shontz, 1977) makes no mention of the trait-state controversy. Instead, the literature indicates that personality structure is remarkably stable even in persons who have sustained severe physical disability or illness. Hundreds of studies indicate that there is no relationship between traits and disability. Shontz (1977), in summarizing research, stated that few of the traditional theories of personality have impacted on rehabilitation. Shontz exhorted researchers to cease examining the hypothesis of relationship between disability and personality and instead to explore the personal meaning of disability to individuals.

Personal meaning theory (Wright, 1960, 1983) focuses on the way disability is perceived by self and significant others and thus stresses attitudes, beliefs, and values. Central to the evolution of personal meaning theory were the field theory of Kurt Lewin (1935) and the self-concept theory of Carl Rogers (1951).

The goal of most rehabilitation psychology research is to examine the multiple external and internal forces, both genetic and interactional, that contribute to situational adaptation and life adjustment.

Psychosocial research on disabled athletes has its roots in both sport and rehabilitation psychology. These parent disciplines both emphasize theory but direct their energies toward different kinds of issues and problems. In contrast, psychosocial research with disabled athletes reflects little awareness of theory and issues. The apparent goal is simply to explore and describe.

Data collection instruments, however, are extensions of theory. Thus assuming psychological inventories are carefully selected, data may be used in theoretically relevant ways and future research suggested. Knowledge about the validity and reliability of instruments and their generalizability to disabled athletes is essential to good research. In this chapter, therefore, studies that appear atheoretical are reviewed under their respective data collection instruments. Studies that begin with a discussion of theory are reviewed under that theory.

Sixteen Personality Factor Questionnaire (16 PF)

The 16 PF (Cattell & Stice, 1957) is the instrument used in the research of Shephard and colleagues at the University of Toronto, Canada (Goldberg & Shephard, 1982; Kofsky & Shephard, unpublished study reported in Shephard, in press). The 16 PF consists of 16 bipolar scales, each of which is defined by 3 to 17 adjectives or descriptive phrases. Cattell claimed that these 16 scales measured *source traits* (i.e., fundamental dimensions) of normal personality functioning as opposed to *surface traits* assessed by most existing personality inventories. These traits are A, reserved vs. outgoing; B, less intelligent vs. more intelligent; C, affected by feelings vs. emotionally stable; E, humble vs. assertive; F, sober vs. happy-go-lucky; G, expedient vs. conscientious; H, shy vs. venturesome; I, tough-minded vs. tender-minded; L, trusting vs. suspicious; M, practical vs. imaginative; N, forthright vs. shrewd; O, self-assured vs. apprehensive; Q1, conservative vs. experimenting; Q2, group-dependent vs. self-sufficient; Q3, undisciplined vs. controlled; and Q4, relaxed vs. tense.

The validity of the 16 PF was established through several factor analytical studies (Buros, 1978). Test reviewers indicate, however, that other types of validity (i.e., known groups) have not been adequately examined. Five forms (A, B, C, D, E) are available, but the use of the combined forms (A + B or C + D) is recommended.

Test-retest reliabilities for the 16 scales of Forms A and B average in the .70s; none are reported for Forms C and D. Test-retest reliabilities for combined

Forms A + B range from .45 to .93 (median, .81) and for C + D, from .67 to .86 (median, .78).

Morgan (1980) pointed out that the 16 PF has been used in physical education research more than any other personality inventory and lies at the heart of the trait psychology controversy. Inherent in this criticism is whether the instrument is used to describe or predict, with most of the antagonism directed at failure of trait inventories to predict more than a small proportion of actual behaviour.

Goldberg and Shephard (1982) administered the 16 PF to 17 males in wheelchairs. Comparing highly active (i.e., athletes) and moderately active subjects, significant differences were found on 3 of 16 scales. High active males were more emotionally stable and venturesome whereas moderate actives were more practical. When subjects were combined (n = 17), there were no significant differences between their scores and the test manual norms (Shephard, in press). When sport classes 1-3 (most severe) were compared with classes 4-6 (least severe), the more severely disabled individuals scored significantly higher on apprehension only (Trait O).

Kofsky and Shephard (Shephard, in press) extended this study to include 163 male and 93 female lower-limb disabled adults. Findings revealed that 12 of the 16 personality scores differed significantly from test manual norms, with most deviations disadvantageous to the wheelchair sample. Significant differences were also found with regard to severity of disability, with high lesion individuals more detached, humble, serious, and resourceful than low lesion subjects. Shephard and colleagues' research is illustrative of trait theory inquiry.

In summary, the 16 PF was used by physical educators more frequently than any other personality inventory prior to 1980. Since then, it has received little attention, presumably because able bodied (AB) research has changed its direction from trait description to prediction and/or examination of performance enhancement and success. Rehabilitation psychology, since the 1970s, has accepted the hypothesis of no relationship between personality traits and disabilities. By selecting the 16 PF to study wheelchair athletes, Shephard and colleagues showed a willingness to deviate from contemporary trends and practices. Their findings that 16 PF scores of disabled athletes did indeed differ significantly from test manual norms suggest a need to re-examine trait theory and perhaps explore ways that it can be interwoven with personal meaning theory.

Profile of Mood States (POMS)

Most of the recent research on the psychological states of disabled athletes has come from French, Sherrill, and Gench (Texas Woman's University), Henschen

(University of Utah), Horvat (University of Georgia), and doctoral students at Texas Woman's University (Mastro, Canabal, Greenwood, Paulsen, and Rainbolt). Two instruments have been used in this research: the Profile of Mood States (POMS) by McNair, Lorr, and Droppleman (1971) and the State-Trait Anxiety Inventory (STAI) of Spielberger, Gorsuch, and Lushene (1970).

The POMS, a 65-item paper-pencil instrument, was developed to meet "the need for a rapid, economical method of identifying and assessing transient, fluctuating affective states" (McNair et al., 1971, p. 1). POMS contains six scales: tension-anxiety, depression-dejection, anger-hostility, psychic vigour-activity, psychic fatigue-inertia, and confusion-bewilderment. Each scale score is derived from the sum of ratings over 7 to 15 adjectives; there is no item overlap among scales. Subjects use a 5-point rating scale to indicate "how you have been feeling during the past week including today?"

The validity and reliability of POMS is excellent (Buros, 1978). Construct validity is supported by five separate factor analyses as well as the known groups method (i.e., ability of the instrument to discriminate between psychiatric outpatients and university students). Internal consistency coefficients range from .84 to .95, and test-retest coefficients range from .65 to .74 for outpatients of a university medical centre psychiatric clinic over a 20-day duration (McNair et al., 1971). Test-retest coefficients for blind subjects over 2 consecutive days ranged from .78 to .95 (Mastro, French, & Hall, 1987a).

The POMS test manual presents T score norms for psychiatric outpatients (n = 1000) and normal college students (n = 856). Significant gender differences are reported for college students, with women scoring higher (i.e., less desirable) than men on tension, depression, and confusion. Correlations between gender and factor scores indicate, however, that 1% or less of the variance is associated with gender. Therefore the test manual norms are based on combined gender data.
Although originally developed for use with psychiatric outpatients, the POMS gained popularity in the 1970s as a major data collection instrument in examining the mental health model of Morgan (1980). This model, which posits that success in sports and positive mental health are directly proportional, is now widely accepted. POMS profile data on the 1972 and 1976 U.S. Olympic Wrestling Teams led Morgan to create the name "iceberg profile" to describe the phenomenon that elite athletes score above the 50th T score on vigour and below the 50th T score on tension, depression, anger, fatigue, and confusion. Morgan (1980) summarized findings of research on elite wrestlers, oarsmen, and distance runners, showing that POMS data on each resulted in the iceberg profile.

Henschen (1984) was the first researcher to report POMS data on disabled athletes (n = 35, no gender indicated). Reanalysed for 33 male wheelchair athletes (Henschen, Horvat, & French, 1984), these data indicated that athletes with lower limb impairments, aged 18 to 35 years, demonstrated similar iceberg profiles to elite, AB athletes. Visual comparison of profiles indicated that wheelchair athletes were closest to the ideal iceberg, manifesting high vigour and low tension, depression, anger, fatigue, and confusion. POMS data were reported as T-score means, and no test of significance was used. Data were collected 1 hour prior to each athlete's first event in a regional track meet that determined qualifiers for the annual national games.

Similar iceberg profiles were reported for 62 female wheelchair basketball players, aged 19 to 37 years, who were members of one of 10 teams in the Tenth Annual U.S. Women's National Wheelchair Basketball Tournament (French, Henschen, & Horvat, 1985). These data and those of the 33 male wheelchair athletes (Henschen et al., 1984) were later subjected to a multivariate analysis (Horvat, French, & Henschen, 1986), which indicated significant gender differences ($p < .05$). Males scored lower on depression, anger, fatigue, and confusion but higher on vigour. Profiles of male and female wheelchair groups were then compared visually with AB athlete groups. Horvat et al. (1986) concluded that Morgan's thesis that athletes possess superior mental and emotional health when compared to the general population can be generalized to wheelchair athletes.

Wheelchair tennis players (77 males and 10 females) in the 1987 Southwest National Wheelchair Tennis Championships also evidenced the iceberg profile (Greenwood, Dzewaltowski, & French, 1988). These individuals, ages 19 to 62 years, $M = 32.6$, were compared with nonsport participants in wheelchairs (32 men and 8 women) of similar ages identified through various state organizations and hospitals. Comparison of POMS measures resulted in significant differences ($p < .001$) between groups, favouring the athletes, on all mood states.

Paulsen (1988), in a similar research design, reported only one significant difference (depression) in a comparison of 26 wheelchair basketball players and 28 wheelchair nonathletes. All subjects were male, had been disabled at least 2 years, and attended a college or university in Texas. The nonathletes (i.e., the group higher in depression) did not exercise on a regular basis. Both disabled groups presented the iceberg profile that has been typically associated only with sport participation. Paulsen also compared the two wheelchair groups with AB varsity basketball players ($n = 11$) and test manual means and standard deviations for male college students ($n = 340$), who presumably were nonathletes. The wheelchair basketball players scored more athletically on all POMS scales than the two AB groups. The wheelchair nonathletes, with one exception--anger, also scored more in the direction of athletic success than the two AB groups.

Most research on wheelchair athletes has been in segregated sport settings. Horvat, Roswal, Jacobs, and Gaunt (1988) investigated whether the findings of these studies would generalize to athletes competing in an integrated meet. Subjects were all wheelchair athletes (10 males and five females) who competed and 15 AB athletes matched by gender, age, experience, and event. No significant difference between athlete groups or genders was found on POMS. Groups exhibited similar iceberg profiles.

Research on blind athletes has been spearheaded by James Mastro, a gold medallist in international blind sports. Mastro's dissertation (1985) was a report of POMS and STAI data on the 33 elite male blind athletes, ages 16 to 32 years, who competed in the 1984 International Games for the Disabled. POMS data were collected 4 days prior to competition and compared with data from 37 elite sighted Greco-Roman wrestlers, ages 17 to 32, collected during the training camp for the 1984 U.S. Olympic team (Silva, Shultz, Haslam, Martin, & Murray, 1985). Mastro was the first POMS researcher to fully describe disabled subjects in terms of sport classification (i.e., degree of blindness, onset of disability (congenital vs. adventitious), and number of years of competition (national and international). The sample included 42% totally blind, 21% light perception, and 36% legally blind. Visual impairment was congenital for 52% of the sample and adventitious for 48%. Multivariate comparison of blind and sighted athletes revealed a significant difference in only one variable, vigour. Blind athletes scored significantly higher (M = 22.58) in vigour than sighted athletes (M = 19.03). POMS data from 15 of the 33 blind male athletes in Mastro's dissertation (1985) were compared with data from the 15 female blind athletes who competed in the same International Games (Mastro, Sherrill, Gench, & French, 1987b). Elite blind male athletes demonstrated the iceberg profile but their female counterparts did not. Multivariate analysis revealed that the males had significantly lower tension, fatigue, and confusion than the females. Mastro et al. (1987b) also reported no significant difference in POMS scores between athletes with congenital vs. adventitious blindness and varying degrees of blindness.

To compare blind and sighted athletes competing together in the same sport, Mastro, Canabal, and French (1988) chose beep baseball, a unique sport in which teams consist of six blind players and two sighted players. The sighted athletes act as pitcher and catcher when their team is up to bat and as spotters (calling out the fielder's name to which the hit ball is coming closest) when their team is in field. Subjects were 81 blind and 39 sighted players representing 21 teams in the 1985 National Beep Baseball Association World Series Tournament. Data were collected within 24 hours of each athlete's first game. Univariate t tests revealed significant differences between blind and sighted players on tension and depression. These differences favoured the sighted athletes. Both groups exhibited the iceberg profile.

Mood states of 6 blind male golfers and their coaches (3 males and 3 females) were reported by Mastro, French, Henschen, and Horvat (1986). Mean ages of the blind golfers and their coaches were 55 and 52.5 years, respectively. POMS data were collected within 12 hours of competition. No statistical analysis was performed. Visual comparison of profiles indicated that coaches demonstrated psychological characteristics closer to the ideal iceberg profile than golfers. Blind golfers scored close to the college student test manual norms except for a lower score on confusion.

POMS data on cerebral palsied (CP) athletes were collected by Sherrill (1986b) as part of a broadly conceived study of the psychosocial dimensions of disability. Differences in mood states by gender and by level of competition (international vs. national) were subsequently examined (Canabal, Sherrill, & Rainbolt, 1987). Subjects were 39 international and 34 national competitors, with mean ages of 26.1 and 27.3, respectively. Sport classes, when combined into wheelchair (Classes 1-4) and ambulatory (Classes 5-8), were about equally distributed. No significant difference between genders was found. Multivariate analysis showed that CP international athletes had significantly higher vigour scores ($M = 22.8$) than CP national athletes ($M = 18.9$), $p = .03$. Correlations between POMS measures and various demographic variables were also examined, revealing four significant but low relationships: (a) vigour with sports class (-.33), with wheelchair athletes scoring higher than ambulatory athletes; (b) vigour with gender (-.29), with males scoring higher than females; (c) anger with sports class (-.27), with wheelchair athletes scoring higher than ambulatory; and (d) confusion with years of competition (-.25), with experienced athletes indicating less confusion than inexperienced ones.

The mood states of Canadian CP athletes, also of international calibre, were studied by Goodbrand (1987) of McGill University. Four groups of subjects ($n = 28$ in each group) were statistically compared: (a) international CP athletes, M age = 24.4; (b) elite AB athletes, M age = 18.3; (c) CP nonathletes, M age = 33; and (d) AB nonathletes, M age = 23.8. Several factorial multivariate analyses were conducted to examine the effects of age, gender, education, sport classification (wheelchair vs. ambulatory), sport type (swimming vs. track and field), and number of years in competition. Among Goodbrand's many conclusions were the following: (a) there are no significant differences between the CP and AB athletes; (b) there are no significant gender differences, and (c) there are no significant differences among sport classifications. Athletes and nonathletes are significantly different, regardless of physical ability.

Sherrill, Gench, Canabal, and Mastro (1988a) compared mood states of elite male CP ($n = 24$), blind ($n = 32$), and AB ($n = 37$) athletes. Multivariate analysis revealed only one significant difference, vigour, with blind athletes scoring higher than AB athletes ($p = .05$) but not CP athletes. All three groups exhibited the ideal athletic iceberg profile.

In summary, 14 studies have been reported on the mood states of disabled athletes: 7 on wheelchair athletes (i.e., lower-limb disability with impairment not specified), 4 on blind athletes, 2 on CP athletes, and 1 on crossdisability comparisons. Data were collected in disability-specific (12 studies) and integrated (2 studies) settings. With two exceptions [elite blind females (Mastro et al., 1987b) and blind golfers (Mastro et al., 1986)], all samples, regardless of gender, type of sport, level of skill, and sport setting, exhibited the iceberg profile. Statistical comparisons of disabled athletes with AB athletes and/or test manual norms were reported in 3 wheelchair athlete studies, 2 blind athlete studies, and both CP athlete studies, with varied findings, probably because extraneous variables were poorly controlled. Overall, disabled athletes appear similar to AB athletes in mood states during athlete training and competition. Significant differences between genders have been found for wheelchair athletes (Horvat et al., 1986) and blind athletes (Mastro et al., 1987b) but not for CP athletes (Canabal et al., 1987; Goodbrand, 1987).

State-Trait Anxiety Inventory

Two theories traditionally have been used to explain the relationship between anxiety and motor performance: drive theory (Hull, 1943; Spence, 1958) and inverted-U theory (Martens & Landers, 1970; Yerkes & Dodson, 1908). Since 1970, sport psychologists have tended to support the inverted-U theory, which posits that moderate levels of arousal (i.e., anxiety) facilitate personal performance whereas both high and low arousal levels tend to adversely affect performance. Individual differences are important in this theory, and coaches are encouraged to explore how much arousal individual athletes need to perform optimally. Throughout the 1970s anxiety theory focused on explaining relationships between motor performance and trait- and state anxiety. A frequently used instrument was the State-Trait Anxiety Inventory (Spielberger et al., 1970), which follows the inverted-U theory. Spielberger (1966) was the first theorist to make a distinction between trait and state anxiety, the construct upon which STAI was based.

The State-Trait Anxiety Inventory (STAI) is recommended as "one of the best standardized of anxiety measures, if not the best" (Buros, 1978, p. 683). Landers (1980), however, criticizes the STAI and similar paper-pencil instruments because they are not situation (i.e., sport) specific and they do not yield separate scores for cognitive and somatic anxiety.

Nevertheless many researchers like the STAI because it permits easy comparison of state anxiety (a transitory condition of perceived tension) and trait anxiety (a relatively stable condition of anxiety proneness). The STAI consists of two one-page forms, each listing 20 phrases. These are rated on a 4-point scale. Some items on the two scales are similar (I feel calm vs. I am "calm, cool, and collected;" I feel content vs. I am content; I am relaxed vs. I feel rested).

Several types of validity are reported (Buros, 1978). The criterion-referenced validity of the STAI-Trait Scale is evidenced by its correlations with existing anxiety scales: IPAT Anxiety Scale, .75; Manifest Anxiety Scale, .80; and Affect Adjective Checklist, .52. Construct validity by the known groups method is reported for the Trait Scale, which statistically discriminates between neuropsychiatric patients and nonpsychiatric patients. Validity of the State Scale has been examined by repeatedly testing the same persons over different conditions and showing that their scores change in the expected directions.

Reliability coefficients vary according to whether test-retest or alpha coefficients are reported. According to Buros (1978), alpha coefficients are more suitable indicators of reliability for state anxiety than test-retest. Alpha coefficients range from .83 to .92 for state scores and .86 to .92 for trait scores. Test-retest coefficients for trait anxiety for males and females, respectively, are .86 and .76 for a 20-day interval and .73 and .77 for a 104-day interval. To determine if verbal administration (as opposed to standardized paper-pencil procedures) influenced reliability, Mastro, French, Henschen, and Horvat (1985) studied 15 elite blind female athletes. The resulting test-retest coefficients were .88 and .90 for the state and trait scales, respectively.

Most research on the state-trait anxiety of disabled athletes is interwoven into research on mood states. Since these studies, with two exceptions, were reviewed in the last section, findings will be reported briefly. Henschen et al. (1984) reported that male wheelchair athletes scored low on state anxiety (M = 41) and average on trait anxiety (M = 34). French et al. (1985) indicated that female wheelchair basketball players also scored low on state anxiety and average on trait anxiety.

STAI findings of Mastro's dissertation (1985) were published by Mastro and French (1986). The rationale for the research was largely a challenge of the oft-repeated statement that blind persons tend to exhibit a higher anxiety level than sighted people when performing physical activities. Findings revealed that international blind male athletes (n = 33) exhibited state (M = 50) and trait (M = 48) anxiety within the range reported for the normative population in the test manual. A comparison of state and trait scores for inventories administered to blind athletes 6 days and 1 day prior to international competition indicated no significant differences between trials. One reason posited for this finding was that permission could not be obtained to collect data within 45 min of the competition as is recommended. Mastro and French also found no significant state anxiety differences between high- and low-trait blind athletes.

Mastro et al. (1986) reported state- and trait-anxiety T scores for blind golfers (n = 6) as 61 and 60. Scores for coaches (n = 6) were 57 and 57. French, Mastro, and Montelione (1987) examined state and trait anxiety of 21 male, blind goalball players in a state tournament. The STAI was administered to athletes within 15 min of the first game, and the state scale was readministered within 5 min of each athlete's completion of his last game. No significant STAI differences were found between successful athletes (on first, second, or third place teams) and unsuccessful athletes (on fourth, fifth, or sixth place teams) and between athletes who won their last game and lost their last game.
In summary, five studies have reported findings on state trait anxiety of disabled athletes. Research on 33 male wheelchair athletes (Henshen et al., 1984) and 66 female wheelchair athletes (French et al., 1985) indicated similar findings: low state anxiety and average trait anxiety. Research on blind athletes with sample sizes of 33, 9, and 21 respectively, revealed no differences between state and trait anxiety scores. Both fell in the average to high range compared to test manual norms. These five studies were relatively atheoretical, with very brief reviews of literature and no mention of theory. Each study appeared supportive of trait theory and the concept that specific personality traits can raise or lower anxiety to a level that impedes optimal athletic performance (Henshen et al., 1984).

The Journal of Sport Psychology and Exercise is a rich resource on sport competition and anxiety (Burton, 1988; Gould, Petlichkoff & Weinberg, 1984). Researchers interested in anxiety and disabled athletes may wish to consider replicating designs used with AB athletes. An exciting new instrument is the Competitive State Anxiety Inventory-2 (CSAI-2).

Self-Actualization

Self-actualization theory serves as the basis of much of the recent research of Sherrill and colleagues. This theory, which is attributed to Maslow (1954), posits that professed values, beliefs, and behaviours (i.e., one's personal orientation in relation to both self and environment) determine self-actualization, the inner drive to become all that one can be. Gill (1986) identified self-actualization theory as organismic theory, the opposite of Freud's psychodynamic theory. A central feature of organismic theory is intrinsic motivation, an inner drive toward achieving optimal mental and physical health. Self-actualization theory is closely associated with the self-concept theory of Carl Rogers; together these two theories are recognized as the conceptual framework of humanistic psychology and/or counselling.

Having interviewed approximately 200 CP and 100 blind athletes at various national and international competitions, Sherrill (1986b) noted that almost all athletes reported coping with stigmatization, stereotyping, and prejudice as part of their lifestyle. Almost all saw sports as a means of affirming their competence, thereby seeking to focus attention on their abilities rather than their disabilities. In spite of the problems confronted daily and the severe disability which characterized some, the athletes seemed to be self-actualizing. Intrigued with this observation, Sherrill designed a number of research studies. The Personal Orientation Inventory (POI) of Shostrom (1966) was the instrument used in each study. Of the many psychological inventories available, the POI is the only one that purports to measure self-actualization (Tosi & Lindamood, 1975). Scores are derived for two major scales (Time Competence, 23 items, and Inner-Directedness, 127 items) which are independent of one another and 10 subscales, each consisting of 9 to 32 items taken from the major scales. These subscales are Self-Actualizing Value (affirmation of values of self-actualizing), Existentiality (ability to react situationally rather than rigidly), Feeling Reactivity (responsiveness to one's needs and feelings), Spontaneity (ability to be oneself), Self-Regard (affirmation of self because of worth or strength), Self-Acceptance (affirmation of self in spite of weaknesses), Nature of Man (constructive view of nature of masculinity/femininity); Synergy (ability to see opposites of life as meaningfully related), Acceptance of Aggression (affirmation of one's natural aggressiveness), and Capacity for Intimate Contact (meaningful relationships with other human beings that are unencumbered by expectations/obligations).

The numerous studies conducted on the validity and reliability of the POI have been summarized by Tosi and Lindamood (1975), who indicated that it has good validity. Stability coefficients over .75 have been reported for all scales except Self-Actualizing Value (.74), Nature of Man (.69), and Synergy (.50). Test-retest reliabilities for blind and CP athletes, respectively, ranged from .80 to .97 and .78 and .92 (Sherrill, Gilstrap, Richir, Gench, & Hinson, 1988b). Crossmodality reliability coefficients (oral vs. written administration) of the POI have been reported as .72 to .92 (Sherrill et al., 1988b).

Early self-actualization research on disabled athletes was conducted by Sherrill and Rainbolt (1987a,b,c). The first two studies entailed visual inspection of POI profiles of elite (i.e., international competitors) CP athletes in relation to AB athlete and test manual profiles. The third paper (Sherrill & Rainbolt, 1987c) was a 2 X 2 (Skill X Gender) MANOVA comparison of four groups of CP athletes: international females (n = 23), national females (n = 29), international males (n = 30), and national males (n = 51). Mean ages of the four groups, respectively, were 27.7, 26.6, 24.9, and 28.2. All eight sport classifications were included in each group. Results indicated no significant difference between genders, while difference between skill levels (i.e., international vs. national) was significant. Univariate F tests indicated that this difference, which favoured the higher skill group, was primarily in Time Competence, Inner-Directedness, Self-Actualizing Value, Feeling Reactivity, and Capacity for Intimate Contact.

To enable comparison of disabled and AB athlete groups, Sherrill (1986c) developed composite profiles, means, and standard deviations for male (n = 265) and female (n = 134) AB athletes. These were used in a study of the self-actualization of elite male CP athletes (Sherrill & Rainbolt, 1988). Statistical analysis revealed significant differences between CP and AB athletes on only three scales: Time Competence, Self-Regard, and Self-Acceptance. These favoured CP athletes.

Individual t-test comparisons of CP athletes with test manual norms revealed that only 4 of 12 dimensions (Existentiality, Self-Regard, Self-Acceptance, and Synergy) were significantly different for males and only 2 (Existentiality and Self-Acceptance) were significantly different for females. Except for Self-Regard, in which CP athletes score high, all significant differences favour adult norms.

Research on self-actualization of blind elite athletes (Sherrill, Gench, Hinson, Gilstrap, Richir & Mastro, in press) also has indicated no significant difference between genders and little deviation from test manual adult norms. Subjects were 26 blind males (M age = 28.6) and 26 blind females (M age = 20.8), most of whom were international competitors in several events. Age was not significantly related to POI scores. Blind male athletes were significantly different from adult norms on two scales (Time Competence and Self-Acceptance), whereas blind female athletes were significantly different on three scales (Existentiality, Self-Regard, and Self-Acceptance). Except for Self-Regard, these differences favoured adult norms.

Self-actualization of elite spinally paralysed and amputee athletes in wheelchairs was studied by Sherrill, Silliman, Gench, and Hinson (in press). The sample was comprised of 48 males (M age = 29.4) and 23 females (M age = 28.9), most of whom were international competitors in track, basketball, and swimming. Statistical analysis revealed no significant difference between genders. When mean scores of these wheelchair athletes were compared statistically with test manual adult means, both male and female athletes scored significantly higher on Spontaneity and Self-Regard. Additionally male athletes scored significantly higher than normal on Self-Actualizing Value and significantly lower than normal on Self-Acceptance.

In summary, self-actualization theory posits 12 areas of personal orientation that influence intrinsic motivation to achieve one's potential. Study of six different samples of athletes (CP, blind, and wheelchair males and females) indicated that all groups except CP females and blind males score significantly higher than test manual norms on Self-Regard. All groups score significantly lower than test manual norms on Self-Acceptance, and three groups score significantly lower on Existentiality. In general, however, there is no significant difference between athletes and normative adults in self-actualization as measured by the POI. Also there are no gender differences.

These findings support Sherrill's observation, based on interviews, that disabled athletes are self-actualizing in that they possess value orientations similar to those of the general population. In disabled persons who become elite athletes the internal drive to achieve one's potential (i.e., to become all that one can become) apparently is not deterred by the disability, congenital or acquired, or by the attitudinal, aspirational, and environmental barriers that disabled individuals must overcome. It should be noted, however, that the disabled athlete population sampled represented the most elite in the U.S.A., and in some instances, the world. One might expect, therefore, that these individuals would have scored significantly above test manual norms on all dimensions of self-actualizing rather than only one (self-regard). Investigation of variables affecting self-actualization might shed insight into how the process of becoming is affected by disability, sport, and the interaction between the two.

Cognitive Psychology Theory

Cognitive psychology, which emphasizes individual differences in cognitive styles and abilities, has dominated sport psychology research on motivation and personality since 1975. Several cognitive theories have been examined in relation to the psychosocial status of disabled athletes: attentional and interpersonal style, perceived ability, attribution, locus of control, and learned helplessness.

Cognitive Styles and Abilities

One approach to examining individual styles and abilities of athletes is the Test of Attentional and Interpersonal Style (TAIS) of Nideffer (1976). The TAIS is a 144-item inventory that yields 17 subscale scores: (a) six reflect attentional processes; (b) two pertain to information processing ability and behaviour or impulse control, and (c) nine describe interpersonal style. Number of items for each scale ranges from 6 to 20. There is some overlapping of items from scale to scale.

Several validity and reliability studies have been conducted (Nideffer, 1976; Vallerand, 1983). Items were assigned rationally to each scale, based on an item analysis. If the correlation between a subscale item and its total subscale score was not significant, the item was dropped. The TAIS discriminates, to some extent, between known groups (males vs. females, 5 subscales; white male police applicants in a large city vs. male college students, 15 subscales). Vallerand (1983), however, criticizes the predictive validity of TAIS in sport settings. Several TAIS subscale correlations with other instruments and/or their scales range from .50 to .64. Test-retest reliabilities range from .60 to .93, with a median of .83. These are based on a 2-week interval.

Roeder and Aufsesser (1986) compared nonwheelchair athletes (21 males and 17 females) with wheelchair athletes (42 males and 5 females) who were finalists in the national wheelchair basketball championships. Mean ages for the two groups were 28.4 and 30.6, respectively. Many wheelchair athletes reported being involved in sports prior to becoming disabled. Nonwheelchair athletes were all college or university students. Significant differences, favouring the athletes, were found on self-esteem, physical orientation, intellectual expression, and control. No significant differences were found on introversion vs. extroversion and negative vs. positive affect levels. Scores of wheelchair athletes in relation to those of 74 able-bodied college varsity swimmers were examined also. Roeder and Aufsesser (1986) concluded, "It appears from the results of this study, that the athletic groups are indeed similar" (p. 32).

Perceived Ability Theory of Roberts (1984)

Roberts (1984) posited that perceived ability is the central construct in sports motivation, an important correlate of the personal meaning (i.e., satisfaction/dissatisfaction) of sports achievement, and a significant factor in sports dropout. Variables that relate to perceived ability in AB athletes include importance of sport in life, training effort, performance expectations, and event outcome (win/lose).

Dummer, Ewing, Habeck and Overton (1987b) used ANOVA procedures to determine whether perceived ability of 168 CP athletes was related to six variables: level of disability, gender, frequency of training sessions, importance of sport in life, performance expectations, and event outcome (win/lose). Only two of six variables were significantly related to perceived ability: event outcome (i.e., winning) and high performance expectation. Similar to the literature of AB sport, there were no gender differences in perceived sport ability. Unlike AB sport literature, perceived ability in CP athletes was not related to training/effort or to rating of importance of sport in life. Likewise, perceived ability did not depend on severity of disability (i.e., sport classification). Further research is needed to determine if these findings are generalizable to other disabled groups. No evidence exists, as yet, that perceived ability is as important in disabled sport as AB competition.

Attribution and Locus of Control

Attribution theory (Weiner, 1972) was applied to CP athletes by Dummer, Ewing, Habeck, and Overton (1987a). To determine the attributions used to explain their win/lose performance in an individual sport event, 147 CP athletes were asked to rate 10 attributions and one affect (I enjoy competition) on a 9-point Likert-type scale. Data were collected within 10 min of finishing an event. Unlike the findings of AB sport literature, there were no gender differences. Discriminant function analysis, however, revealed a significant difference between sport classifications 1, 2, 6 and 3, 4, 5, 7, and 8. The more severely disabled athletes revealed more external locus of control by often explaining their performance as luck and task difficulty rather than ability and effort. Overall, responses of CP athletes were about evenly divided between stable and unstable attributions. Dummer et al. (1987a) posited that the use of unstable attributions was related to lack of motor control experienced by persons with abnormal reflex activity.

Attributions of CP athletes were also examined in relation to performance outcome (win/lose) and overall personal satisfaction with performance. Unlike AB athletes who generally choose internal attributions to explain both winning and personal satisfaction, CP event winners used all attributions to a greater degree than CP event losers.

To determine the relationship between personal satisfaction and win/lose status, four groups were compared: satisfied winners (n = 26), satisfied losers (n = 18), dissatisfied winners (n = 2), and dissatisfied losers (n = 20). The results indicated different attributional responses by satisfied winners and losers vs. dissatisfied losers. This finding was inconsistent with AB athlete research, which has shown that internal attributions are associated with clear outcomes (i.e., satisfied winners and dissatisfied losers) and external attributions are associated with ambiguous outcomes (i.e., dissatisfied winners and satisfied losers).

Cognitive characteristics may be different for CP and AB athletes. Dummer et al. (1987a) concluded that winning may not be the primary motivator for CP athletes. The most important determinant of persistence in CP athletes is satisfaction with performance. Satisfaction is associated with using the right strategy, enjoying competition, and realistic assessment of ability.

Locus of control has been researched also in high and moderate activity paraplegic males (Goldberg & Shephard, 1982) and in lower-limb disabled males and females (Kofsky & Shephard in Shephard, in press). Data in both studies were collected using Nowicki and Strickland's (1973) Locus of Control Scale. Goldberg and Shephard described the locus of control (LOC) of their subjects (n = 17) as external. There was no difference in LOC scores between high activity (M = 21.9) and moderate activity (M = 22.9) subjects, nor between more severely (M = 22) and less severely (M = 22.5) disabled individuals. The high activity subjects in this study were wheelchair athletes.

In contrast, Kofsky and Shephard reported an internal locus of control (10.7 and 12.7) for lower-limb disabled men and women, respectively. LOC was not related to level of lesion or to physical activity habits. This high internal LOC may have been related to subjects' initiative in becoming involved in exercise training (i.e., the sampling design).

Research on LOC that relates to rehabilitation of spinal cord injured persons was reviewed by Trieschmann (1980). Among the points highlighted were the following. Low socioeconomic persons tend to score more as externals; thus research on LOC should include examination of socioeconomic status. Race also has been found to be related to LOC, with blacks having a more external LOC than whites. Severity of disability, however, is not correlated with LOC.

Response to spinal cord injury is believed dependent upon preinjury LOC, but this hypothesis is difficult to test. It has been shown that persons exhibiting internal LOC after injury show less tension and depression than external LOC persons (Trieschmann, 1980). External LOC persons score lower on knowledge tests about their condition than internals and typically exert little personal effort toward overcoming barriers. Overall, rehabilitation is more complete and life satisfaction greater in internals than externals.

LOC and/or motivation to work toward optimal health and function is not exclusively a personality characteristic (Seligman, 1975). Environment is a critical element. If a person has learned that there is no contingency between his/her behaviours (efforts) and outcomes, then the use of rewards to enhance motivation will not be effective. Spinal cord injury, as well as chronic illness and numerous other injuries, may contribute to the expectancy that nothing can be done to change the situation. This belief, called learned helplessness, characterizes many disabled persons. Trieschmann (1980) posited that LOC may be the variable that best explains individual differences in susceptibility to the learned helplessness phenomenon. In studying disabled persons it is essential therefore to examine not only the person but also the rewards and punishments available in past and present environments.

Future Directions

Quantity and quality of research on the psychosocial status of disabled athletes will increase in the future. Youth sports, in particular, will become a fruitful area of study. Existing research has been conducted mainly by physical education specialists concerned with special populations but who have little formal training in sport and/or rehabilitation psychology research. As sport for disabled persons increases, there will be more multi- and interdisciplinary study and collaboration. Researchers will become increasingly knowledgeable about the psychology of disability (i.e., individual differences) and of sport, and resulting research will parallel that of both rehabilitation psychology (Bolton & Parker, 1987; Trieschmann, 1980) and sport psychology (Landers, 1983). This means that research will become increasingly theoretical with considerably more time devoted to rationale, review of the AB athlete literature, and resolution of design problems that prevent or minimize generalization.

Research concerning disabled populations is intricately linked with advocacy in regard to rights and opportunities of disabled persons. Many of the studies reviewed in this paper were more concerned with examining the hypothesis of similarity between disabled and AB athletes than with testing traditional theories. Findings seem substantial enough to posit similarity theory: athletes, whether disabled or able, are similar in traits, states, personal orientations, attentional and interpersonal styles, and attributions. Implicit in this theory is the belief that athletes who are similar should have identical rights, opportunities, and responsibilities and that research can be a viable approach to information dissemination in relation to changing society's attitudes toward disabled persons.

For quantity and quality to increase, physical educators must initiate communication with sport and rehabilitation psychologists, and psychologists like Ogilvie (1985) and Asken (1987) must continue their endeavors to interest colleagues in research on disabled persons. Advocacy must be directed also toward leaders and coaches in the sport for disabled movement to increase their awareness of the importance of sport psychology and research and to encourage their cooperation. Athletes must find their roles as subjects meaningful and productive, with data collectors becoming more accountable and ethical in terms of sharing findings with subjects and submitting work for publication.

Quality of research will improve as professional organizations raise standards for conference presentations and journals impose more stringent publication criteria. Population description, sampling design, and use of tests of significance are particular areas of needed improvement. Comparisons must incorporate control of relevant variables across groups, and much exploratory research is needed to learn which personal and situational variables relate to sport performance, personal growth, and self-actualization. If sport classification is found relevant, then samples should be representative of the population in this regard. Data collection instruments and protocol need validity/reliability study for use with disabled samples (Mastro et al., 1985; Mastro et al., 1987a; Sherrill et al., 1988b), and normative comparative groups must be examined in terms of appropriateness.

Just as AB sport psychology was exploratory and descriptive for many years, likewise for disabled athlete research. Exploratory research, however, should follow the scientific method, using both deduction and induction. Each theory that is being studied with AB athletes should be explored with disabled athletes, findings generalized when appropriate, and theories reformulated as necessary. Cognitive psychology theory, with its focus on individual differences in training and competition styles, abilities, attributions, and motivations, will provide the conceptual basis for most future research although humanistic theory will continue to attract some scholars.

Summary

In this review of psychosocial research on disabled athletes, 32 studies completed since 1984 were identified as relating to seven theories: (1) Cattell's trait theory, (2) state theory in conjunction with Morgan's Mental Health Model, 14 (3) Spielberger's state-trait anxiety theory, (4) Maslow's self-actualization theory, (5) Nideffer's attentional and interpersonal style theory, (6) Robert's perceived ability theory, (7) and Weiner's attribution and locus of control theory. The five most frequently used data collection instruments were reviewed, based on the belief that quality of research is determined largely by validity and reliability of instruments. The status of disabled athlete research in relation to AB scholarly inquiry was discussed, emphasizing the trend from atheoretical to theoretical. Speculations about future directions centered on the need to improve quantity and quality of research and to parallel theory development and testing in sport and rehabilitation psychology.

Conclusion

Psychosocial research on disabled athletes, now in the exploratory stage of inquiry, will require many years and much work to progress to the explanatory stage in which emphasis is on theory development and testing. Multi- and interdisciplinary study of sport and rehabilitation psychology will enhance the research competence, theory awareness, and idea generation of adapted physical educators. Cognitive psychology theory is worthy of much attention but should be held in balance with humanistic theory.

Author Notes

1. Send requests for reprints to Claudine Sherrill, Department of Kinesiology, Texas Women's University, P.O. Box 23717, Denton, Texas, USA, 76204.

References

Asken, M. (1987, March). *Sport psychology: Psychological effects of sport participation in physically disabled individuals.* Paper presented at U.S. Olympic Committee Conference on Sports Medicine and Disabled Athletes, Mt. Washington Valley, NH.

Asken, M. & Goodling, M. (1986). Sport psychology: An undeveloped discipline from among the sport sciences for disabled athletes. *Adapted Physical Activity Quarterly, 3,* 312-319.

Bolton, B., & Parker, R. (1987). Research in rehabilitation counseling. In R. Parker (Ed.), *Rehabilitation counseling: Basics and beyond* (pp. 157-187). Austin, TX: Pro.Ed.

Buros, O. (Ed.). (1978). *The eighth mental measurements yearbook (Vol. 1).* Highland Park, NJ: The Gryphon Press.

Burton, D. (1988). Do anxious swimmers swim slower? Reexamining the elusive anxiety-performance relationship. *Journal of Sport Psychology and Exercise, 10*(1), 45-61.

Canabal, M., Sherrill, C., & Rainbolt, W. (1987). Psychological mood profiles of elite cerebral palsied athletes. In M. Berridge & G. Ward (Eds.), *International perspectives on adapted physical activity* (pp. 157-163). Champaign, IL: Human Kinetics.

Cattell, R., & Stice, G. (1957). *Handbook for the sixteen personality factor questionnaire.* Champaign, IL: Institute for Personality and Ability Testing.

Cook, D. (1987). Psychosocial impact of disability. In R. Parker (Ed.), *Rehabilitation counseling* (pp. 97-120). Austin, TX: Pro. Ed.

DePauw, K. (1988). Sport for individuals with disabilities: Research opportunities. *Adapted Physical Activity Quarterly, 5*(2), 80-89.

Dickinson, J., & Perkins, D. (1985). Socialization into physical activity for disabled populations. *Canadian Association for Health, Physical Education, and Recreation Journal, 51,* 4-12.

Dummer, G., Ewing, M., Habeck, R., & Overton, S. (1987a). Attributions of athletes with cerebral palsy. *Adapted Physical Activity Quarterly, 4*(4), 278-292.

Dummer, G., Ewing, M., Habeck, R., & Overton, S. (1987b). Perceived ability in sport by persons with physical disabilities. *Abstracts of Research Papers.* Reston, VA: American Alliance for Health, Physical Education, Recreation, and Dance.

Endler, N., & Hunt, J. (1984). *Personality and the behaviorial disorders: Volume 1* (2nd ed.). New York, NY: John Wiley & Sons.

French, R., Henschen, K., & Horvat, M. (1985). The psychological characteristics of female wheelchair basketball players. *Abstracts of Research Papers.* Reston, VA: American Alliance for Health, Physical Education, Recreation, & Dance.

French, R., Mastro, J., & Montelione, T. (1987). State and trait anxiety and athletic performance of visually impaired athletes. *Abstracts of Research Papers.* Reston, VA: American Alliance for Health, Physical Education, Recreation, and Dance.

Fridhandler, B. (1986). Conceptual note on state, trait, and the state-trait distinction. *Journal of Personality and Social Psychology, 50*(1), 169-174.

Gill, D. (1986). *Psychological dynamics of sport.* Champaign, IL: Human Kinetics.

Goldberg, G., & Shephard, R. (1982). Personality profiles of disabled individuals in relation to physical activity patterns. *Journal of Sports Medicine and Physical Fitness, 22,* 477-484.

Goodbrand, S. (1987). *A comparison of the psychological mood profiles of elite cerebral palsied athletes and cerebral palsied nonathletes.* Unpublished master's thesis, McGill University, Montreal, Quebec.

Goodling, M., & Asken, M. (1987). Sport psychology and the physically disabled athlete. In J. May & M. Asken (Eds.), *Sport psychology: The psychological health of the athlete* (pp. 117-133). New York, NY: PMA Publishing Corp.

Gould, D., Petlichkoff, L., & Weinberg, R. (1984). Antecedents of temporal changes in and relationships between CSAI-2 subcomponents. *Journal of Sport Psychology, 6,* 289-304

Greenwood, M., Dzewaltowski, D., & French, R. (1988). Self-efficacy and psychological well-being of wheelchair tennis participants and wheelchair nontennis participants. *Abstracts of Research Papers.* Reston, VA: American Alliance for Health, Physical Education, Recreation, and Dance.

Hall, C., & Lindzey, G. (1978). *Theories of personality* (3rd ed.). New York, NY: John Wiley & Sons.

Henschen, K. (1984). Wheelchair athletes have more of what able-bodied athletes are looking for? *Abstracts of Research Papers*. Reston, VA: American Alliance for Health, Physical Education, Recreation, and Dance.

Henschen, K., Horvat, M., & French, R. (1984). A visual comparison of psychological profiles between able-bodied and wheelchair athletes. *Adapted Physical Activity Quarterly, 1*(2), 118-124.

Horvat, M., French, R., & Henschen, K. (1986). A comparison of the psychological characteristics of male and female able-bodied and wheelchair athletes. *Paraplegia, 24*, 115-122.

Horvat, M., Roswal, G., Jacobs, D., & Gaunt, S. (1988). Psychological characteristics of able-bodied and disabled athletes. *Abstracts of Research Papers*. Reston, VA: American Alliance for Health, Physical Education, Recreation, and Dance.

Hull, C. L. (1943). *Principles of behavior*. New York, NY: Appleton-Century Crofts.

Kane, J. (1980). Personality research: The current controversy and implications for sports studies. In W. Straub (Ed.), *Sport psychology: An analysis of athlete behavior* (pp. 340-352). Ithaca, NY: Mouvement Publications.

Kennedy, M. J. (1980). *Sport role socialization and attitudes toward physical activity of wheelchair athletes*. Unpublished master's thesis, University of Oregon, Eugene.

Landers, D. (1980). The arousal-performance relationship revisited. *Research Quarterly for Sport and Exercise, 51*(1), 77-90.

Landers, D. (1983). Whatever happened to theory testing in sport psychology? *Journal of Sport Psychology, 5*(2), 135-151.

Lewin, K. (1935). *A dynamic theory of personality*. New York, NY: McGraw Hill.

Maslow, A. (1954). *Motivation and personality*. New York, NY: Harper.

Martens, R., & Landers, D. (1970). Motor performance under stress: A test of the inverted-U hypothesis. *Journal of Personality and Social Psychology, 16*, 29-37.

Mastro, J. (1985). *Psychological characteristics of elite male visually impaired and sighted athletes.* Unpublished doctoral dissertation, Texas Woman's University, Denton.

Mastro, J., Canabal, M., & French, R. (1988). Psychological mood profiles of sighted and unsighted beep baseball players. *Research Quarterly for Exercise and Sport, 59*(3), 262-264.

Mastro, J., & French, R. (1986). Sport anxiety and blind athletes. In C. Sherrill (Ed.), *Sport and disabled athletes* (pp. 203-208). Champaign, IL: Human Kinetics.

Mastro, J., French, R., Henschen, K., & Horvat, M. (1985). Use of the state trait anxiety inventory for visually impaired athletes. *Perceptual and Motor Skills, 61,* 775-778.

Mastro, J., French, R., Henschen, K., & Horvat, M. (1986). Selected psychological characteristics of blind golfers and their coaches. *American Corrective Therapy Journal, 40,* 111-114.

Mastro, J., French, R., & Hall, M. (1987a). Test-retest reliability of the profile of mood states using visually impaired athletes. *Perceptual and Motor Skills, 65,* 593-594.

Mastro, J., Sherrill, C., Gench, B., & French, R. (1987b). Psychological characteristics of elite visually impaired athletes: The iceberg profile. *Journal of Sport Behavior, 10*(1), 39-46.

McNair, D., Lorr, M., & Droppleman, L. (1971). *Manual for profile of mood states.* San Diego, CA: Educational and Industrial Testing Service.

Morgan, W. (1980). The trait psychology controversy. *Research Quarterly in Exercise and Sport, 51*(1), 50-76.

Nideffer, R. (1976). Test of attentional and interpersonal style. *Journal of Personality and Social Psychology, 34*(3), 394-404.

Nowicki, S., & Strickland, B. R. (1973). A locus of control scale for children. *Journal of Consulting Clinical Psychology, 40*(1), 148-154.

Ogilvie, B. (1985). Sports psychologists and the disabled athlete. *Palaestra, 1*(4), 36-40, 43.

Paulsen, P. (1988). *Comparison of wheelchair athletes and nonathletes on selected mood states.* Unpublished master's thesis, Texas Woman's University, Denton.

Price, R. (1986). The status of international activity in recreation, sports, and cultural activities with disabled persons, Part II. *Palaestra, 3*(1), 32-37.

Reid, G. (1987). Motor behaviour and psychosocial correlates in young handicapped performers. In D. Gould & M. Weiss (Eds.), *Advances in pediatric sport sciences* (Vol. 2, pp. 235-258). Champaign, IL: Human Kinetics.

Roberts, G. (1984). Toward a new theory of motivation in sport: The role of perceived ability. In J. Silva & R. Weinberg (Eds.), *Psychological foundations of sport* (pp. 214-228). Champaign, IL: Human Kinetics.

Roeder, L., & Aufsesser, P. (1986). Selected attentional and interpersonal characteristics of wheelchair athletes. *Palaestra, 2*(2), 28-32, 43-44.

Rogers, C. (1951). *Client-centered therapy.* Boston, MA: Houghton Mifflin.

Seligman, M. (1975). *Helplessness: On depression, development, and death.* San Francisco, CA: W. H. Freeman and Co.

Shephard, R. (in press). *Physical activity in special populations.* Champaign, IL: Human Kinetics.

Sherrill, C. (1986a). *Adapted physical education and recreation: A multidisciplinary approach* (3rd ed.). Dubuque, IA: Wm C. Brown.

Sherrill, C. (1986b). Social and psychological dimensions of sports for disabled athletes. In C. Sherrill (Ed.), *Sport and disabled athletes* (pp. 21-33). Champaign, IL: Human Kinetics.

Sherrill, C. (1986c). *Composite self-actualization profiles of male and female able-bodied athletes.* Unpublished manuscripts, Texas Woman's University, Denton, Texas.

Sherrill, C., & Rainbolt, W. (1987a, March). *Self-actualization profiles of elite male cerebral palsied athletes.* Paper presented at U.S. Olympic Committee Conference on Sports Medicine and Disabled Athletes, Mt. Washington Valley, NH.

Sherrill, C., & Rainbolt, W. (1987b, April). Self-actualization profiles of able bodied and cerebral palsied female athletes. *Abstracts of Research Papers.* Reston, VA: American Alliance for Health, Physical Education, Recreation, and Dance.

Sherrill, C., & Rainbolt, W. (1987c, June). *Self-actualization of adult cerebral palsied athletes: Gender and skill level differences.* Paper presented at International Federation of Adapted Physical Activity. Brisbane, Australia.

Sherrill, C., & Rainbolt, W. (1988). Self-actualization profiles of male able bodied and elite cerebral palsied athletes. *Adapted Physical Activity Quarterly, 5,* 108-119.

Sherrill, C., Gench, B., Canabal, M., & Mastro, J. (1988a). *Mood state profiles of elite male cerebral palsied, blind, and able-bodied athletes.* Manuscript submitted for publication.

Sherrill, C., Gilstrap, T., Richir, K., Gench, B., & Hinson, M. (1988b). Use of the personal orientation inventory with disabled athletes. *Perceptual and Motor Skills, 67,* 263-266.

Sherrill, C., Gench, B., Hinson, M., Gilstrap, T., Richir, K., & Mastro, J. (in press). Self-actualization of elite blind athletes. *Journal of Visual Impairment and Blindness.*

Sherrill, C., Silliman, L., Gench, B. & Hinson, M. (in press). Self-actualization of elite spinally paralysed and amputee athletes. *Paraplegia.*

Shontz, F. (1977). Physical disability and personality: Theory and recent research. In J. Stubbins (Ed.), *Social and psychological aspects of disability* (pp. 333-353). Baltimore, MD: University Park Press.

Shostrom, E. (1966). *Manual for personal orientation inventory.* San Diego, CA: Educational and Industrial Testing Service.

Silva, J., Shultz, B., Haslam, R., Martin, T., & Murray, D. (1985). Discriminating characteristics of contestants at the United States olympic training trials. *International Journal of Sport Psychology, 16,* 79-102.

Spence, K. (1958). A theory of emotionally based drive and its relation to performance in simple learning situations. *American Psychologist, 13,* 131-141.

Spielberger, C. D. (1966). Theory and research on anxiety. In C. D. Spielberger (Ed.), *Anxiety and behavior* (pp. 3-20). New York, NY: Academic Press.

Spielberger, C. D., Gorsuch, R., & Lushene, R. (1970). *STAI manual.* Palo Alto, CA: Consulting Psychologists Press.

Szyman, R. J. (1980). The effect of participation in wheelchair sports. *Dissertation Abstracts International, 41,* 804A-805A. (University Microfilms No. 8018209).

Tosi, D., & Lindamood, C. (1975). The measurement of self-actualization: A critical review of the Personal Orientation Inventory. *Journal of Personality Assessment, 39*(3), 215-223.

Trieschmann, R. (1980). *Spinal cord injuries: Psychological, social, and vocational adjustment.* New York, NY: Pergamon Press.

Vallerand, R. (1983). Attention and decision making: A test of the predictive validity of the test of attentional and interpersonal style (TAIS) in a sport setting. *Journal of Sport Psychology, 5,* 449-459.

Weiner, B. (1972). *Theories of motivation: From mechanism to cognition.* New York, NY: Rand McNally.

Wright, B. (1960). *Physical disability: A psychological approach.* New York, NY: Harper & Row.

Wright, B. (1983). *Physical disability: A psychosocial approach* (2nd ed.). New York, NY: Harper & Row.

Yerkes, R., & Dodson, J. (1980). The relation of strength of stimulus to rapidity of habit formation. *Journal of Comparative Neurology of Psychology, 18,* 459-482.

AUTHOR INDEX

- C -

- D -

- H -

- T -

SUBJECT INDEX

- N -

- OP -

www.ingramcontent.com/pod-product-compliance
Ingram Content Group UK Ltd.
Pitfield, Milton Keynes, MK11 3LW, UK
UKHW020232290926
15470UKWH00002B/489

9 780444 880932